AF524840

# Acetabular Revision Surgery in Major Bone Defects

Eduardo García-Rey • Eduardo García-Cimbrelo
Editors

# Acetabular Revision Surgery in Major Bone Defects

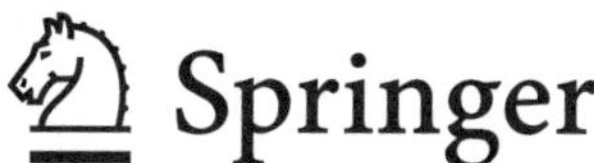

*Editors*
Eduardo García-Rey
Orthopaedic Surgery Department
Hospital Universitario La Paz-IdiPaz
Madrid
Spain

Eduardo García-Cimbrelo
Orthopaedic Surgery Department
Hospital Universitario La Paz-IdiPaz
Madrid
Spain

ISBN 978-3-319-98595-4 ISBN 978-3-319-98596-1 (eBook)
https://doi.org/10.1007/978-3-319-98596-1

Library of Congress Control Number: 2018957994



This Springer imprint is published by the registered company Springer Nature Switzerland AG
The registered company address is: Gewerbestrasse 11, 6330 Cham, Switzerland

# Preface

Total hip arthroplasty (THA) has been recognised as one of the most important surgical advances during the last five decades. End-hip arthritis is probably the most disabling condition to affect daily life activities not only in elderly but also in young patients. The older population is increasing in most countries worldwide, and they are more active than ever during the last decades so cartilage aging plus more physical and social demands in the more developed societies are strongly increasing THA indications. Thus, in young patients diagnoses other than primary arthritis, such as avascular necrosis, post-traumatic conditions, rheumatologic diseases and congenital hip diseases or other developmental sequelae, influence THA outcome together with the possibility of loosening and wear at long term. All these issues contribute to a greater number of THA revision procedures.

Nowadays, both cemented and cementless bone fixation can provide excellent long-term survival when using most contemporary implants. Most current femoral components have a survivorship higher than 95% more than 10 and 15 years after surgery. In fact, the THA revision procedure that is increasing is acetabular revision, and, as is reflected in most National Registries and clinical studies, the most frequent indication for THA revision surgery is related to the acetabular side. Indications for acetabular revision surgery at short term include dislocation, infection or, more rarely, fractures. To date, recent problems related to newer, not-very well studied, implants have also increased the number of revision procedures due to newer complications. At long term, the most frequent reasons for hip revision surgery are wear and loosening with the appearance of osteolysis. During last years, the appearance of late dislocation in older patients has become of interest. Nevertheless, in an indication for acetabular revision surgery, the most challenging issue is the existence of bone defect. Proper hip reconstruction during surgery to allow the closest distance to the hip rotation centre and the longest duration of the implant is the main purpose of the treatment.

First, a hip surgeon must be familiar with the basic science that can affect bone biology and changes associated to implants. A better understanding of all these changes related to bearing surfaces and bone interfaces facilitates clinical management when facing a patient with THA. Biological processes secondary to wear particles and different reactions to all kinds of polyethylenes, metallic particles, ceramics and cement contribute to silent osteolysis until there is significant bone destruction or implant loosening. The hip surgeon must also be familiar with advances in research that may improve clinical management. Second, it is necessary to classify the bone defects in every patient. Different imaging techniques can nowadays improve preoperative diagnosis, while newer surgical tools and tricks can diminish bone loss during explantation of the failed acetabular component.

Appropriate surgical planning is critical before starting an acetabular revision procedure. Recommendations in young patients presenting severe polyethylene wear with osteolysis and fixed implants are different than in other patients with loosened cups. The surgical team needs to be familiar with revision implants, techniques and bone graft use. Understanding the biology of the latter, particularly of allografts, improves the clinical and radiological outcome. Despite the surgical choice, the surgeon must keep in mind that bone defect determines surgical technique. From conventional cementless cups to cages, bone impaction grafting or reinforcement rings, adequate hip rotation centre reconstruction in stable construction will affect the clinical and radiological outcome of these patients. Independent industry-unrelated high-quality studies are the most reliable way to review all the different clinical choices. Finally, all issues associated to different complications, such as dislocation or infection, must be addressed for proper management.

Acetabular revision surgery in the presence of bone defect continues to be of concern for the patient and the surgeon. In this book all the most critical topics are covered beginning with the basic science, trying to clarify some newer research findings, continuing with established reconstruction techniques with or without the use of bone graft are reviewed. Continuing high-quality clinical studies to evaluate this complex problem and improve our understanding of the concepts will allow us to reliably improve outcomes for our patients.

Madrid, Spain Eduardo García-Rey
Madrid, Spain Eduardo García-Cimbrelo

# Contents

# Chapter 1
# Osteolysis After Total Hip Arthroplasty: Basic Science

**G. Vallés and N. Vilaboa**

## Total Hip Replacement: Clinical Need and Demand

Total hip arthroplasty (THA) represents the most successful and revolutionary intervention achieved in orthopedic surgery in the last century [1–3]. This surgery is performed to restore the injured or degenerated joint function when conservative treatment options have failed and pain, stiffness and other limitations drastically reduce the patient's quality of life. The clinical settings in which hip arthroplasty is indicated involve acute and chronic underlying joint-related diseases, mostly degenerative osteoarthritis and rheumatoid arthritis but also other arthropathies including avascular necrosis, developmental and congenital disorders, neoplasias, fractures and post-traumatic degenerative arthritis [4]. In 2010, the number of individuals bearing hip implants in USA was estimated in more than 2.5 millions [5]. In Europe, countries with high incidence are Germany, Switzerland and Belgium with ratios, of 296, 287 and 240 THA procedures per 100,000 inhabitants, respectively, while in US and UK the frequencies are 184 and 194 [3].

Early hip failure (within 5 years of implantation) is mainly associated to instability, aseptic loosening (AL), infections, wear and fracture and has a decreasing trend due to improvements in surgery techniques and advances in the biomaterials field. However, an alarming prevalence has been detected in some cohorts, especially in patients with metal-on metal (MoM) bearings [6, 7]. In the long-term, the survival rate (endpoint at revision) of prosthesis after 10–15 years of implantation has been estimated about a 90–95% [8–10] although percentages of only 58–62% or even less have been also reported after longer service periods [10–12].

G. Vallés · N. Vilaboa (✉)
Hospital Universitario La Paz-IdiPaz, Madrid, Spain

Centro de Investigación Biomédica en Red de Bioingeniería, Biomateriales y Nanomedicina, CIBER-BBN, Madrid, Spain
e-mail: nuria.vilaboa@salud.madrid.org

 
E. García-Rey, E. García-Cimbrelo (eds.), *Acetabular Revision Surgery in Major Bone Defects*, https://doi.org/10.1007/978-3-319-98596-1_1

Demographic changes and lifestyle habits, with a younger and more active population suffering from disabling joint diseases, have led to a significant raise in the number of THA performed [4, 5, 13]. While THA was initially intended for elderly patients with limited activity, current candidates include young and middle-age patients as well as physically active elderly individuals [3, 13]. As a consequence, the incidence of total hip replacements (THR) increased by a 25% during the period 2000–2009 and is expected to increase annually at a rate of approximately a 5% per year in the coming years, to such an extent that in the period 2005–2030 THA procedures will increase a 174% [4, 14]. Approximately half of the joint replacements currently performed in USA are made in patients younger than 65 years. In Europe, 42% of men and 31% of women who underwent THA in England and Wales were in this age group [15]. By 2030, 52% of THR might be performed in these patients [16, 17]. Given the limited expected time of service of prosthesis in patients younger than 50 years, the revision rates will dramatically increase in coming years [17, 18].

## Implant Failure: Aseptic Loosening

Implant failure is still a major complication of joint arthroplasty with severe consequences for the patient that impact the health-care system [8, 16, 19–21]. Failure, origined by mechanical and/or biological factors, can arise from multifactorial causes such as implant design, surgical technique, method of fixation or infection but the main factor limiting the longevity of THAs is AL secondary to periprosthetic osteolysis [3, 13, 15, 17]. Specifically, implant loosening due to aseptic osteolysis accounts for over 70% of total hip revisions while infections, recurrent dislocations, periprosthetic fractures and surgical errors contribute to about a 20% of the reported failures [21–23]. Instability and infection are complications frequently diagnosed in the early postoperative period, while osteolysis and AL usually appear in the medium to long-term [18]. Revision surgery is a procedure technically more challenging than primary arthroplasty and often associated with poorer prognosis and higher risk of failure [24, 25]. The late development and diagnosis of AL, usually asymptomatic in early stages, and its association to severe periprosthetic bone defects are factors that compromise the revision surgery procedure [18, 26]. Patients for revision surgery are typically in their 70s and 80s, and age-associated issues including morbidity and mortality risks undermine the intervention. The exponential growth in the number of primary total joint replacement procedures is associated to a concomitant increase in the number of revision operations. In this regard it has been estimated that the revision burden (ratio of revision/primary THA) will be about 17% in 2030 [27, 28]. Statistical data have shown that 10 years after of the primary hip arthroplasty, 24% of cases develop osteolysis and about a 15% of recipients require further surgical intervention due to AL [17, 29]. In young patients, under 30 years, the percentage of cases which requires revision surgery can reach rates up to 33% while in older patients range from 7% to 15% [30]. Regarding components, the acetabular cup is revised more frequently than the femoral stem [30, 31]. Currently, 40,000 hip revision procedures due to loosening are performed annually in USA and it is expected to increase about a 137% for 2030 [14, 32].

AL is characterized by areas of osteolysis at the bone-implant interface, identified radiographically as radiolucent zones, which can result in displacement of the prosthetic component [3, 33]. Progression of peri-prosthetic bone loss as assessed by radiology is very slow. Osteolytic lesions often appear many years after the primary surgery and can be associated to mechanically stable implants [34]. Clinical symptoms associated to bone tissue destruction may not be clearly apparent or even remain silenced.

Several factors determine the longevity of hip implants. Apart from the importance of a correct surgical technique (orientation and alignment of prosthetic components, prosthesis stability, anchorage and osteointegration of the implant …) there are significant differences regarding prosthesis- (e.g. type of bearing material, prosthesis design, shape of prosthesis, surface technology, type of fixation …) and patient- related factors (e.g. age, co-morbidities, level of activity and differences in mechanical loading,…) wich influence the host response to the implant and therefore its success or failure [17, 35]. In this regard, Engh et al. found that implant wear and patient-specific propensity equally contribute to the degree of osteolysis and might account for the extent of the area affected by periprosthetic bone loss [36]. Research efforts have attempted to identify clinical risk factors and individual susceptibility to periprosthetic osteolysis in order to predict the outcome and prevent, or at least attenuate, the ensuing complications of THA [37]. Over the last years, the influence of parameters such as gender, body mass index, and age [21, 37, 38], as well as the contribution of genetic factors to the development and progression of AL [15, 37, 38] have been considered. Regarding age and gender, young male patients show high risk of developing osteolysis [38]. Considering other factors, genetic variations affecting molecules involved in inflammation and bone turnover may play a role in the predisposition to AL of patients with THA. Particularly, polimorphisms in genes encoding proteins such as tumor necrosis factor-α (TNF-α), interleukin-6 (IL-6), transforming growth factor-β (TGF-β), interleukin-1 receptor antagonist (IL-1 Ra), matrix metalloproteinase-1 (MMP-1), osteoprotegerin (OPG) or receptor activator for nuclear factor kappa-B ligand (RANKL), have been associated with susceptibility to osteolysis and/or short prosthesis longevity [15, 20, 39–41]. These proteins are powerful mediators in the biological response to particulate wear debris and the periprosthetic bone loss around THR.

Other risk factor associated to predisposition to osteolysis is the preoperative diagnosis, which might influence the host response to the biomaterial. While some authors have observed higher rates of loosening in patients who underwent THA due to inflammatory arthritis, post-traumatic arthritis, developmental dysplasia or osteonecrosis as compared to primary osteoarthritis, others have not found significant differences between these groups [15, 42].

## The Enemy: Wear Debris Particles

Osteolysis is the long-term consequence of the biological response to wear debris and products derived from corrosion of implants [3, 33, 43]. Particulate wear debris, mainly generated by articulating motion at the bearing surfaces but also by non-articular surfaces, are the primary causes of periprosthetic bone loss and implant loosening [44, 45]. Locally, continous exposure to prosthetic debris combined to repetitive mechanical stresses triggers an inflammatory chronic response which is highly influenced by the intrinsic properties of wear debris particles. The type of prosthesis determines the characteristics of the resultant wear debris particles and therefore the magnitude of the host response [33]. Articulating bearings in THA are hard-on-hard material such as MoM or ceramic-on-ceramic (CoC) and hard-on-soft material (metal-on-polymer) couples, being the most satisfactory the combination of a cobalt chrome femoral head articulating on an ultra high molecular weight polyethylene (UHMWPE) acetabular component [33, 46]. Wear occurs through five major mechanisms: adhesion, abrasion, third body, fatigue, and corrosion. Third body wear damage is considered a relevant source of particles in which metal, polymer, cement or even cortical bone debris are entrapped between the UHMWPE acetabular component and the hard bearing surface contributing to accelerated deterioration of the implant [3, 47]. Research in materials manufacturing and tribology has focused on identifying alternative bearing surfaces that reduce the production of wear particles debris [3, 46]. These new materials might give rise to wear particles with unknown characteristics.

In general, the standing paradigm of AL states that implant-derived-particles stimulate periprosthetic cells to release factors which affect cell functions through autocrine and/or paracrine mechanisms [13, 18, 33, 48]. Potentially, all cell types at the periprosthetic tissue are targets of wear debris but macrophages are critically involved [17, 29, 33, 45]. Macrophages activated by particles produce an array of inflammatory, chemotactic and bone-resorbing factors such as chemokines, growth factors, cytokines, degradative enzymes and reactive oxygen radicals, among others, triggering and perpetuating the periprosthetic osteolytic cascade [3, 24, 43, 48]. As result of the inflammatory response, a granulomatous pseudomembrane generates at the bone-implant interface, which further compromises the interface stability and osseointegration of the device. Altered-load bearing effects contribute to abnormal wear processes and production of particles in the implant bed, leading in advanced stages of periprosthetic osteolysis to further anomalous mechanical loading [45]. Although osteolysis due to wear debris initiates as a localized phenomenon, joint fluid can transport wear debris, cells and molecules to adjacent bone sites extending the affected bone-implant interface. Morever, high fluid production and altered loading increase periprosthetic pressure in the peri-implant region [34, 49]. Moreover, the extent of the inflammatory reaction to wear particles is not confined to joint and adjacent tissues since wear debris, mainly metal particles, have been detected in remote organs including the spleen, liver, kidney and lung [3, 45]. Whether systemic dissemination of wear particles may cause side effects, e.g. toxicity and carcinogenicity, is a matter of debate.

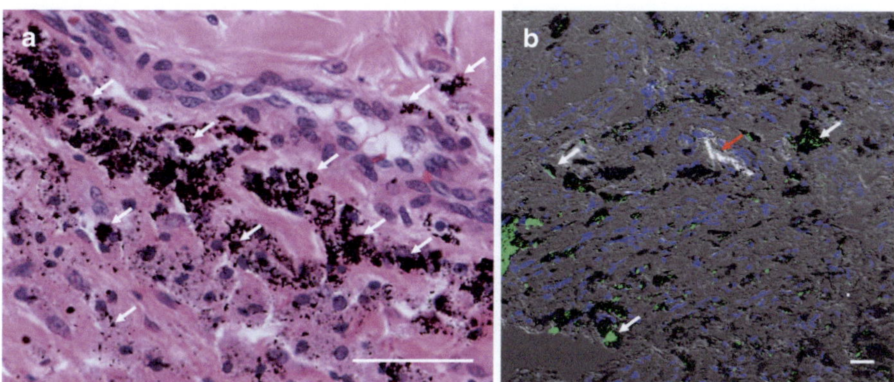


**Fig. 1.1** Periprosthetic membrane retrieved from a patient undergoing revision surgery due to hip aseptic loosening. (**a**) Optical microscopy imaging. Hematoxylin-eosin staining showing characteristic features of the foreign body reaction induced by wear debris particles, with infiltration of inflammatory cells. High amounts of metal particles are found, indicated by white arrows. (**b**) Transmitted polarized light and confocal microscopy imaging. Nuclei of cells in the tissue were counterstained with DAPI (blue). UHMWPE particles were detected by polarized light as bright areas (indicated by a red arrow) and metal particles were detected by transmitted light (black, white arrows) and by reflection (green false colour labelled). Scale bar: 100 μm

Histological examination of periprosthetic tissues retrieved during revision surgery has revealed significant amounts of prosthesis-derived particles (Fig. 1.1) and a multi-cellular composition characterised by the presence, among other cells, of macrophages, multinucleated foreign body giant cells containing engulfed particles, lymphocytes, fibroblasts and osteoclasts in association to elevated levels of pro-inflammatory cytokines, such as TNF-α, interleukin-1β (IL-1β), prostaglandin-E2 ($PGE_2$) and RANKL [33, 50].

The phagocytosable range size of particles able to induce an in vitro inflammatory response has been established in less than 10 μm [33]. In general, nanometer-sized particles with diameters lower than 150 nm can be internalized through endocytosis or pinocytosis, while particles sized between 150 nm and 10 μm utilize a phagocytosis-mediated process and particles higher than 20 μm induce multinucleated giant cell formation [33, 51]. The greater the particle load of phagocytosable particles, the higher is the local inflammatory response. Regarding shape, elongated particles are more reactive than round particles [23].

Originally coined as "cement disease", as osteolysis due to AL was thought to be a response to particles of polymethylmethacrylate (PMMA), later it was observed that osteolysis also occurs with cementless implants and potentially all kind of particles (metals, PE, ceramics, and bone cement) can elicit a biological response in joint tissues [3, 33, 43]. Particle chemistry plays an important role [3, 13, 33]. In general, metal particles are more pro-inflammatory and/or toxic than polymers or ceramics [3, 52–54]. An overview of the most relevant and recent findings about the cellular events and molecular pathways modulated by the different types of wear debris is presented in the following sections.

## *Polyethylene Particles*

Analyses of periprosthetic tissues retrieved during revision surgery have shown that UHMWPE wear debris originated from the acetabular liner are the most frequent types of debris, standing for 70–90% of the debris load independently if implants are cemented or not [3, 17]. Probably due to their abundance, UHMWPE particles are considered as key players in the stimulation of periprosthetic bone loss and implant loosening. Traditionally, the most used bearing couple was UHMWPE articulating against a metallic ball [3]. With hundreds of thousands of UHMWPE particles generated in a single step in the periprosthetic space, about 500 billion of particles produced per year, and a total amount of trillions of particles during the lifetime of a prosthesis, osteolysis was associated to a threshold of $2.16 \times 10^9$ and polyethylene (PE) particles per gram of interfacial tissue and a wear rate greater than 0.1 mm/year of the UHMWPE acetabular liner [3, 17, 23, 55].

Histological examination of periprosthetic tissues have revealed that UHMWPE debris appears as small particles or large shards, and exhibit birefringence under polarized light [45]. Once isolated from membranes, UHMWPE particles display an irregular surface with a predominant globular shape, although other irregular shapes are also observed especially in those of larger size, being 90% smaller than 1 μm [3, 17]. The different sizes and shapes observed have been related to the specific wear mode as well as to the implantation period [3, 45]. Small particles can be detected within macrophages while large particles are usually included within foreign body multinucleated giant cells [45].

Bacterial lipopolysaccharide (LPS), possibly derived from subclinical infections or systemic sources, may bind to particles and contribute further to the inflammatory reaction [56, 57]. Some evidence suggests that macrophages might not be able to induce an inflammatory response if adsorbed endotoxins are not present on UHMWPE particles [58]. Proteins present in the physiological fluids, including type I collagen, aggrecan proteoglycans, immunoglobulin, fibronectin and albumin, can also be adsorbed on UHMWPE surfaces [59]. The interaction of adsorbed proteins and cell surface receptors, such as integrins, has a remarkable role in the macrophage interactions with biomaterials. Specifically, integrins participate in receptor-mediated phagocytosis of wear particles of different composition, including UHMWPE. The downstream effects of integrin-mediated interactions result in the production of pro-inflammatory cytokines and osteoclast activation, as shown by Zaveri et al. who have recently reported that Mac-1 integrin and RGD-binding integrins are involved in osteolysis induced by UHMWPE particles [59]. Macrophage activation can occur not only by phagocytosis of UHMWPE particles but also by cell contact through receptor-mediated mechanisms, including Toll-like receptors (TLRs), and the cluster of differentiation molecules CD11b and CD14 [60]. Thus, Maitra et al. reported that UHMWPE particles stimulate in vitro TLR1/2 and activate phagocytosis [61]. In a PE particle-induced osteolysis murine calvarial model, TLR2 and TLR4 were found highly expressed in macrophages [60]. TLRs act primarily through the adapter protein myeloid differentiation primary response protein

(MyD88) and induce activation of nuclear factor kappa-B (NF-κB), mitogen-activated protein kinases (MAPK) and interferon-regulatory factors (IRFs), leading to the release of pro-inflammatory cytokines, growth factors and chemokines [22, 24]. TLRs are activated by pathogen- or damage-associated molecular patterns in response to infection or tissue damage. Oxidative stress, e.g. oxygen intermediates and free radicals, may provoke degradation of UHMWPE resulting in products as alkane polymers. These degradation products could influence the "original" inmunogenecity of particles, altering their binding affinity to TLRs or other molecules in the cells surfaces and thereby activating endogenous signaling systems. Moreover, particulate debris affects the host tissue integrity by increasing cell death, which generates danger signals such as heat shock proteins that further increase TLR activation [51].

The inflammasome has been recently involved in the cellular activation by wear particles [17, 61]. Inflammasome activation depends on reactive oxygen species (ROS), enzymes release and other danger signals. Upon phagocytosis of UHMWPE particles, endosomal and lysosomal damage results in release of cathepsins which trigger the inflammasome activation. If particles are larger that 20 μm, multinucleated giant cells may activate also NADPH oxidases and generate ROS, also contributing to its activation [51].

After the initial interaction with macrophages, particles induce an active infiltration of inflammatory cells into the periprosthetic area. Migration is mediated through chemotactic factors such as interleukin-8 (IL-8), macrophage chemotactic protein-1 (MCP-1), and macrophage inflammatory protein-1 (MIP-1) released by inflammatory and mesenchymal cells, among others, upon challenging with particles [62]. Thus, the pro-resorptive environment is created not only by locally activated cells but also by migration of macrophages and osteoclast precursors, i.e. monocytes. In this regard, in vivo studies employing UHMWPE particles have shown the contribution of chemotactic factors released by macrophages and mesenchymal stem cells (MSCs) to cell recruitment [60]. Specifically, the CCR2/MCP-1 and the CCR1/MIP-1α ligand/receptor axes are involved in the systemic recruitment of macrophages and MSCs, respectively, in the presence of UHMWPE particles [60, 63].

The most active field of research during the last decade has been focused in the identification of factors associated to the destruction of the bone tissue when UHMWPE particles are present. For instance, in vitro stimulation of macrophages with these particles increases the expression of genes involved in inflammation and osteoclastogenesis such as MMP9 (coding for matrix metalloproteinase-9), CTSK (coding for cathepsin K protein), CALCR (coding for calcitonin receptor) and TNFRSF11A (coding for receptor activator of nuclear factor kappa-B protein (RANK)). In vivo, calvarial models of PE particle-induced osteolysis have corroborated these findings [16].

Production of factors involved in bone destruction depends on the size and concentration of wear particles. Green et al. showed that, for a given tested concentration, PE particles of 0.24 μm in length induce higher production of TNF-α, IL-1β,

IL-6, and $PGE_2$ in macrophages than larger particles. Dose- and size-dependent effects were also reported, as sizes range between 0.45 and 1.71 μm were the most reactive when higher concentrations were tested [51]. A recent study has shown that treatment of peripheral blood mononuclear cells with UHMWPE particles below 50 nm does not induce the release of TNF-α, IL-1β, IL-6 and IL-8 [64]. Regarding concentration, UHMWPE particles showed a dose-dependent induction in the production of TNF-α, IL-1β and IL-6 in macrophages, and in the production of RANKL in osteoblasts [16, 51, 65]. PE particles are able to regulate proliferation and function of osteoblastic or bone-forming cells, through induced expression of pro-osteoclastogenic factors RANKL, IL-6, IL-8, $PGE_2$ and macrophage colony-stimulating factor (M-CSF) and also through the interference in the regulation of matrix synthesis proteins such as collagen or alkaline phosphatase (ALP) [16, 66, 67]. Differentiation of osteoblastic cells into a mature, osteocyte-like phenotype is tighly regulated by several genes including runt-related ranscription factor-2 (Runx2), sclerostin (SOST) and osterix (Osx) whose expression is also altered in the presence of PE particles. In osteoprogenitor cells, UHMWPE particles inhibit in a dose-dependent manner proliferation and osteogenic differentiation [67]. Effects of PE particles on osteoblasts are further influenced by their maturation state [66]. A recent study has detected increased expression of catabolic markers incuding matrix metalloproteinase-13 (MMP-13), carbonic anhydrase 2 (CA2), cathepsin K, and tartrate resistant acid phosphatase (TRAP) in human primary osteocyte-like cultures exposed to PE particles [68]. Moreover, in vitro exposure of macrophages to these particles induces spontaneous differentiation into mature and active osteoclasts [69]. In other coexisting cells in the periprosthetic bone bed, studies are scarce. For instance, in fibroblasts, dominant cell type in the interfacial membrane, PE particles induce the expression of the pro-inflammatory cytokine IL-6 [16]. The role of these cells in wear-induced osteolysis has been mainly attributed to their interaction and cooperation with macrophages to amplify inflammation, fibrosis and osteoclast activation [51]. Macrophages and fibroblasts in the interfacial tissues overexpress macrophage migration inhibitory factor (MIF), which can up-regulate the expression of pro-inflamatory factors and matrix metalloproteinases (MMPs) involved in the periprosthetic bone tissue destruction [70]. New lines of evidence have addressed the role of dendritic cells (DCs) in UHMWPE particles-induced osteolysis, with a similar role than macrophages [51].

Research efforts have recently focused in how to fit the paradigm of polarization of macrophages when exposed to wear particles. Wear particles contribute to the creation of a periprosthetic environment in which macrophages can be polarized to M1 (pro-inflammatory) and M2 (anti-inflammatory) phenotypes. Both phenotypes have been observed and extensively characterized [17, 60]. Polarization of uncommitted M0 or M1 macrophages toward the M2 phenotype, that promotes bone healing, has been proposed as therapeutic strategy to decrease the local inflammation. In a calvaria model employing UHMWPE particles, bone resorption was reduced after administration of the M2 phenotype inducer interleukin-4 (IL-4) [71].

Broad-scale expression profiling of human macrophages challenged to UHMWPE particles revealed changes in the expression of genes related to inflammatory response, cell proliferation, cytokine-mediated signaling, response to stress, cell migration and death [24]. Among others, particles modulated the transcript levels of genes encoding factors with remarkable roles in osteoclastogenesis and bone resorption such as IL-8, MIP-1α, MIP-1β, macrophage inflammatory protein-3 alpha (MIP-3α), interleukin-23 (IL-23), M-CSF, IL-1α and vascular endothelial growth factor (VEGF); and cell surface receptors involved in the recognition of particles such as β-integrins, protein-coupled receptors, intercellular adhesion molecules, TNF receptor superfamily members and TLRs-signaling. Moreover significant up-regulation of the expression of genes encoding MMPs, including MMP-1 and MMP-19, was also found.

Overall, these findings show that inflammation and osteoclastogenesis-related mechanisms activated by UHMWPE particles are main processes involved in the pathogenesis of wear-induced osteolysis. The introduction of highly crosslinked polyethylene (HXLPE) to reduce wear and osteolysis in total joint arthroplasty has attracted great interest. Moreover, as compared to polymeric and metallic particles, HXLPE particles induce a moderate degree of peri-implant osteolysis [72].

## *Metallic Particles*

Metal particles are massively generated from the bearing surfaces of MoM hip replacements, which were conceived as alternative to metal-on-polyethylene (MoP). However, adverse long-term effects are associated to MoM, including a higher rate of failure as compared to other bearing surfaces [46]. Metals are susceptible to degradation upon exposure to extracellular tissue fluids, and therefore the clinical outcome and durability of implants are affiliated to particulate corrosion and wear products. Metal wear particles arise mainly from the bearing surfaces but also from the metal back and fixation screws of the acetabular cup [45, 73]. Under the optical microscope, they appear as black to brownish colored entities, with amorphous or irregular shapes (flakes or needles) and sharp edges, and sizes ranging from 0.1 to 5 μm [3]. Ultrastructural methods showed that the majority of metal particles retrieved from periprosthetic tissues and joint simulators are in the nanometric range [3, 74]. These nanoparticles have a greater relative surface area than microparticles and are potentially more chemically and biologically reactive [45]. About $6–250 \times 10^{12}$ metal particles are released per year from a MoM articulating surface [3]. As particles with other compositions, metallic particles stimulate inflammation and bone resorption in detriment of bone formation [75]. Resorption areas associate to metal particles and periprosthetic tissues are characterized by express inflammatory mediators including IL-8, IL-1β, macrophage inflammatory protein-2 alpha (MIP-2α), stromal cell-derived factor 1 (SDF-1) and its receptor CXCR4 [9, 76, 77].

In vitro, exposure to Ti particles induces macrophages to release TNF-α, IL-6, IL-1β and $PGE_2$ in a process mediated by tyrosine phosphorylation and MAPK pathway [9]. A recent factor associated to induced inflammation by Ti particles is the cannabinoid receptor type 2 (CB2), inductor of osteoclastogenesis [78]. Similar to described in PE particles, dose- and size-dependent responses have been observed and the release of pro-inflammatory factors can occur independently of phagocytosis-dependent mechanisms. Concentration-dependent effects have been detected for TNF-α, IL-1β and IL-6 [54]. Apart from inflammatory factors, the expression of genes encoding osteoclastogenic markers can be induced by Ti particles, including TRAP, nuclear factor of activated T-cells 1 (NFATC1, also termed NFAT2), cathepsin K and RANK, as well as nitric oxide synthase 2 (NOS2), NF-κB and MMP-9. By regulating the expression of genes involved in the superoxide dismutase pathways, Ti particles also modulate oxidative stress [16]. Regarding chemotactic factors, in vitro exposure of primary human monocytes/macrophages to Ti particles increased the production of MIP-1α, resulting in increased monocyte migration. Other chemokines induced upon exposure to Ti particles in osteoblasts and osteoclasts are CCL17 and CCL22. Interestingly, the expression of the gene encoding CCR4, receptor of both chemokines, is up-regulated in osteoclast precursors exposed to Ti particles which accounts for macrophage recruitment and bone loss [79].

In osteoblastic cells, metal particles modulate the expression of genes encoding pro-inflammatory and bone-resorbing factors. In vitro studies have shown that Ti particles decrease OPG and induce IL-6 production, effects associated to increased nuclear factor IL-6 (NF-IL-6) and NF-κB activation while production of MMP-2 increases through p38 signaling [9, 16, 80]. Ti particles severely impact on the viability and osteogenic potential of osteoblast precursors [16, 81]. Moreover, Ti particles produce adverse effects in MSCs that include toxicity and increased IL-8 production. Induction of genes encoding pro-apoptotic proteins and down-regulation of those encoding anti-apoptotic and osteogenic factors has been detected in MSCs challenged with Ti particles [16]. Altogether, these findings indicate that Ti particles impair the viability, proliferation and differentiation ability of MSCs. Exposure of fibroblasts to Ti-based particles induce the expression and/or production of RANKL, IL-6 and MCP-1 in a dose-dependent manner and stimulates the release of osteolytic enzymes as stromelysin and collagenase [3, 9, 16]. In human synovial cells, Ti particles increase MMP-2 activity [82].

Bacterial endotoxins are detected frequently and in a significant amount adsorbed to metallic wear particles [57, 75]. In macrophages, exposure to Ti particles adsorbed to LPS results in the regulation of TLRs-mediated responses and the stimulation in the production of the proinflammatory cytokines TNF-α, IL-1β and IL-6 [75]. Nonetheless, endotoxin-free Ti particles activate TLRs-mediated pathways and induce the expression of same genes [83]. However, comparative studies have shown that endotoxin-free Ti particles induce inflammation and osteolysis to a lower extent than those with adsorbed bacterial debris [84]. As observed with UHMWPE particles, NALP3 inflammasome can be activated upon Ti particles internalization and subsequent cathepsin release [17].

In response to implant metal debris challenge, macrophages adopt a pro-inflammatory M1 phenotype [16, 79]. In a study to clarify whether macrophage phenotypes are equally sensitive to Ti particles, these cells were polarized towards phenotype M0, M1 and M2 and then incubated with Ti particles. While no significant effects were observed in M2-macrophages after Ti particle challenge, M1-macrophages experienced drastic changes both at the transcriptome and the proteome levels, with a notable increase in the production of inflammatory chemokines (e.g. MCP-1, MIP-1α, IL-8), cytokines (TNF-α, IL-1β) and growth factors (e.g. granulocyte-macrophage colony-stimulating factor (GM-CSF), granulocyte-colony stimulating factor (G-CSF) and epidermal growth factor (EGF)) [85]. This study supports again the notion that the local microenvironment, which determines the macrophage phenotype, notably influences the response to particles.

Changes in mechanotransduction and adhesive properties of cells treated with metal particles have also been addressed in in vitro studies. For example, Preedy et al. observed that Ti particles increase osteoblast elasticity [86].

In vivo studies employing calvaria or air pouch models have corroborated the in vitro findings regarding Ti particles induction of TNF-α, cyclooxygenase-2 (COX-2), IL-1β, MMP-9, MCP-1, RANK, RANKL, NFATC1, VEGF and CB2 expression and/or production [9, 16]. Similar results were observed when Ti-alloy particles were investigated [16].

Concerns about wear debris derived from CoCr are mainly based on ions release. Co and Cr ions can travel through lymh and blood with harmful consequences for heart, brain and thyroid, spleen or liver [9]. CoCr alloy particles have been histologically identified in necrotic areas with infiltrating macrophages and lymphocytes [87]. In the local tissues, Co-Cr alloy particles and ions impair the expression of proteins related with osteoblastic differentiation (OPG, Osx and osteocalcin (OCN)) and increase those related with inflammation and osteoclastogenesis (IL-6, RANKL, MCP-1 and NFATC1) [16]. Co ions affect osteoblasts and neutrophils functions and stimulate chemokine secretion in both cell types [88]. Ions released from a CoCr alloy (CoCr29Mo6) induced necrosis in osteoblasts and peripheral blood mononuclear cells (PBMCs) and also stimulated IL-6, IL-8, and MMP-1 expression in these cell types [89]. Co and Cr ions are highly cytotoxic for macrophages and lymphocytes, inducing apoptosis [9]. Exposure to CoCr particles, increase expression and/or production of pro-inflammatory factors (IL-1α, IL-6, interleukin-10 (IL-10), IL-8, GM-CSF and $PGE_2$) in monocyte-macrophage lineage cells, reduce viability in histiocytes and fibroblasts and affect osteogenic differentiation in MSCs [9, 16, 90]. Treatment of THP-1 cells with a CoCr alloy (ASTM F75) particles increase the production of TNF-α, IL-1β and IL-8 through TLR4 signaling pathway [91]. In fibroblasts, CoCr nanoparticles increase the production of ROS and induce apoptosis [9, 92]. Regarding size, CoCr nanoparticles release more ions and are more cytotoxic than CoCr microparticles [93].

After being phagocytosed by macrophages metal nanoparticles trigger endoplasmic reticule (ER) stress. Periprosthetic tissues express large amounts of ER stress-associated molecules ($Ca^{2+}$, IRE1-α, GRP78/Bip, CHOP, cleaved Caspase-4, and JNK). It has been speculated that apoptosis in macrophages challenged to metal particles might be mediated by ER stress pathways, also linked to inflammation and osteoclastogenesis [94]. Similar to UHMWPE particles, chemical changes in metal particles surface altere the recognition of particles by cells and their subsequent effects [9, 95]. Also, release of endogenous alarmins has been proposed to contribute to positive feedback mechanisms in the periprosthetic tissue challenged with metallic debris [84, 18].

Several studies report a scarce number of T-lymphocytes in periprosthetic tissues, concluding that osteolysis occurs independently of these cells [51]. However, lymphocytes play a key role in hypersensitivity reactions leading to early osteolysis [45, 51]. Hypersensitivity or allergy to metallic components is a matter of concern to orthopaedic surgeons. This reaction is usually a cell-mediated (type-IV delayed hypersensitivity) response, characterized by activation of delayed-type hypersensitivity T lymphocytes by haptenic antigen and cytokine release which leads to recruitment of cytotoxic T-cells and macrophages activation. Activated macrophages mediate delayed-type hypersensitivity T lymphocytes activation, self-perpetuating the inflammatory response [9, 79]. Another adverse local tissue reaction is the aseptic lymphocyte-dominated vasculitis-associated lesions (ALVaL). This response is similar to the type IV hypersensitivity response, characterized by inflammation accompanied by lymphocytic infiltration, accumulation of plasma cells and macrophages and soft tissue necrosis [3, 9, 96]. Pseudotumors, mainly affecting soft tissues, are another complication of metal THA. Pseudotumors are identified as a solid or cystic mass-forming tissue characterized by necrosis areas, mononuclear cell infiltration and giant multinucleated cells, with high degree of perivascular lymphocytic aggregation. The prevalence of pseudotumors in hip implanted patients is a controversial issue. While some authors estimated a low frequency, just about a 1% within 5 years of MoM implantation, others have found a much higher incidence, up to 60% [3, 9, 97]. This absence of consensum may be explained due to the asymptomatic nature in some cases and the similarity with other adverse reactions. In this regard, Catelas et al. have stated relevant differences in the proteome of pseudotumors and osteolytic tissues which correlate with predominant adaptive immune responses in patients with pseudotumors and innate immune responses in patients with periprosthetic osteolysis [98]. One molecular mechanism which might explain the local soft tissue growing around the implant (fibro-pseudotumors) is the induction of hypoxia and angiogenesis by metal debris, which increases the levels of transcription factor hypoxia inducible factor 1 alpha (HIF-1$\alpha$) and VEGF [79]. Finally, some studies suggested an association between MoM implants and risk for developing cancer but epidemiological studies have not been able to prove increased incidence of cancer in patients with these implants [9, 99].

In summary, existing data employing metal and metal-alloys wear debris and their byproducts indicate their involvement in the induction of adverse local tissue reactions, based not only in the activation of inflammation and bone resorption-related mechanisms but also in the induction of the oxidative stress and cytotoxicity. These effects are mainly dose- and concentration-dependents which, in the context of metal particles exhibiting submicrometric and nanometric sizes and being released in high amounts to the periprosthetic space, represent a clear threat to tissue homeostasis.

## *Ceramic Particles*

Ceramics present chemical and mechanical advantageous properties for the manufacturing of orthopaedic devices, especially for young patients, including biochemical inertness, hardness, high-strength and corrosion and wear resistance [3, 100, 101]. Currently, the most used ceramic materials in clinical practice are alumina ($AL_2O_3$) and zirconia ($ZrO_2$) [3]. Hip implant revisions of $Al_2O_3$-based components have been associated to their brittleness and the subsequent risk of catastrophic failures due to deficiencies in the manufacture [3, 102]. A great variability in the frequency of ceramics fracture rate has been reported but in general, incidence is small [3, 103]. Wear volume of ceramic bearing couples is lower than that of metallic and therefore a lower risk of revision is expected [3, 104]. Moreover, PE component exhibits a lower linear wear in CoP (0.034 mm/year) than in MoP (0.1 mm/year) bearings. On crosslinked PE, ceramics display a wear rate of 0.019 mm/year compared to 0.03 for metals [3]. Relative inertness and low abundance of ceramic wear debris in the periprosthetic space imply limited adverse biologic reactions and risk of osteolysis associated to this type of material.

Ceramic debris appears as fine greyish-brown particles ($ZrO_2$) and brown, brownish-green or black granules ($Al_2O_3$) [45, 105, 106]. Regarding size, ceramic particles are similar to metal particles, and ten times smaller than polymeric particles. More in detail, some studies have shown a range from 0.13 to 7.2 μm in tissues around loosened CoC hip implants and others have reported a bimodal size distribution, with most of them in the nanometric-order (5–90 nm) and submicron- to micron-scale for the rest (up to 3.2 μm) [3, 106, 107].

Manufacturing defects, instability or mal position of hip prosthesis components are main factors involved in the generation of ceramic particles, which once produced are "potential" inducers of periprosthetic osteolysis [3, 60, 108]. In fact, production of ceramic debris associated to occasional osteolytic areas has been considered as the consequence of mechanical instability rather than the origin of failure [108]. Typical foreign body reaction was only observed in association to large amounts of wear particles [109]. The cellular mechanisms involved in the biological response to ceramic particles are a controversial issue, not fully elucidated. While some authors state that ceramics are able to activate cells in a similar manner to metallic debris due to their comparable size, others express doubts about the involvement of the same mechanisms. In fact, studies in retrieved tissues have shown a differential cellular response to accumulated ceramic wear debris [110]. Biocompatibility of $ZrO_2$ particles seems to be greater than that of Ti particles since induction of pro-inflammatory gene expression was significantly lower in macrophages challenged with $ZrO_2$. In vivo experiments support these findings, with higher extent of inflammation and bone resorption induced by Ti or PE particles than ceramics [83, 111]. Bylski et al. exposed THP-1 macrophage-like cells to different concentrations of $Al_2O_3$ and Ti particles and found that, regardless of particle size and time exposure, ceramic caused only minor up-regulations of RANK, TNF-α and OPG mRNA levels while Ti highly stimulated the expression these genes and led to cytotoxic effects in a dose- and time-dependent manner [107]. Also, minor induction in the production of pro-inflammatory proteins such as IL-1β and MCP-1 has been reported after exposure of primary human macrophages to $Al_2O_3$ particles [112]. In a comparative study using murine macrophage cells treated with PE or ceramic particles, the latter led to lower release of TNF-α [113].

The negligible in vitro effects of $Al_2O_3$ particles on cell viability and cytokines production may account for the low incidence of osteolysis in patients with CoC prosthesis [60]. Once again, particle size, composition and concentration are relevant factors to consider [114, 115, 116]. Regarding induction of pro-inflammatory cytokines, neither $Al_2O_3$ or $ZrO_2$ particles induced IL-1 or IL-6 production in human fibroblast-like synoviocytes isolated from patients with osteoarthritis or rheumatoid arthritis [117]. $Al_2O_3$ and $ZrO_2$ are susceptible of internalization in J774 cells, inducing both type of particles the release of TNF-α at same extent [118].

Exposure of human macrophages to $ZrO_2$ or $TiO_2$ nanoparticles upregulated the expression of TLR7 and TLR10 [119]. Moreover, $ZrO_2$ nanoparticles induced IL-1β production and IL-1Ra synthesis while in LPS-treated macrophages IL-1Ra release is reduced, therefore promoting the creation of a pro-inflammatory environment, amplifying the M1 macrophage-effector functions.

A recent study has evaluated the $ZrO_2$ effects on osteoclasts, whose recruitment and activation are directly involved in the periarticular osteolysis [120]. Exposure of osteoclasts to $ZrO_2$ increased cell fusion and expression of osteoclast function- and bone matrix-related proteins including vitronectin receptor (VNR), TRAP, RANK and cathepsin K without stimulating osteoclast bone resorptive capacity. Moreover, higher expression of MMP-1 and an impaired production of the tissue inhibitor of this metalloproteinase were observed.

$AL_2O_3$ particles can be internalized by osteoblastic MG-63 cells which resulted in decreased proliferation, ALP activity and TGF-β1 secretion [121]. In contrast, exposure of these cells to $ZrO_2$ stimulated proliferation and ALP activity. Interestingly, both types of particles induced the production of $PGE_2$ in a dose-dependent manner. Treatment of primary human osteoblasts with $Al_2O_3$ induced the expression and secretion of IL-6 [122] and affected the osteoblastic function by decreasing the C-terminal type I procollagen (PICP) secretion and ALP activity [123]. The paracrine interactions between macrophages and osteoblasts were also affected by treatment of these cell types with $Al_2O_3$ particles which resulted in increased production of IL-6 and GM-CSF as assessed in a a co-culture in vitro model [124]. Another study examined the cross talk between macrophages and osteoblasts in the presence of $Al_2O_3$ particles employing media conditioned by osteoblasts exposed to particles in which a slight decrease in OPG-to-RANKL ratio was detected [125]. In this study, secretion of TNF-α, IL-6 and GM-CSF by PBMCs was not induced by culturing these cells with media conditioned by osteoblast exposed to $Al_2O_3$. Osteoclasts formation assays showed an increase in TRAP-positive aggregates which suggested the activation of osteoclastogenesis although osteoclast generation was not enhanced in PBMC cultures exposed to conditioned medium of osteoblasts challenged with $Al_2O_3$.

In summary, although ceramics present advantages in comparison to other materials, they still seem able to elicit an adverse local reaction. However, the moderate wear rate of ceramic components together with the limited effects of ceramic particles-induced biological responses may significantly account for the low incidence of osteolysis in patients bearing this type of prosthesis.

## Cement Particles

PMMA debris arise from the fragmentation of the cement used to fix components of THA [3, 126]. Bone cement is frequently applied to the femoral stem but also the acetabular shell may be fixed to the adjacent bone. PMMA-based bone cement was introduced by Charnley as an effective mean to achieve stable fixation between the bone bed and the implant, and later as matrix for local delivery of antibiotics [126]. Apart from favouring formation of a fibrous interfacial tissue, PMMA experiences brittleness and shrinkage, lack of adherence to the bone and during its application, the in situ exothermic polymerization reaction can damage the adjacent bone tissue. In general, cemented prostheses are not options for young and active patients, with good bone stock quality, as PMMA can cause third body wear and secondary loosening of the hip components [127]. PMMA third-body abrasive particles originated from the failure of the cement mantle can induce surface damage, especially relevant in PE and Ti-based components [3, 128]. $ZrO_2$ and $BaSO_4$ are used as radio-opaque contrast media in bone cement, and therefore disintegration of the cement mantle can produce PMMA and/or $ZrO_2$ or $BaSO_4$ particles which can contribute to direct cell responses and also to third-body wear [3, 126].

Acrylic particles found in the capsular tissue present a size range from 1–2 μm to several hundreds of microns. Several shapes have been observed, being the smallest particles similar to dust granules and the largest ones like pearls clusters or grapes bunch [3]. Under light microscopy, particles present a size between 0.5 and 2 μm with grey or yellow brown colour and under polarized light, they show slight white birefringence [129].

Localized areas of osteolysis exhibiting foreign body response to cement particles are frequently observed [60]. PMMA, $ZrO_2$ and $BaSO_4$ particles of phagocytosable size can be internalized and stored within macrophages while the non-phagocytosable large cement fragments are surrounded by foreign body giant cells. Aggressive granulomatous lesions as well as non-granulomatous AL around cemented total hip prostheses have been observed. PMMA particles are also able to activate the lymphocyte-mediated immune response [3].

Cell surface receptor complement receptor 3 (CR3) is involved in the phagocytosis and activation of signaling pathways of macrophages exposed to PMMA [48]. Production of inflammatory mediators is also mediated by TLRs in a manner partly dependent on MyD88 signaling pathway, since inhibition of this adaptor molecule decreased the induced production of TNF-α in RAW 264.7 murine macrophages exposed to PMMA [22]. As described for polymeric and metallic particles, PMMA particles activate the NALP3 inflammasome [130]. Phagocytosed cement particles induce caspase-1 activation in monocyte/macrophage cells and the release of downstream effectors IL-1β and TNF-α, both involved in the amplification of osteoclastogenesis mediated by RANKL.

In vitro studies suggest that PMMA particles may have more potent osteolytic effects than high density PE particles [131]. In fact, the activation of macrophages by PMMA particles has long been considered as a key mechanism in wear-induced osteolysis of cemented implants [3, 48]. Apart from peri-implant resident cell activation, PMMA particles are also able to recruit peripheral monocyte/macrophages, promoting the systemic trafficking of macrophages to the site of inflammation [3], as observed after PMMA injection in the medullary canal of nude mice and the intravenous administration of RAW264.7 macrophages stably expressing a bioluminescent reporter gene [132]. This finding was corroborated using a severe combined immunodeficiency mouse chimera model, in which fragments of periprosthetic granulomatous tissues and bone chips retrieved during revision surgery in loosened patients were implanted in mice [133]. PBMCs isolated from patients during revision surgery were fluorescently labeled and cultured with cement particles before intraperitoneal injection. Fluorescent-labeled PBMCs challenged with PMMA particles and a high number of TRAP-positive cells accumulated in transplanted periprosthetic tissues.

The chemotactic effects induced by PMMA particles leading to migration of human monocyte and MSCs have been studied in in vitro studies [60, 79]. Macrophages challenged with cement particles increase MCP-1 release. Like MCP-1, MIP-1α is expressed in periprosthetic tissues and produced by cells of the monocytic/macrophagic lineage after priming with PMMA particles [22]. Moreover, neutralizing antibody to MIP-1α lessened the migration of monocytes induced by media conditioned by macrophages exposed to PMMA particles [134]. An independent study confirmed the involvement of MCP-1 and MIP-1α induced by PMMA particles in the homing of monocytes and MSCs, suggesting the involvement of various chemokines in the recruitment of macrophages and MSCs [135]. Fibroblasts, a cell source of chemokines, increase MCP-1 release upon exposure to PMMA particles [136].

Exposure of macrophages to PMMA increases the expression of pro-inflammatory cytokines, via activation of the NF-κB pathway [137, 138]. Among other macrophage-releated cell types, dose- and time-dependent induction of the secretion of IL-1 and $PGE_2$ has been observed in peritoneal macrophages [60] while induction in the release of IL-1β and TNF-α was described in bone marrow macrophages [139]. In line with this, Pearle and colleagues performed microarrays profiling of monocytes and unfractionated PBMCs exposed to PMMA and Ti particles to assess, respectively, the activation of the innate immune system and the innate and adaptive immune system [140]. Exposure of monocytes to PMMA induced the transcript levels of TNF-α, IL-1α, IL-1β, IL-6, IL-8 and COX-2, key regulator of $PGE_2$ synthesis, as well as the chemokines MIP-3α and CCL11. Similar data were obtained in PBMC exposed to PMMA. Comparison with data obtained from cells exposed to Ti particles suggested that PMMA-inflammatory effects are mediated by the activation of the innate immune system, i.e., monocytes, in a T cell-independent manner, while lymphocytes are not essential mediators in PMMA-induced osteolysis.

Apart from the induction in the inflammatory response, PMMA particles contribute to mononuclear phagocytes and macrophages differentiation into TRAP-positive cells with resorptive capacity [131, 141]. Other osteoclastic phenotypic markers might be regulated by PMMA particles, as murine RAW264.7 cells exposed to PMMA upregulated cathepsin K and RANK expression [142]. PMMA particles stimulate osteoclastogenesis, at least in part, by induction of RANKL and TNF-α expression and by activation of NF-κB [143]. Signaling pathways that cooperate with RANKL-induced during differentiation of macrophages into osteoclasts, like MAPK pathway, are also activated. Expression and activity of the transcription factor NFAT2, involved critically in osteoclast lineage commitment, increases in osteoclast precursors exposed to PMMA particles [144]. PMMA-derived effects on the osteoclastic lineage seem to be dependent on their stages of development, increasing the number of osteoclasts precursors and enhancing the number and bone resorption capacity of mature cells [145].

As mentioned before, macrophages exhibit functional plasticity in order to adapt to the dynamic periprosthetic microenvironment. Macrophages challenged by PMMA particles exhibit characteristics of M1 phenotype [146]. However, macrophages may evolve from M1 to M2 phenotype as proven in in vitro experiments in which M1 macrophages were treated with IL-4 prior to exposure to PMMA particles or were simultaneously treated with IL-4 and particles [139].

Exposure to PMMA particles impairs viability, proliferation and osteogenic differentiation of osteoprogenitor cells. Transcript levels of the transcription factors Runx2, Osx and Dlx5 that orchestrate osteogenic differentiation, and OCN decrease after exposure of MC3T3-E1 to PMMA particles [138, 147]. Effects on osteoprogenitor proliferation and differentiation have been found to be dose-dependent [148]. The more potent inhibitory effects of PMMA particles have been detected in the early phase of osteoprogenitor differentiation, as shown in cultures of murine bone marrow cells [148, 149]. PMMA-induced inhibition of osteoblastic differentiation is characterized by altered expression of genes encoding bone morphogenetic protein 3 (BMP3) and SOST, which are negative regulators of bone formation [150].

Regarding mature bone-forming cells, proliferation and collagen synthesis of osteoblastic cells exposed to PMMA were reported to be inhibited whereas OCN and IL-6 production were stimulated [151]. Additionally, apoptotic rates and MMP-1 expression were enhanced in osteoblasts exposed to PMMA [152]. As observed with other types of particles, the mechanisms involved in osteoblasts dysfunction after exposure to PMMA particles are not totally understood. Among other participating mechanisms, inhibition of MAPK activity and reduced TGF-β1 production, which play an essential role in differentiation and the response to environmental stress, have been proposed [150]. A recent study has addressed the consequences of the physical stress stimuli that PMMA particles impose to osteoblasts that include an increase in the elastic modulus with time, production of calcium and changes in cytoskeleton organisation which influence cell behaviour and function [86]. Addition of radio-opaque agents favors macrophage-osteoclast differentiation and their resorptive activity, being more resorptive PMMA containing $BaSO_4$ than $ZrO_2$ [153]. Moreover, exposure of osteoblastic cells to cements containing these radio-opaque agents increased the expression ratio RANKL/OPG [154]. Such imbalance might be related to stimulation of osteoclast differentiation and inhibition of osteoclast apoptosis.

Collected evidence indicates that cement-derived wear particles elicit important adverse cellular reactions that lead to to periprosthetic osteolysis. Cement particles are found in high proportion in the periprosthetic bone bed which facilitates their direct action and severe effects on bone and immune cells.

## Perspectives

Research efforts in THR have been oriented toward the improvement of the tribology of materials used in prostheses manufacturing as well as to the elucidation of the biological processes triggered by wear particles [26]. Important advances in orthopaedic materials concerning their microstructure, surface characteristics and/or design have been made and multiple biomaterials have been generated as promising alternatives including advanced composites and hybrid materials [155–157]. Among others, coatings of the material surfaces with bioceramics or functionalization with extracellular matrix proteins, biological peptides or growth factors are expected to stimulate physiological mechanisms that counterbalance the development of osteolysis [50, 158]. However, novel materials still face issues regarding their long-term performance and biological response to wear and corrosion debris. Moreover, a deeper understanding of the local and systemic biological responses to materials is needed. The identification of signaling pathways and cellular and molecular mediators that contribute to periprosthetic osteolysis will facilitate not only the generation of mimetic, self-diagnosing and multifunctional materials but also the development of targeted and personalized therapeutic strategies. Innovations in genotyping, pharmacogenomics and large-scale molecular phenotyping will facilitate the identification of the mechanisms involved in the pathogenesis of osteolysis that then will be used to design strategies for the diagnosis, prevention and treatment of AL [24, 159]. For instance, recent progresses in the understanding of the signaling pathways that integrate ER stress, apoptosis, inflammation or osteoclastogenesis have been proposed as promising therapeutic targets to mitigate wear particle-induced osteolysis [94, 160]. Acting upstream of the inflammatory cascade activated by wear particles might lead to better therapeutic control of the local process, in opposition to systemic management which might be associated to adverse side-effects. Three main events triggered by the presence of particles can be targeted: cellular chemotaxis, polarization of macrophages and NF-κB signaling [60, 85, 161, 162]. Protein phosphatase 2A, a major serine-threonine phosphatase involved in NF-κB and c-Jun N-terminal kinase signaling pathways has been proposed as new target for pharmacological intervention in Ti-induced osteolysis [163]. Inhibition of the glycogen synthetase kinase 3 beta, regulator in the canonical Wnt signaling pathway which is essential in the maintenance of normal bone mass, has been suggested as a target of molecules to treat wear-debris induced osteolysis [164]. Other proposed targets explored are bone morphogenetic proteins [165] and protein kinase C [166]. Therefore, the more we know about intracellular signaling activated by wear particles, the more options we have to develop therapeutic interventions for aseptic implant loosening.

Other therapeutic intervention has focused in controlling the levels of RANKL and OPG [50]. Specific materials, such as biosilica and microstructured Ti surfaces, are able to stimulate the endogenous production of OPG. Treatments with anti-resorptive bisphosphonates (e.g. alendronate and zolendronate), RANKL antibodies or OPG-like molecules have been proposed. Some of these drugs have proven their efficacy in pathologies associated to catabolic bone disorders, but might have an important impact at systemic level. Unwanted side effects have been also associated to anti-inflammatory drugs as corticosteroids or TNF-α antagonists or IL-1 antagonists, which have been suggested to treat wear-induced osteolysis [51]. Other pharmacological agents assayed include the synthetic molecules OA-14 ((N-(3-(dodecylcarbamoyl)phenyl)-1H-indole-2-carboxamide)) [167] and methotrexate [168] or the ursolic acid [169].

An active research has been performed testing agents able to modulate the NF-κB signaling pathway, including natural bioactive compounds such as triptolide, notoginsenoside R1 or sophocarpine [170–172], antibiotics as rifampin [173], bioflavonoids such as anthocyanin or amentoflavone, [174, 175], components of the omega-3 fatty acids such as the docosahexanoic acid [176] or the probiotic *Lactobacillus casei* [177]. In this search of modulators of NF-κB, the hormone melatonin has been reported as candidate for the treatment of wear debris-induced osteolysis [178]. Sirtuin 1, NAD(+)-dependent histone deacetylase which regulates the transcriptional activity of NF-κB, has been considered as a pharmacological target in osteoblast and macrophages challenged to metal particles [179, 180]. Statins such as simvastatin and pitavastatin, employed as lipid-lowering medication, have been also proposed for the prevention and/or treatment in wear particle-induced bone resorption. Our group reported that simvastatin down-regulates IL-6 secretion in osteoblastic cells cultured in isolation or co-cultured with macrophages and exposed to Ti particles [181]. In order to improve the local efficacy of anti-inflammatory and/or anti-osteolytic therapeutic agents different methods to concentrate the drug preferentially into the inflammatory area have been proposed, avoiding or reducing systemic exposure. In this regard, local delivery of dexamethasone conjugated to the copolymer HPMA or covalently conjugated to $TiO_2$ particles has been assayed [182, 183].

Gene therapy has also emerged as a potential therapeutic avenue. For instance, in vitro and in vivo models have shown the effectiveness of viral gene delivery of IL-10, IL-1Ra and OPG in Ti- and UHMWPE-induced osteolysis models [184–189]. Other therapeutic experimental approaches employed small interfering RNA to silence TNF-α, the catalytic subunit of phosphoinositide 3-kinase (PI3K) p110β or the chemokine receptor CXCR2 [190–192]. Although promising preliminary results have been achieved, the implementation of gene therapy into orthopaedic practice is still a distant possibility.

Other important aspect to consider is the early diagnosis of wear particles-induced osteolysis. Therefore, efforts are focused in the search of biomarkers as diagnostic and prognostic tools to monitor the progression of the disease. Different biomarkers in synovial fluid, urine and serum have been proposed, but still none have proved relevant clinical utility [193, 194]. In this regard, our group has been focused during the last years in the identification of serum proteins with potential to be regarded as biomarkers.

## Concluding Remarks

Wear particles-induced osteolysis is one of the major challenges for orthopedic surgeons due to the absence of clinical signs and symptoms until late stages of destruction and failure. The increasing demand of hip arthroplasties and the growing incidence in young patients, with predictions pointing to a substantial increase in revision surgeries, highlights that this issue has to be seriously considered. Currently, strategies are focused on improving the implant behaviour and limiting the biological response to its degradation products. Despite intense research efforts in the materials field, the long-term performance of novel biomaterials is still unknown. In the biomedical field, it is imperative to unravel the cellular and molecular mechanisms triggered by wear debris to establish effective medical interventions. Too many questions that still remain not answered and become major challenges for basic research groups.

## References

1. Learmonth ID, Young C, Rorabeck C. The operation of the century: total hip replacement. Lancet. 2007;370:1508–19.
2. Apostu D, Lucaciu O, Berce C, Lucaciu D, Cosma D. Current methods of preventing aseptic loosening and improving osseointegration of titanium implants in cementless total hip arthroplasty: a review. J Int Med Res. 2017; https://doi.org/10.1177/0300060517732697.
3. Bitar D, Parvizi J. Biological response to prosthetic debris. World J Orthop. 2015;6:172–89. https://doi.org/10.5312/wjo.v6.i2.172.
4. Singh JA. Epidemiology of knee and hip arthroplasty: a systematic review. Open Orthop J. 2011;5:80–5. https://doi.org/10.2174/1874325001105010080.

5. Kremers HM, Larson DR, Crowson CS, Kremers WK, Washington RE, Steiner CA, et al. Prevalence of total hip and knee replacement in the United States. J Bone Joint Surg Am. 2015;97:1386–97. https://doi.org/10.2106/JBJS.N.01141.
6. Dobzyniak M, Fehring TK, Odum S. Early failure in total hip arthroplasty. Clin Orthop Relat Res. 2006;447:76–8.
7. Melvin JS, Karthikeyan T, Cope R, Fehring TK. Early failures in total hip arthroplasty – a changing paradigm. J Arthroplast. 2014;29:1285–8. https://doi.org/10.1016/j.arth.2013.12.024.
8. Cherian JJ, Jauregui JJ, Banerjee S, Pierce T, Mont MA. What host factors affect aseptic loosening after THA and TKA? Clin Orthop Relat Res. 2015;473:2700–9. https://doi.org/10.1007/s11999-015-4220-2.
9. Gibon E, Amanatullah DF, Loi F, Pajarinen J, Nabeshima A, Yao Z, et al. The biological response to orthopaedic implants for joint replacement: part I: metals. J Biomed Mater Res B Appl Biomater. 2017;105:2162–73. https://doi.org/10.1002/jbm.b.33734.
10. Jansen P, Mumme T, Randau T, Gravius S, Hermanns-Sachweh B. Endoglin (CD105) expression differentiates between aseptic loosening and periprosthetic joint infection after total joint arthroplasty. Springerplus. 2014;3:561. https://doi.org/10.1186/2193-1801-3-561.
11. Mäkelä KT, Eskelinen A, Pulkkinen P, Paavolainen P, Remes V. Results of 3,668 primary total hip replacements for primary osteoarthritis in patients under the age of 55 years. Acta Orthop. 2011;82:521–9. https://doi.org/10.3109/17453674.2011.618908.
12. Landgraeber S, Jäger M, Jacobs JJ, Hallab NJ. The pathology of orthopedic implant failure is mediated by innate immune system cytokines. Mediat Inflamm. 2014;2014:185150. https://doi.org/10.1155/2014/185150.
13. Sukur E, Akman YE, Ozturkmen Y, Kucukdurmaz F. Particle disease: a current review of the biological mechanisms in periprosthetic osteolysis after hip arthroplasty. Open Orthop J. 2016;10:241–51. https://doi.org/10.2174/1874325001610010241.
14. Pajarinen J, Lin TH, Nabeshima A, Jämsen E, Lu L, Nathan K, et al. Mesenchymal stem cells in the aseptic loosening of total joint replacements. J Biomed Mater Res A. 2017;105:1195–207. https://doi.org/10.1002/jbm.a.35978.
15. MacInnes SJ, Gordon A, Wilkinson JM. Risk factors for aseptic loosening following Total hip arthroplasty. Recent Adv Arthroplast. 2012; https://doi.org/10.5772/26975.
16. Veronesi F, Tschon M, Fini M. Gene expression in osteolysis: review on the identification of altered molecular pathways in preclinical and clinical studies. Int J Mol Sci. 2017;25:18. https://doi.org/10.3390/ijms18030499.
17. Nich C, Takakubo Y, Pajarinen J, Ainola M, Salem A, Sillat T, et al. Macrophages-key cells in the response to wear debris from joint replacements. J Biomed Mater Res A. 2013;101:3033–45. https://doi.org/10.1002/jbm.a.34599.
18. Gallo J, Goodman SB, Konttinen YT, Raska M. Particle disease: biologic mechanisms of periprosthetic osteolysis in total hip arthroplasty. Innate Immun. 2013;19:213–24. https://doi.org/10.1177/1753425912451779.
19. Camuzard O, Breuil V, Carle GF, Pierrefite-Carle V. Targeting autophagy to inhibit wear debris-induced osteolysis. AME Med J. 2017;2:5.
20. Yan Y, Hu J, Lu H, Wang W. Genetic susceptibility to total hip arthroplasty failure: a case-control study on the influence of MMP 1 gene polymorphism. Diagn Pathol. 2014;9:177. https://doi.org/10.1186/s13000-014-0177-9.
21. Towle KM, Monnot AD. An assessment of gender-specific risk of implant revision after primary total hip arthroplasty: a systematic review and meta-analysis. J Arthroplast. 2016;31:2941–8. https://doi.org/10.1016/j.arth.2016.07.047.
22. Gu Q, Shi Q, Yang H. The role of TLR and chemokine in wear particle-induced aseptic loosening. J Biomed Biotechnol. 2012;2012:596870. https://doi.org/10.1155/2012/596870.
23. Hallab NJ, Jacobs JJ. Biologic effects of implant debris. Bull NYU Hosp Jt Dis. 2009;67:182–8.
24. Terkawi MA, Hamasaki M, Takahashi D, Ota M, Kadoya K, Yutani T, et al. Transcriptional profile of human macrophages stimulated by ultra-high molecular weight polyethylene partic-

ulate debris of orthopedic implants uncovers a common gene expression signature of rheumatoid arthritis. Acta Biomater. 2018;65:417–25. https://doi.org/10.1016/j.actbio.2017.11.001.

25. Ulrich SD, Seyler TM, Bennett D, Delanois RE, Saleh KJ, Thongtrangan I, et al. Total hip arthroplasties: what are the reasons for revision? Int Orthop. 2008;32:597–604.
26. Howie DW, Neale SD, Haynes DR, Holubowycz OT, McGee MA, Solomon LB, et al. Periprosthetic osteolysis after total hip replacement: molecular pathology and clinical management. Inflammopharmacology. 2013;21:389–96. https://doi.org/10.1007/s10787-013-0192-6.
27. Iorio R, Robb WJ, Healy WL, Berry DJ, Hozack WJ, Kyle RF, et al. Orthopaedic surgeon workforce and volume assessment for total hip and knee replacement in the United States: preparing for an epidemic. J Bone Joint Surg Am. 2008;90:1598–605.
28. McGrory BJ, Etkin CD, Lewallen DG. Comparing contemporary revision burden among hip and knee joint replacement registries. Arthroplast Today. 2016;2:83–6. https://doi.org/10.1016/j.artd.2016.04.003.
29. Nich C, Goodman SB. Role of macrophages in the biological reaction to wear debris from joint replacements. J Long-Term Eff Med Implants. 2014;24:259–65.
30. Girard J, Glorion C, Bonnomet F, Fron D, Migaud H. Risk factors for revision of hip arthroplasties in patients younger than 30 years. Clin Orthop Relat Res. 2011;469:1141–7. https://doi.org/10.1007/s11999-010-1669-x.
31. McGonagle L, Siney PD, Raut VV. Fate of the unrevised cemented stem following cup only revision: 227 hips at an average of 6 years follow-up. Orthop Traumatol Surg Res. 2015;101:781–4. https://doi.org/10.1016/j.otsr.2015.08.005.
32. Magone K, Luckenbill D, Goswami T. Metal ions as inflammatory initiators of osteolysis. Arch Orthop Trauma Surg. 2015;135:683–95. https://doi.org/10.1007/s00402-015-2196-8.
33. Jiang Y, Jia T, Wooley PH, Yang SY. Current research in the pathogenesis of aseptic implant loosening associated with particulate wear debris. Acta Orthop Belg. 2013;79:1–9.
34. Pajarinen J, Gallo J, Takagi M, Goodman SB, Mjöberg B. Particle disease really does exist. Acta Orthop. 2018;89:133–6. https://doi.org/10.1080/17453674.2017.1402463.
35. Bordini B, Stea S, De Clerico M, Strazzari S, Sasdelli A, Toni A. Factors affecting aseptic loosening of 4750 total hip arthroplasties: multivariate survival analysis. BMC Musculoskelet Disord. 2007;24(8):69.
36. Engh CA, Ho H, Powers CC, Huynh C, Beykirch SE, Hopper RH Jr. Osteolysis propensity among bilateral total hip arthroplasty patients. J Arthroplast. 2011;26:555–61. https://doi.org/10.1016/j.arth.2010.05.014.
37. Stelmach P, Kauther MD, Fuest L, Kurscheid G, Gehrke T, Klenke S, et al. Relationship between GNAS1 T393C polymorphism and aseptic loosening after total hip arthroplasty. Eur J Med Res. 2017;22:29. https://doi.org/10.1186/s40001-017-0271-z.
38. MacInnes SJ, Del Vescovo E, Kiss-Toth E, Ollier WE, Kay PR, Gordon A, et al. Genetic variation in inflammatory and bone turnover pathways and risk of osteolytic responses to prosthetic materials. J Orthop Res. 2015;33:193–8. https://doi.org/10.1002/jor.22755.
39. Kolundzić R, Orlić D, Trkulja V, Pavelić K, Troselj KG. Single nucleotide polymorphisms in the interleukin-6 gene promoter, tumor necrosis factor-alpha gene promoter, and transforming growth factor-beta1 gene signal sequence as predictors of time to onset of aseptic loosening after total hip arthroplasty: preliminary study. J Orthop Sci. 2006;11:592–600.
40. Gallo J, Mrazek F, Petrek M. Variation in cytokine genes can contribute to severity of acetabular osteolysis and risk for revision in patients with ABG 1 total hip arthroplasty: a genetic association study. BMC Med Genet. 2009;10:109. https://doi.org/10.1186/1471-2350-10-109.
41. Malik MH, Jury F, Bayat A, Ollier WE, Kay PR. Genetic susceptibility to total hip arthroplasty failure: a preliminary study on the influence of matrix metalloproteinase 1, interleukin 6 polymorphisms and vitamin D receptor. Ann Rheum Dis. 2007;66:1116–20.
42. Kremers HM, Lewallen EA, van Wijnen AJ, Lewallen DG. Clinical factors, disease parameters, and molecular therapies affecting osseointegration of orthopedic implants. Curr Mol Biol Rep. 2016;2:123–32. https://doi.org/10.1007/s40610-016-0042-6.

43. Ollivere B, Wimhurst JA, Clark IM, Donell ST. Current concepts in osteolysis. J Bone Joint Surg Br. 2012;94:10–5. https://doi.org/10.1302/0301-620X.94B1.28047.
44. Ries MD, Link TM. Monitoring and risk of progression of osteolysis after total hip arthroplasty. J Bone Joint Surg Am. 2012;94:2097–105.
45. Revell PA. The combined role of wear particles, macrophages and lymphocytes in the loosening of total joint prostheses. J R Soc Interface. 2008;5:1263–78. https://doi.org/10.1098/rsif.2008.0142.
46. Kumar N, Arora GN, Datta B. Bearing surfaces in hip replacement – evolution and likely future. Med J Armed Forces India. 2014;70:371–6. https://doi.org/10.1016/j.mjafi.2014.04.015.
47. Callaghan JJ, Pedersen DR, Johnston RC, Brown TD. Clinical biomechanics of wear in total hip arthroplasty. Iowa Orthop J. 2003;23:1–12.
48. Noordin S, Masri B. Periprosthetic osteolysis: genetics, mechanisms and potential therapeutic interventions. Can J Surg. 2012;55:408–17. https://doi.org/10.1503/cjs.003711.
49. Sundfeldt M, Carlsson LV, Johansson CB, Thomsen P, Gretzer C. Aseptic loosening, not only a question of wear: a review of different theories. Acta Orthop. 2006;77:177–97.
50. Kapasa ER, Giannoudis PV, Jia X, Hatton PV, Yang XB. The effect of RANKL/OPG balance on reducing implant complications. J Funct Biomater. 2017;8(4):E42. https://doi.org/10.3390/jfb8040042.
51. Kandahari AM, Yang X, Laroche KA, Dighe AS, Pan D, Cui Q. A review of UHMWPE wear-induced osteolysis: the role for early detection of the immune response. Bone Res. 2016;4:16014. https://doi.org/10.1038/boneres.2016.14.
52. Vallés G, Gil-Garay E, Munuera L, Vilaboa N. Modulation of the cross-talk between macrophages and osteoblasts by titanium-based particles. Biomaterials. 2008;29:2326–35. https://doi.org/10.1016/j.biomaterials.2008.02.011.
53. Vallés G, González-Melendi P, Saldaña L, Rodriguez M, Munuera L, Vilaboa N. Rutile and titanium particles differentially affect the production of osteoblastic local factors. J Biomed Mater Res A. 2008;84:324–36.
54. Vallés G, González-Melendi P, González-Carrasco JL, Saldaña L, Sánchez-Sabaté E, Munuera L, et al. Differential inflammatory macrophage response to rutile and titanium particles. Biomaterials. 2006;27:5199–211.
55. Kobayashi A, Freeman MA, Bonfield W, Kadoya Y, Yamac T, Al-Saffar N, et al. Number of polyethylene particles and osteolysis in total joint replacements. A quantitative study using a tissue-digestion method. J Bone Joint Surg Br. 1997;79:844–8.
56. Lähdeoja T, Pajarinen J, Kouri VP, Sillat T, Salo J, Konttinen YT. Toll-like receptors and aseptic loosening of hip endoprosthesis-a potential to respond against danger signals? J Orthop Res. 2010;28:184–90. https://doi.org/10.1002/jor.20979.
57. Xing Z, Pabst MJ, Hasty KA, Smith RA. Accumulation of LPS by polyethylene particles decreases bone attachment to implants. J Orthop Res. 2006;24:959–66.
58. Alley C, Haggard W, Smith R. Effect of UHMWPE particle size, dose, and endotoxin on in vitro macrophage response. J Long-Term Eff Med Implants. 2014;24:45–56.
59. Zaveri TD, Dolgova NV, Lewis JS, Hamaker K, Clare-Salzler MJ, Keselowsky BG. Macrophage integrins modulate response to ultra-high molecular weight polyethylene particles and direct particle-induced osteolysis. Biomaterials. 2017;115:128–40. https://doi.org/10.1016/j.biomaterials.2016.10.038.
60. Gibon E, Córdova LA, Lu L, Lin TH, Yao Z, Hamadouche M, et al. The biological response to orthopedic implants for joint replacement. II: polyethylene, ceramics, PMMA, and the foreign body reaction. J Biomed Mater Res B Appl Biomater. 2017;105:1685–91. https://doi.org/10.1002/jbm.b.33676.
61. Maitra R, Clement CC, Scharf B, Crisi GM, Chitta S, Paget D, et al. Endosomal damage and TLR2 mediated inflammasome activation by alkane particles in the generation of aseptic osteolysis. Mol Immunol. 2009;47:175–84. https://doi.org/10.1016/j.molimm.2009.09.023.
62. Goodman SB, Ma T. Cellular chemotaxis induced by wear particles from joint replacements. Biomaterials. 2010;31:5045–50. https://doi.org/10.1016/j.biomaterials.2010.03.046.

63. Gibon E, Ma T, Ren PG, Fritton K, Biswal S, Yao Z, et al. Selective inhibition of the MCP-1-CCR2 ligand-receptor axis decreases systemic trafficking of macrophages in the presence of UHMWPE particles. J Orthop Res. 2012;30:547–53. https://doi.org/10.1002/jor.21548.
64. Liu A, Richards L, Bladen CL, Ingham E, Fisher J, Tipper JL. The biological response to nanometre-sized polymer particles. Acta Biomater. 2015;23:38–51. https://doi.org/10.1016/j.actbio.2015.05.016.
65. Kauther MD, Xu J, Wedemeyer C. Alpha-calcitonin gene-related peptide can reverse the catabolic influence of UHMWPE particles on RANKL expression in primary human osteoblasts. Int J Biol Sci. 2010;6:525–36.
66. Atkins GJ, Welldon KJ, Holding CA, Haynes DR, Howie DW, Findlay DM. The induction of a catabolic phenotype in human primary osteoblasts and osteocytes by polyethylene particles. Biomaterials. 2009;30:3672–81. https://doi.org/10.1016/j.biomaterials.2009.03.035.
67. Chiu R, Ma T, Smith RL, Goodman SB. Ultrahigh molecular weight polyethylene wear debris inhibits osteoprogenitor proliferation and differentiation in vitro. J Biomed Mater Res A. 2009;89:242–7. https://doi.org/10.1002/jbm.a.32001.
68. Ormsby RT, Cantley M, Kogawa M, Solomon LB, Haynes DR, Findlay DM, Atkins GJ. Evidence that osteocyte perilacunar remodelling contributes to polyethylene wear particle induced osteolysis. Acta Biomater. 2016;33:242–51. https://doi.org/10.1016/j.actbio.2016.01.016.
69. Sartori M, Vincenzi F, Ravani A, Cepollaro S, Martini L, Varani K, et al. RAW 264.7 co-cultured with ultra-high molecular weight polyethylene particles spontaneously differentiate into osteoclasts: an in vitro model of periprosthetic osteolysis. J Biomed Mater Res A. 2017;105:510–20. https://doi.org/10.1002/jbm.a.35912.
70. Pan X, Mao X, Cheng T, Peng X, Zhang X, Liu Z, et al. Up-regulated expression of MIF by interfacial membrane fibroblasts and macrophages around aseptically loosened implants. J Surg Res. 2012;176:484–9. https://doi.org/10.1016/j.jss.2011.09.047.
71. Rao AJ, Nich C, Dhulipala LS, Gibon E, Valladares R, Zwingenberger S, et al. Local effect of IL-4 delivery on polyethylene particle induced osteolysis in the murine calvarium. J Biomed Mater Res A. 2013;101:1926–34. https://doi.org/10.1002/jbm.a.34486.
72. Du Z, Zhu Z, Wang Y. The degree of peri-implant osteolysis induced by PEEK, CoCrMo, and HXLPE wear particles: a study based on a porous Ti6Al4V implant in a rabbit model. J Orthop Surg Res. 2018;13:23. https://doi.org/10.1186/s13018-018-0736-y.
73. Vallés G, García-Cimbrelo E, Vilaboa N. Involvement of extracellular Hsp72 in wear particle-mediated osteolysis. Acta Biomater. 2012;8:1146–55. https://doi.org/10.1016/j.actbio.2011.12.001.
74. Vaculova J, Gallo J, Hurnik P, Motyka O, Goodman SB, Dvorackova J. Low intrapatient variability of histomorphological findings in periprosthetic tissues from revised metal/ceramic on polyethylene joint arthroplasties. J Biomed Mater Res B Appl Biomater. 2017; https://doi.org/10.1002/jbm.b.33990.
75. Hirayama T, Tamaki Y, Takakubo Y, Iwazaki K, Sasaki K, Ogino T, et al. Toll-like receptors and their adaptors are regulated in macrophages after phagocytosis of lipopolysaccharide-coated titanium particles. J Orthop Res. 2011;29:984–92. https://doi.org/10.1002/jor.21369.
76. Dapunt U, Giese T, Lasitschka F, Reinders J, Lehner B, Kretzer JP, et al. On the inflammatory response in metal-on-metal implants. J Transl Med. 2014;12:74. https://doi.org/10.1186/1479-5876-12-74.
77. Drynda A, Singh G, Buchhorn GH, Awiszus F, Ruetschi M, Feuerstein B, et al. Metallic wear debris may regulate CXCR4 expression in vitro and in vivo. J Biomed Mater Res A. 2015;103:1940–8. https://doi.org/10.1002/jbm.a.35330.
78. Geng D, Xu Y, Yang H, Wang J, Zhu X, Zhu G, et al. Protection against titanium particle induced osteolysis by cannabinoid receptor 2 selective antagonist. Biomaterials. 2010;31:1996–2000. https://doi.org/10.1016/j.biomaterials.2009.11.069.
79. Hallab NJ, Jacobs JJ. Chemokines associated with pathologic responses to orthopedic implant debris. Front Endocrinol (Lausanne). 2017;8:5. https://doi.org/10.3389/fendo.2017.00005.

80. Chen M, Chen PM, Dong QR, Huang Q, She C, Xu W. p38 signaling in titanium particle-induced MMP-2 secretion and activation in differentiating MC3T3-E1 cells. J Biomed Mater Res A. 2014;102:2824–32. https://doi.org/10.1002/jbm.a.34956.
81. Qiu S, Zhao F, Tang X, Pei F, Dong H, Zhu L, et al. Type-2 cannabinoid receptor regulates proliferation, apoptosis, differentiation, and OPG/RANKL ratio of MC3T3-E1 cells exposed to titanium particles. Mol Cell Biochem. 2015;399:131–41. https://doi.org/10.1007/s11010-014-2240-y.
82. Fu C, Xie J, Hu N, Liang X, Chen R, Wang C, et al. Titanium particles up-regulate the activity of matrix metalloproteinase-2 in human synovial cells. Int Orthop. 2014;38:1091–8. https://doi.org/10.1007/s00264-013-2190-0.
83. Obando-Pereda GA, Fischer L, Stach-Machado DR. Titanium and zirconia particle-induced pro-inflammatory gene expression in cultured macrophages and osteolysis, inflammatory hyperalgesia and edema in vivo. Life Sci. 2014;97:96–106. https://doi.org/10.1016/j.lfs.2013.11.008.
84. Greenfield EM, Beidelschies MA, Tatro JM, Goldberg VM, Hise AG. Bacterial pathogen-associated molecular patterns stimulate biological activity of orthopaedic wear particles by activating cognate Toll-like receptors. J Biol Chem. 2010;285:32378–84. https://doi.org/10.1074/jbc.M110.136895.
85. Pajarinen J, Kouri VP, Jämsen E, Li TF, Mandelin J, Konttinen YT. The response of macrophages to titanium particles is determined by macrophage polarization. Acta Biomater. 2013;9:9229–40. https://doi.org/10.1016/j.actbio.2013.06.027.
86. Preedy EC, Perni S, Prokopovich P. Cobalt, titanium and PMMA bone cement debris influence on mouse osteoblast cell elasticity, spring constant and calcium production activity. RSC Adv. 2015;5:83885–98.
87. Howie DW, Vernon-Roberts B. Synovial macrophage response to aluminium oxide ceramic and cobalt-chrome alloy wear particles in rats. Biomaterials. 1988;9:442–8.
88. Devitt BM, Queally JM, Vioreanu M, Butler JS, Murray D, Doran PP, et al. Cobalt ions induce chemokine secretion in a variety of systemic cell lines. Acta Orthop. 2010;81:756–64. https://doi.org/10.3109/17453674.2010.537806.
89. Jonitz-Heincke A, Tillmann J, Klinder A, Krueger S, Kretzer JP, Høl PJ, et al. The impact of metal ion exposure on the cellular behavior of human osteoblasts and PBMCs: in vitro analyses of osteolytic processes. Materials (Basel). 2017;10:E734. https://doi.org/10.3390/ma10070734.
90. Rakow A, Schoon J, Dienelt A, John T, Textor M, Duda G, Perka C, Schulze F, Ode A. Influence of particulate and dissociated metal-on-metal hip endoprosthesis wear on mesenchymal stromal cells in vivo and in vitro. Biomaterials. 2016;98:31–40. https://doi.org/10.1016/j.biomaterials.2016.04.023.
91. Potnis PA, Dutta DK, Wood SC. Toll-like receptor 4 signaling pathway mediates proinflammatory immune response to cobalt-alloy particles. Cell Immunol. 2013;282:53–65. https://doi.org/10.1016/j.cellimm.2013.04.003.
92. Raghunathan VK, Devey M, Hawkins S, Hails L, Davis SA, Mann S, et al. Influence of particle size and reactive oxygen species on cobalt chrome nanoparticle-mediated genotoxicity. Biomaterials. 2013;34:3559–70. https://doi.org/10.1016/j.biomaterials.2013.01.085.
93. Papageorgiou I, Brown C, Schins R, Singh S, Newson R, Davis S, Fisher J, Ingham E, Case CP. The effect of nano- and micron-sized particles of cobalt-chromium alloy on human fibroblasts in vitro. Biomaterials. 2007;28:2946–58.
94. Liu G, Guo T, Zhang Y, Liu N, Chen J, Chen J, Zhang J, Zhao J. Apoptotic pathways of macrophages within osteolytic interface membrane in periprosthestic osteolysis after total hip replacement. APMIS. 2017;125:565–78. https://doi.org/10.1111/apm.12679.
95. Lewis AC, Ladon D, Heard PJ, Peto L, Learmonth I. The role of the surface chemistry of CoCr alloy particles in the phagocytosis and DNA damage of fibroblast cells. J Biomed Mater Res A. 2007;82:363–72.
96. Athanasou NA. The pathobiology and pathology of aseptic implant failure. Bone Joint Res. 2016;5:162–8. https://doi.org/10.1302/2046-3758.55.BJR-2016-0086.

97. Daniel J, Holland J, Quigley L, Sprague S, Bhandari M. Pseudotumors associated with total hip arthroplasty. J Bone Joint Surg Am. 2012;94:86–93. https://doi.org/10.2106/JBJS.J.01612.
98. Catelas I, Lehoux EA, Ning Z, Figeys D, Baskey SJ, Beaulé PE. Differential proteomic analysis of synovial fluid from hip arthroplasty patients with a pseudotumor vs. periprosthetic osteolysis. J Orthop Res. 2018; https://doi.org/10.1002/jor.23858.
99. McCarthy CL, Uchihara Y, Vlychou M, Grammatopoulos G, Athanasou NA. Development of malignant lymphoma after metal-on-metal hip replacement: a case report and review of the literature. Skelet Radiol. 2017;46:831–6. https://doi.org/10.1007/s00256-017-2612-y.
100. Gallo J, Goodman SB, Lostak J, Janout M. Advantages and disadvantages of ceramic on ceramic total hip arthroplasty: a review. Biomed Pap Med Fac Univ Palacky Olomouc Czech Repub. 2012;156:204–12. https://doi.org/10.5507/bp.2012.063.
101. Mehmood S, Jinnah RH, Pandit H. Review on ceramic-on-ceramic total hip arthroplasty. J Surg Orthop Adv. 2008;17:45–50.
102. Tateiwa T, Clarke IC, Williams PA, Garino J, Manaka M, Shishido T, Yamamoto K, Imakiire A. Ceramic total hip arthroplasty in the United States: safety and risk issues revisited. Am J Orthop (Belle Mead NJ). 2008;37:E26–31.
103. Howard DP, Wall PDH, Fernandez MA, Parsons H, Howard PW. Ceramic-on-ceramic bearing fractures in total hip arthroplasty: an analysis of data from the National Joint Registry. Bone Joint J. 2017;99-B:1012–9. https://doi.org/10.1302/0301-620X.99B8.BJJ-2017-0019.R1.
104. Lee YK, Yoon BH, Choi YS, Jo WL, Ha YC, Koo KH. Metal on metal or ceramic on ceramic for cementless total hip arthroplasty: a meta-analysis. J Arthroplast. 2016;31:2637–45. https://doi.org/10.1016/j.arth.2016.04.014.
105. Mochida Y, Boehler M, Salzer M, Bauer TW. Debris from failed ceramic-on-ceramic and ceramic-on-polyethylene hip prostheses. Clin Orthop Relat Res. 2001;389:113–25.
106. Hatton A, Nevelos JE, Nevelos AA, Banks RE, Fisher J, Ingham E. Alumina-alumina artificial hip joints. Part I: a histological analysis and characterisation of wear debris by laser capture microdissection of tissues retrieved at revision. Biomaterials. 2002;23:3429–40.
107. Bylski D, Wedemeyer C, Xu J, Sterner T, Löer F, von Knoch M. Alumina ceramic particles, in comparison with titanium particles, hardly affect the expression of RANK-, TNF-alpha-, and OPG-mRNA in the THP-1 human monocytic cell line. J Biomed Mater Res A. 2009;89:707–16. https://doi.org/10.1002/jbm.a.31956.
108. Savarino L, Baldini N, Ciapetti G, Pellacani A, Giunti A. Is wear debris responsible for failure in alumina-on-alumina implants? Acta Orthop. 2009;80:162–7. https://doi.org/10.3109/17453670902876730.
109. Man K, Jiang LH, Foster R, Yang XB. Immunological responses to total hip arthroplasty. J Funct Biomater. 2017;8:E33. https://doi.org/10.3390/jfb8030033.
110. Wooley PH. How has the introduction of new bearing surfaces altered the biological reactions to byproducts of wear and modularity? Clin Orthop Relat Res. 2014;472:3699–708. https://doi.org/10.1007/s11999-014-3725-4.
111. Warashina H, Sakano S, Kitamura S, Yamauchi KI, Yamaguchi J, Ishiguro N, et al. Biological reaction to alumina, zirconia, titanium and polyethylene particles implanted onto murine calvaria. Biomaterials. 2003;24:3655–61.
112. Kaufman AM, Alabre CI, Rubash HE, Shanbhag AS. Human macrophage response to UHMWPE, TiAlV, CoCr, and alumina particles: analysis of multiple cytokines using protein arrays. J Biomed Mater Res A. 2008;84:464–74.
113. Petit A, Catelas I, Antoniou J, Zukor DJ, Huk OL. Differential apoptotic response of J774 macrophages to alumina and ultra-high-molecular-weight polyethylene particles. J Orthop Res. 2002;20:9–15.
114. Germain MA, Hatton A, Williams S, Matthews JB, Stone MH, Fisher J, et al. Comparison of the cytotoxicity of clinically relevant cobalt-chromium and alumina ceramic wear particles in vitro. Biomaterials. 2003;24:469–79.

115. Gutwein LG, Webster TJ. Increased viable osteoblast density in the presence of nanophase compared to conventional alumina and titania particles. Biomaterials. 2004;25:4175–83.
116. Lerouge S, Huk O, Yahia LH, Sedel L. Characterization of in vivo wear debris from ceramic-ceramic total hip arthroplasties. J Biomed Mater Res. 1996;32:627–33.
117. Liagre B, Moalic S, Vergne P, Charissoux JL, Bernache-Assollant D, Beneytout JL. Effects of alumina and zirconium dioxide particles on arachidonic acid metabolism and proinflammatory interleukin production in osteoarthritis and rheumatoid synovial cells. J Bone Joint Surg Br. 2002;84:920–30.
118. Catelas I, Huk OL, Petit A, Zukor DJ, Marchand R, Yahia L. Flow cytometric analysis of macrophage response to ceramic and polyethylene particles: effects of size, concentration, and composition. J Biomed Mater Res. 1998;41:600–7.
119. Lucarelli M, Gatti AM, Savarino G, Quattroni P, Martinelli L, Monari E, et al. Innate defence functions of macrophages can be biased by nano-sized ceramic and metallic particles. Eur Cytokine Netw. 2004;15:339–46.
120. Pasold J, Markhoff J, Tillmann J, Krogull M, Pisowocki P, Bader R. Direct influence of titanium and zirconia particles on the morphology and functionality of mature human osteoclasts. J Biomed Mater Res A. 2017;105:2608–15. https://doi.org/10.1002/jbm.a.36114.
121. Lohmann CH, Dean DD, Köster G, Casasola D, Buchhorn GH, Fink U, Schwartz Z, Boyan BD. Ceramic and PMMA particles differentially affect osteoblast phenotype. Biomaterials. 2002;23:1855–63.
122. Rodrigo AM, Martinez ME, Saldaña L, Vallés G, Martinez P, González-Carrasco JL, et al. Effects of polyethylene and alpha-alumina particles on IL-6 expression and secretion in primary cultures of human osteoblastic cells. Biomaterials. 2002;23:901–8.
123. Rodrigo AM, Martínez ME, Martínez P, Escudero ML, Ruíz J, Saldaña L, et al. Effects of MA 956 superalloy and alpha-alumina particles on some markers of human osteoblastic cells in primary culture. J Biomed Mater Res. 2001;54:30–6.
124. Rodrigo A, Vallés G, Saldaña L, Rodríguez M, Martínez ME, Munuera L, Vilaboa N. Alumina particles influence the interactions of cocultured osteoblasts and macrophages. J Orthop Res. 2006;24:46–54.
125. Granchi D, Ciapetti G, Amato I, Pagani S, Cenni E, Savarino L, Avnet S, Peris JL, Pellacani A, Baldini N, Giunti A. The influence of alumina and ultra-high molecular weight polyethylene particles on osteoblast-osteoclast cooperation. Biomaterials. 2004;25:4037–45.
126. Vaishya R, Chauhan M, Vaish A. Bone cement. J Clin Orthop Trauma. 2013;4:157–63. https://doi.org/10.1016/j.jcot.2013.11.005.
127. Saleh KJ, El Othmani MM, Tzeng TH, Mihalko WM, Chambers MC, Grupp TM. Acrylic bone cement in total joint arthroplasty: a review. J Orthop Res. 2016;34:737–44. https://doi.org/10.1002/jor.23184.
128. Sagbas B, Durakbasa MN. Third-body wear behavior of orthopedic biopolymers. Int J Min Mater Metall Eng (IJMMME). 2016;2:1–7.
129. Morawietz L, Classen RA, Schröder JH, Dynybil C, Perka C, Skwara A, et al. Proposal for a histopathological consensus classification of the periprosthetic interface membrane. J Clin Pathol. 2006;59:591–7.
130. Burton L, Paget D, Binder NB, Bohnert K, Nestor BJ, Sculco TP, Santambrogio L, Ross FP, Goldring SR, Purdue PE. Orthopedic wear debris mediated inflammatory osteolysis is mediated in part by NALP3 inflammasome activation. J Orthop Res. 2013;31:73–80. https://doi.org/10.1002/jor.22190.
131. Pandey R, Quinn J, Joyner C, Murray DW, Triffitt JT, Athanasou NA. Arthroplasty implant biomaterial particle associated macrophages differentiate into lacunar bone resorbing cells. Ann Rheum Dis. 1996;55:388–95.
132. Ren PG, Lee SW, Biswal S, Goodman SB. Systemic trafficking of macrophages induced by bone cement particles in nude mice. Biomaterials. 2008;29:4760–5. https://doi.org/10.1016/j.biomaterials.2008.09.004.

133. Yang SY, Zhang K, Bai L, Song Z, Yu H, McQueen DA, et al. Polymethylmethacrylate and titanium alloy particles activate peripheral monocytes during periprosthetic inflammation and osteolysis. J Orthop Res. 2011;29:781–6. https://doi.org/10.1002/jor.21287.
134. Nakashima Y, Sun DH, Trindade MC, Chun LE, Song Y, Goodman SB, Schurman DJ, Maloney WJ, Smith RL. Induction of macrophage C-C chemokine expression by titanium alloy and bone cement particles. J Bone Joint Surg Br. 1999;81:155–62.
135. Huang Z, Ma T, Ren PG, Smith RL, Goodman SB. Effects of orthopedic polymer particles on chemotaxis of macrophages and mesenchymal stem cells. J Biomed Mater Res A. 2010;94:1264–9. https://doi.org/10.1002/jbm.a.32803.
136. Yaszay B, Trindade MC, Lind M, Goodman SB, Smith RL. Fibroblast expression of C-C chemokines in response to orthopaedic biomaterial particle challenge in vitro. J Orthop Res. 2001;19:970–6.
137. Lin TH, Tamaki Y, Pajarinen J, Waters HA, Woo DK, Yao Z, Goodman SB. Chronic inflammation in biomaterial-induced periprosthetic osteolysis: NF-κB as a therapeutic target. Acta Biomater. 2014;10:1–10. https://doi.org/10.1016/j.actbio.2013.09.034.
138. Shen Y, Wang W, Li X, Markel DC, Ren W. Mitigative effect of erythromycin on PMMA challenged preosteoblastic MC3T3-E1 cells. Sci World J. 2014;2014:107196. https://doi.org/10.1155/2014/107196.
139. Antonios JK, Yao Z, Li C, Rao AJ, Goodman SB. Macrophage polarization in response to wear particles in vitro. Cell Mol Immunol. 2013;10:471–82. https://doi.org/10.1038/cmi.2013.39.
140. Pearle AD, Crow MK, Rakshit DS, Wohlgemuth J, Nestor BJ. Distinct inflammatory gene pathways induced by particles. Clin Orthop Relat Res. 2007;458:194–201.
141. Sabokbar A, Pandey R, Quinn JM, Athanasou NA. Osteoclastic differentiation by mononuclear phagocytes containing biomaterial particles. Arch Orthop Trauma Surg. 1998;117:136–40.
142. Li N, Xu Z, Wooley PH, Zhang J, Yang SY. Therapeutic potentials of naringin on polymethylmethacrylate induced osteoclastogenesis and osteolysis, in vitro and in vivo assessments. Drug Des Devel Ther. 2013;8:1–11. https://doi.org/10.2147/DDDT.S52714.
143. Yamanaka Y, Abu-Amer Y, Faccio R, Clohisy JC. Map kinase c-JUN N-terminal kinase mediates PMMA induction of osteoclasts. J Orthop Res. 2006;24:1349–57.
144. Yamanaka Y, Abu-Amer W, Foglia D, Otero J, Clohisy JC, Abu-Amer Y. NFAT2 is an essential mediator of orthopedic particle-induced osteoclastogenesis. J Orthop Res. 2008;26:1577–84. https://doi.org/10.1002/jor.20714.
145. Zhang H, Ricciardi BF, Yang X, Shi Y, Camacho NP, Bostrom MG. Polymethylmethacrylate particles stimulate bone resorption of mature osteoclasts in vitro. Acta Orthop. 2008;79:281–8. https://doi.org/10.1080/17453670710015166.
146. Rao AJ, Gibon E, Ma T, Yao Z, Smith RL, Goodman SB. Revision joint replacement, wear particles, and macrophage polarization. Acta Biomater. 2012;8:2815–23. https://doi.org/10.1016/j.actbio.2012.03.042.
147. Chiu R, Smith KE, Ma GK, Ma T, Smith RL, Goodman SB. Polymethylmethacrylate particles impair osteoprogenitor viability and expression of osteogenic transcription factors Runx2, osterix, and Dlx5. J Orthop Res. 2010;28:571–7. https://doi.org/10.1002/jor.21035.
148. Chiu R, Ma T, Smith RL, Goodman SB. Polymethylmethacrylate particles inhibit osteoblastic differentiation of bone marrow osteoprogenitor cells. J Biomed Mater Res A. 2006;77:850–6.
149. Chiu R, Ma T, Smith RL, Goodman SB. Kinetics of polymethylmethacrylate particle-induced inhibition of osteoprogenitor differentiation and proliferation. J Orthop Res. 2007;25:450–7.
150. Ma GK, Chiu R, Huang Z, Pearl J, Ma T, Smith RL, et al. Polymethylmethacrylate particle exposure causes changes in p38 MAPK and TGF-beta signaling in differentiating MC3T3-E1 cells. J Biomed Mater Res A. 2010;94:234–40. https://doi.org/10.1002/jbm.a.32686.
151. Zambonin G, Colucci S, Cantatore F, Grano M. Response of human osteoblasts to polymethylmetacrylate in vitro. Calcif Tissue Int. 1998;62:362–5.

152. Lochner K, Fritsche A, Jonitz A, Hansmann D, Mueller P, Mueller-Hilke B, et al. The potential role of human osteoblasts for periprosthetic osteolysis following exposure to wear particles. Int J Mol Med. 2011;28:1055–63. https://doi.org/10.3892/ijmm.2011.778.
153. Sabokbar A, Fujikawa Y, Murray DW, Athanasou NA. Radio-opaque agents in bone cement increase bone resorption. J Bone Joint Surg Br. 1997;79:129–34.
154. Granchi D, Cenni E, Savarino L, Ciapetti G, Forbicini G, Vancini M, et al. Bone cement extracts modulate the osteoprotegerin/osteoprotegerin-ligand expression in MG63 osteoblast-like cells. Biomaterials. 2002;23:2359–65.
155. Pezzotti G, Yamamoto K. Artificial hip joints: the biomaterials challenge. J Mech Behav Biomed Mater. 2014;31:3–20. https://doi.org/10.1016/j.jmbbm.2013.06.001.
156. Ghalme SG, Mankar A, Bhalerao Y. Biomaterials in hip joint replacement. Int J Mater Sci Eng. 2016;4:113–25. https://doi.org/10.17706/ijmse.2016.4.2.113-125.
157. Grieco PW, Pascal S, Newman JM, Shah NV, Stroud SG, Sheth NP, Maheshwari AV. New alternate bearing surfaces in total hip arthroplasty: a review of the current literature. J Clin Orthop Trauma. 2018;9:7–16. https://doi.org/10.1016/j.jcot.2017.10.013.
158. Zhang BG, Myers DE, Wallace GG, Brandt M, Choong PF. Bioactive coatings for orthopaedic implants-recent trends in development of implant coatings. Int J Mol Sci. 2014;15:11878–921. https://doi.org/10.3390/ijms150711878.
159. Cooper HJ. Emerging applications of proteomics in hip and knee arthroplasty. Expert Rev Proteomics. 2014;11:5–8. https://doi.org/10.1586/14789450.2014.865522.
160. Zhang L, Tian Z, Li W, Wang X, Man Z, Sun S. Inhibitory effect of quercetin on titanium particle-induced endoplasmic reticulum stress (ERS)-related apoptosis and in vivo osteolysis. Biosci Rep. 2017;37:BSR20170961. https://doi.org/10.1042/BSR20170961.
161. Goodman SB, Gibon E, Pajarinen J, Lin TH, Keeney M, Ren PG, et al. Novel biological strategies for treatment of wear particle-induced periprosthetic osteolysis of orthopaedic implants for joint replacement. J R Soc Interface. 2014;11:20130962. https://doi.org/10.1098/rsif.2013.0962.
162. Mahon OR, O'Hanlon S, Cunningham CC, McCarthy GM, Hobbs C, Nicolosi V, et al. Orthopaedic implant materials drive M1 macrophage polarization in a spleen tyrosine kinase- and mitogen-activated protein kinase-dependent manner. Acta Biomater. 2018;65:426–35. https://doi.org/10.1016/j.actbio.2017.10.041.
163. Wang L, Guo X, Zhou W, Ding Y, Shi J, Wu X, et al. Protein phosphatase 2A as a new target for downregulating osteoclastogenesis and alleviating titanium particle-induced bone resorption. Acta Biomater. 2018; https://doi.org/10.1016/j.actbio.2018.04.013.
164. Geng D, Wu J, Shao H, Zhu S, Wang Y, Zhang W, et al. Pharmaceutical inhibition of glycogen synthetase kinase 3 beta suppresses wear debris-induced osteolysis. Biomaterials. 2015;69:12–21. https://doi.org/10.1016/j.biomaterials.2015.07.061.
165. Nam JS, Sharma AR, Jagga S, Lee DH, Sharma G, Nguyen LT, et al. Suppression of osteogenic activity by regulation of WNT and BMP signaling during titanium particle induced osteolysis. J Biomed Mater Res A. 2017;105:912–26. https://doi.org/10.1002/jbm.a.36004.
166. Drynda A, Ren Q, Buchhorn GH, Lohmann CH. The induction of CXCR4 expression in human osteoblast-like cells (MG63) by CoCr particles is regulated by the PLC-DAG-PKC pathway. J Biomed Mater Res B Appl Biomater. 2017;105:2326–32. https://doi.org/10.1002/jbm.b.33770.
167. Tian B, Jiang T, Shao Z, Zhai Z, Li H, Fan Q, et al. The prevention of titanium-particle-induced osteolysis by OA-14 through the suppression of the p38 signaling pathway and inhibition of osteoclastogenesis. Biomaterials. 2014;35:8937–50. https://doi.org/10.1016/j.biomaterials.2014.06.055.
168. Mediero A, Perez-Aso M, Wilder T, Cronstein BN. Brief report: methotrexate prevents wear particle-induced inflammatory osteolysis in mice via activation of adenosine A2A receptor. Arthritis Rheumatol. 2015;67:849–55. https://doi.org/10.1002/art.38971.
169. Jiang C, Xiao F, Gu X, Zhai Z, Liu X, Wang W, et al. Inhibitory effects of ursolic acid on osteoclastogenesis and titanium particle-induced osteolysis are mediated primarily via

suppression of NF-κB signaling. Biochimie. 2015;111:107–18. https://doi.org/10.1016/j.biochi.2015.02.002.

170. Huang J, Zhou L, Wu H, Pavlos N, Chim SM, Liu Q, et al. Triptolide inhibits osteoclast formation, bone resorption, RANKL-mediated NF-½B activation and titanium particle-induced osteolysis in a mouse model. Mol Cell Endocrinol. 2015;399:346–53. https://doi.org/10.1016/j.mce.2014.10.016.
171. Zhao S, Yan L, Li X, Zhang Z, Sun Y, Wang J. Notoginsenoside R1 suppresses wear particle-induced osteolysis and RANKL mediated osteoclastogenesis in vivo and in vitro. Int Immunopharmacol. 2017;47:118–25. https://doi.org/10.1016/j.intimp.2017.03.018.
172. Zhou CH, Shi ZL, Meng JH, Hu B, Zhao CC, Yang YT, et al. Sophocarpine attenuates wear particle-induced implant loosening by inhibiting osteoclastogenesis and bone resorption via suppression of the NF-κB signalling pathway in a rat model. Br J Pharmacol. 2018;175:859–76. https://doi.org/10.1111/bph.14092.
173. Zhu L, Kang H, Guo CA, Fan WS, Wang YM, Deng LF, et al. Rifampin suppresses osteoclastogenesis and titanium particle-induced osteolysis via modulating RANKL signaling pathways. Biochem Biophys Res Commun. 2017;484:64–70. https://doi.org/10.1016/j.bbrc.2017.01.071.
174. Li Y, Li J, Li B, Qin H, Peng X, Zhao Y, et al. Anthocyanin suppresses CoCrMo particle-induced osteolysis by inhibiting IKKα/β mediated NF-κB signaling in a mouse calvarial model. Mol Immunol. 2017;85:27–34. https://doi.org/10.1016/j.molimm.2017.02.003.
175. Zhang Z, Zhao S, Li X, Zhuo X, Zhang W, Nie Q, et al. Amentoflavone inhibits osteoclastogenesis and wear debris-induced osteolysis via suppressing NF-κB and MAPKs signaling pathways. Planta Med. 2018;84:759–67. https://doi.org/10.1055/s-0043-124594.
176. Kim HJ, Ohk B, Yoon HJ, Kang WY, Seong SJ, Kim SY, et al. Docosahexaenoic acid signaling attenuates the proliferation and differentiation of bone marrow-derived osteoclast precursors and promotes apoptosis in mature osteoclasts. Cell Signal. 2017;29:226–32. https://doi.org/10.1016/j.cellsig.2016.11.007.
177. Wang Z, Xue K, Bai M, Deng Z, Gan J, Zhou G, et al. Probiotics protect mice from CoCrMo particles-induced osteolysis. Int J Nanomedicine. 2017;12:5387–97. https://doi.org/10.2147/IJN.S130485.
178. Ping Z, Wang Z, Shi J, Wang L, Guo X, Zhou W, et al. Inhibitory effects of melatonin on titanium particle-induced inflammatory bone resorption and osteoclastogenesis via suppression of NF-κB signaling. Acta Biomater. 2017;62:362–71. https://doi.org/10.1016/j.actbio.2017.08.046.
179. Deng Z, Wang Z, Jin J, Wang Y, Bao N, Gao Q, et al. SIRT1 protects osteoblasts against particle-induced inflammatory responses and apoptosis in aseptic prosthesis loosening. Acta Biomater. 2017;49:541–54. https://doi.org/10.1016/j.actbio.2016.11.051.
180. Deng Z, Jin J, Wang Z, Wang Y, Gao Q, Zhao J. The metal nanoparticle-induced inflammatory response is regulated by SIRT1 through NF-κB deacetylation in aseptic loosening. Int J Nanomedicine. 2017;12:3617–36. https://doi.org/10.2147/IJN.S124661.
181. Vallés G, Pérez C, Boré A, Martín-Saavedra F, Saldaña L, Vilaboa N. Simvastatin prevents the induction of interleukin-6 gene expression by titanium particles in human osteoblastic cells. Acta Biomater. 2013;9:4916–25. https://doi.org/10.1016/j.actbio.2012.08.027.
182. Ren K, Dusad A, Yuan F, Yuan H, Purdue PE, Fehringer EV, et al. Macromolecular prodrug of dexamethasone prevents particle-induced peri-implant osteolysis with reduced systemic side effects. J Control Release. 2014;175:1–9. https://doi.org/10.1016/j.jconrel.2013.11.024.
183. Rodrigues M, Perni SD, Sloan A, Prokopovich PD. Dexamethasone-loaded TiO2 nanoparticles to locally target wear-debris induced inflammation. Front Bioeng Biotechnol. Conference Abstract: 10th World Biomaterials Congress. 2016; https://doi.org/10.3389/conf.FBIOE.2016.01.01681.
184. Carmody EE, Schwarz EM, Puzas JE, Rosier RN, O'Keefe RJ. Viral interleukin-10 gene inhibition of inflammation, osteoclastogenesis, and bone resorption in response to titanium particles. Arthritis Rheum. 2002;46:1298–308.

185. Yang SY, Wu B, Mayton L, Mukherjee P, Robbins PD, Evans CH, et al. Protective effects of IL-1Ra or vIL-10 gene transfer on a murine model of wear debris-induced osteolysis. Gene Ther. 2004;11:483–91.
186. Ulrich-Vinther M, Carmody EE, Goater JJ, S balle K, O'Keefe RJ, Schwarz EM. Recombinant adeno-associated virus-mediated osteoprotegerin gene therapy inhibits wear debris-induced osteolysis. J Bone Joint Surg Am. 2002;84-A:1405–12.
187. Yang SY, Mayton L, Wu B, Goater JJ, Schwarz EM, Wooley PH. Adeno-associated virus-mediated osteoprotegerin gene transfer protects against particulate polyethylene-induced osteolysis in a murine model. Arthritis Rheum. 2002;46:2514–23.
188. Wang H, Jia TH, Zacharias N, Gong W, Du HX, Wooley PH, et al. Combination gene therapy targeting on interleukin-1β and RANKL for wear debris-induced aseptic loosening. Gene Ther. 2013;20:128–35. https://doi.org/10.1038/gt.2012.1.
189. Langlois J, Hamadouche M. New animal models of wear-particle osteolysis. Int Orthop. 2011;35:245–51. https://doi.org/10.1007/s00264-010-1143-0.
190. Qin CQ, Huang DS, Zhang C, Song B, Huang JB, Ding Y. Lentivirus-mediated short hairpin RNA interference targeting TNF-alpha in macrophages inhibits particle-induced inflammation and osteolysis in vitro and in vivo. BMC Musculoskelet Disord. 2016;17:431.
191. Huang JB, Ding Y, Huang DS, Zeng WK, Guan ZP, Zhang ML. rna interference targeting p110β reduces tumor necrosis factor-alpha production in cellular response to wear particles in vitro and osteolysis in vivo. Inflammation. 2013;36:1041–54. https://doi.org/10.1007/s10753-013-9636-9.
192. Wang C, Liu Y, Wang Y, Li H, Zhang RX, He MS, et al. Adenovirus-mediated siRNA targeting CXCR2 attenuates titanium particle-induced osteolysis by suppressing osteoclast formation. Med Sci Monit. 2016;22:727–35.
193. Mertens MT, Singh JA. Biomarkers in arthroplasty: a systematic review. Open Orthop J. 2011;5:92–105. https://doi.org/10.2174/1874325001105010092.
194. Illingworth KD, Wachter N, Maloney WJ, Paprosky WG, Ries MD, Saleh KJ. Advances in acetabular osteolysis: biomarkers, imaging, and pharmacologic management. Instr Course Lect. 2014;63:177–8.

# Chapter 2
# Bone Defects in Acetabular Revision Surgery. Imaging and Classifications

**Eduardo García-Rey**

## Introduction

Prosthetic component loosening leads to bone loss and complicating the reconstruction of the hip during a revision surgery. Osteolytic lesions may develop from a biological reaction to wear debris, most frequently polyethylene and metal debris, or by bone erosion produced by repeated movement secondary to component loosening [1]. This biological reaction produces an osteoclastic resorption that can be seen on radiographs as cystic lesions or radiolucent lines around the prosthetic components.

Osteolysis of the pelvis is found associated with both cemented and cementless cups. However, its pattern will differ depending on the type of hip fixation. These differences are related to the path of least resistance for particle-laden joint fluid [2]. Access to the implant-bone interface is related to the type of fixation, subsequent remodeling and implant design. With cemented acetabular components, the subcondral bone can be reamed at the time of surgery, but it usually reconstitutes itself. Sclerotic bone is a relative barrier for the ingress of joint fluid and wear particles into the trabecular bone of the supracetabular region [3]. As a consequence, bone resorption occurs most frequently in a linear manner, resulting in degradation of the bone at the cement-bone interface and loosening of the implant over the time. A soft tissue membrane develops and compromises stability as the cutting wedge of bone resorption progresses toward the dome of the cemented acetabular component. In contrast, with cementless cups, the pattern of bone remodeling and the path of least resistance for joint fluid and wear particles around a cementless porous-coated cup are different. Both tend to ingrow into the porous coating in a limited fashion. The areas that develop ingrowth become osteointegrated and are resistant to fluid and

E. García-Rey
Orthopaedic Surgery Department, Hospital Universitario La Paz-IdiPaz, Madrid, Spain



E. García-Rey, E. García-Cimbrelo (eds.), *Acetabular Revision Surgery in Major Bone Defects*, https://doi.org/10.1007/978-3-319-98596-1_2

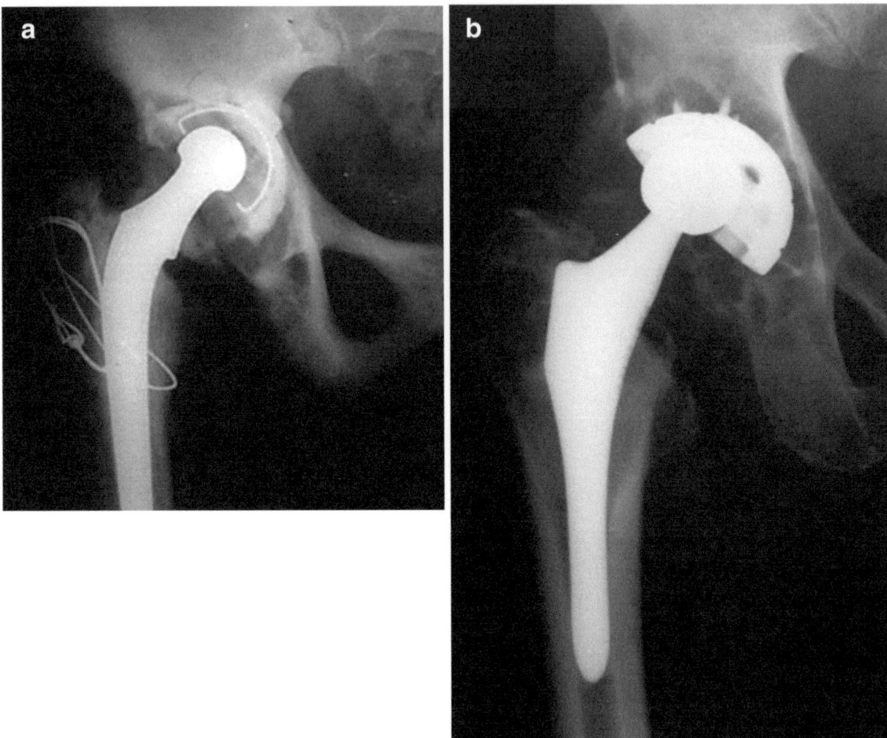


**Fig. 2.1** (**a**) Anteroposterior radiograph of the hip showing acetabular osteolysis around a cemented cup. Bone resorption occurs in a linear manner, resulting in degradation of the bone at the cement-bone interface and loosening of the implant over the time. (**b**) Anteroposterior radiograph of the hip showing acetabular osteolysis around a cementless cup. The areas that develop ingrowth become osseointegrated and are resistant to fluid and particles migrating along the interface. Extensive bone loss can occur without affecting implant stability

particles migrating along the interface. However, areas without ingrowth are potential access channels for joint fluid to be pumped into the supracetabular region [4]. Acetabular osteolysis destroys lateral and anterior acetabular walls while the cup migrates medially, affecting the acetabular roof and the medial wall and producing segmental defects. Acetabular osteolytic lesions develop around the dome or screw holes of the acetabular component and near the cup rim, where particulate debris from the bearing surface tend to migrate [5–7]. Extensive bone loss can occur without affecting implant stability (Fig. 2.1). These patients can be clinically asymptomatic despite significant destruction of the pelvic bone [8] and detected only with radiographs or other imaging diagnosis techniques. Osteolysis is associated with pain if the bone loss results in decreased mechnical support for the acetabular component.

Although the osteolytic pattern around cemented and cementless components is different, histologic evaluation shows the membrane is similar regardless of the type

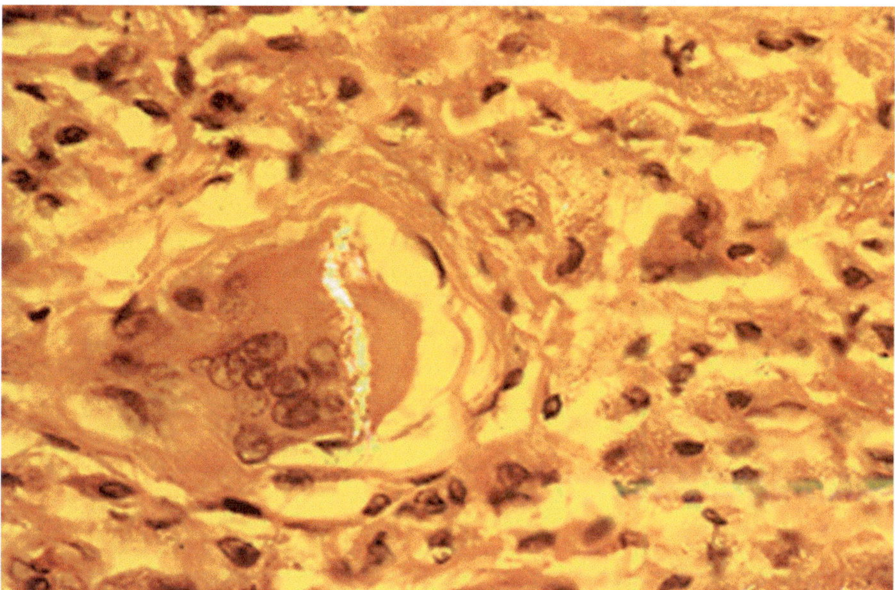

**Fig. 2.2** Microphotography of an osteolytic cavity showing abundant macrophages in association with intra- and extracellular wear debris. In the presence of larger polyethylene particles, giant cells are common

of implant fixation or the pattern of osteolysis. Histologically, we can find abundant macrophages in association with intra- and extracelular wear debris. In the presence of larger particles of polyethylene, giant cells are common [2, 3, 9, 10] (Fig. 2.2).

Diagnosis and treatment of osteolysis of the pelvis presents challenging and controversial problems. It is often asymptomatic and does not present symptoms until considerable bone loss and loosening of the acetabular socket occur. Reconstructive hip surgery in cases with major bone deficiency is more complex and takes longer than a standard total replacement. In order to avoid complications and having to abandon the planned reconstruction, preoperative planning must meticulous. Planning must be include patient evaluation, detailed imaging assessment of the bone defects and the proposed surgical reconstruction.

## Patient Evaluation

The severity of the patient' hip problems will inform decision on whether the patient can benefit from a long and potentially dangerous operation. A detailed orthopedic history should be obtained, including characteristics of the pain, function, range of motion, limb length discrepancies, hip musculature, ambulatory capacity, ability to climb stairs, to sit, etc. The surgeon must be sure that subjective complaints in the hip region are caused by hip pathology and are not referred from the lumbar spine, retroperitoneum, inguinal hernias or femoral neuropathies. Assessing whether some pathology in joints other than the hip or impairment of cardiac, pulmonary or neurologic systems might compromise results.

The white blood cell count, erythrocyte sedimentation rate, and C-reactive protein level should be part of the standard workup before revision surgery, given their high sensitivity and specificity for infections when these tests are combined [11]. Patient evaluation also requires detection of any preoperative anemia, which is frequent in patients undergoing primary and revision surgery [12]. It is well known that preoperative anemia is a risk factor for allogenic blood transfusion [13], and transfusion is associated with a higher risk for longer stays, infection, and an increased mortality rate [14]. So, any preoperative anemia must be treated before surgery to avoid intra and postoperative complications. Different studies support the use of recombinant human erythropoietin and oral and intravenous iron supplementation in the patients [12, 15].

## Imaging Assessment

### *Radiographic Evaluation*

Diagnosis of osteolysis and aseptic loosening is made based on serial radiographs. Osteolytic lesions on radiographs appears as well-demarcated, scalloped areas of bone loss, depending on the type of fixation and subsequent bone remodeling. These lesions are differentiated from loss from stress-shielding bone loss, which causes more diffuse trabecular thinning. A proper technique is important for accurate interpretation of the radiographs [16]. A true anteroposterior (AP) view must be taken with the patient in supine position (or standing), with the tube-to-image distance of 120 cm and the beam centered on the pubic symphysis. The radiographic assessment options include: (1) AP of the pelvis with hips in neutral rotation and neutral abduction. (2) Oblique view of the pelvis. (3) True lateral view of the involved hip. (4) AP and rotational views of the femur.

1. **AP radiograph of the pelvis with hips in neutral rotation and neutral abduction.** A true AP X-ray of the pelvis with both hips in neutral rotation and abduction should be obtained for every patient. It is important to include the contralateral hip to allow comparison between the two hips and to make a preliminary assessment of leg length discrepancy. Subtle as well as large medial wall defects can be identified. The AP pelvis X-ray allows assessment of the roof and floor of the acetabulum, superior rim. A high center of rotation of the failed hip is indicative of a deficiency in the acetabular roof or superior rim. Penetration of the implant more medially than the Köhler' line suggests a deficient acetabulum floor. Loss of integrity of the teardrop indicates that the medial wall is damaged. The quality of the bone stock can be compared with the other

hip. If there is marked superior migration on the AP X-ray, anterior and posterior wall deficiency should be anticipated because the ilium becomes very thin above the area where the true acetabulum should be. However, the AP radiograph provides only limited information regarding the integrity of the anterior and posterior columns because these structures are superimposed and partly obscured by the implant. The presence of ischial lysis can suggest significant posterior column deficiency [17].

A true AP radiograph of the acetabulum allows accurate acetabular templating. However patients with significant flexion deformities will often end up with an inlet view if their standard AP X-ray is taken with their hips in extension. This view can be misleading when tempalting the acetabulum and it is better to flex the hip to make a normal AP X-ray of the pelvis.

2. **Oblique radiograph of the pelvis**. Iliac and obturator oblique views described by Judet el al. [18] provide additional information. The AP X-ray may suggest that there is adequate lateral coverage of the acetabular component. However superior migration should make one suspicious of a posterior wall (deficiency). An obturator oblique view can reveal the extent of the superior rim or posterior wall deficiency. The AP view may suggest superior rim deficiency, an iliac oblique view may be of value to demonstrate superior coverage anteriorly but can be misleading when estimating acetabular volume. The obturator oblique films should help reveal the true magnitude of the superior and posterior rim deficiency.
3. **True lateral of the involved hip**. A true lateral view can be helpful in assessing bone stock of both prosthetic components. On the acetabular side this view allows assessment of the thickness of the posterior intra-acetabular segment. This segment is defined on X-ray by the apex of the sciatic notch and the mid-posterior arch of the subchondral bony condensation.
4. **AP and rotational views of the femur**. Rotational views make it possible to check the integrity of the femur and bone quality. The frog lateral view (external rotation) also allows assessment of the femoral canal alignment which can be distorted following protrusion of a long-stem prosthesis.

Because radiographs show only a two-dimensional image of a three-dimensional structure, a comparison of different X-ray series with computed tomography (CT) images found higher specificity than sensitivity when assessing with CT [7, 19–21]. The use of oblique radiographs increased sensitivity compared to the use of only and AP X-ray [20, 22, 23].

## *Computed Tomography*

Acetabular bone defects determine the type of acetabular revision surgery, but potential treatment can be complicated by difficulties in the presurgical evaluation when plain radiographs provide limited information regarding the existence and location of lysis that consequently results in an underestimation of the lesions [21–23]. CT can be used to supplement information for radiographic assessment. CT and MRI can provide cross-sectional images of osteolytic lesions, especially when radiographs do not provide adequate visualization of the lesion size, location or progression. However, CT and MRI images can be distorted by metal artifacts from the adjacent prosthetic components. Metal artifact reduction protocols permit acceptable visualization of osteolysis. CT images are preferred if osteolytic lesions do not affect soft tissue. CT images are grossly distorted around cobalt-chromium and stainless steel implants, whereas artifacts around titanium implants are mild [5].

Initially, the value of CT images for evaluating bone adjacent to metal implants was limited, but the use of metal artifact suppression protocols has improved the quality of the images [24]. New techniques using volumetric computed tomography (CT) scanning with three-dimensional reconstruction and artifact minimization are believed to accurately determine the volume and location of osteolytic cavities in failed THAs. Multislice CT scanners produce images in a continuous fashion as the table and patient move through the gantry. Because the multislice CT technique provides sequential images of lytic defects, the total volume of lytic bone loss can be determined. The area of the lytic lesion can be calculated from each tracing by determining the number of pixels per square centimeter. Volumes are calculated automatically by the measurement software. Horizontal and vertical measurements of the cup are determined on the coronal CT planes. The volume between adjacent cuts is calculated by averaging the areas between adjacent cuts multiplied by the distance between the cuts. Summation of the volumes of each of these cuts is used to determine the total volume of bone loss produced by lysis [21].

These CT techniques with three-dimensional reconstruction and artifact minimization have been used and validated for diagnosing and measuring pelvic osteolysis and have demonstrated the volume and location of osteolytic cavities in patients with failed cups more accurately than plain radiographs. Since the bone loss is almost always more extensive than seen on radiographs alone, CT is very useful in planning acetabular revision [6, 21, 25–27]. In hemipelvis retrieved at autopsy, Leung et al. [28] report plain radiographs identified 52% of the lesions, whereas CT scans identified 87% of the lesions. Garcia-Cimbrelo et al. [27] reported, in a series of 33 hips with osteolysis on the radiographs and the 52 hips with osteolysis on CT, that radiographs had a sensitivity of 61.5% with and a specificity of 87.5% when using the CT findings as the gold standard. Claus et al. [19] reported overall sensitivity for osteolysis detection with a single radiograph as 41.5%, depending on the location and size of the lysis. They found that sensitivity ranged from 72% for lesions in the ilium to 15% for lesions in the ischium and acetabular rim, and that the detection rate for lesions with a volume greater than 10 $cm^3$ was higher than the for smaller lesions. The best concordance between radiographic and CT findings was in the ilium [19, 27]. However, the pubic region can have more artifacts than other periacetabular areas as a result of streak artifacts from double hip implants and this could mask pubic lesions [25, 27].

Because of the higher irradiation associated with CT, it is unlikely this technique will replace radiographs, and it should only be used in a single instance and to improve the evaluation of the osteolytic cavities and help in planning a difficult revision surgery, but it is not needed for regular controls. Despite the radiation, CT is useful in two scenarios. The first is in the research setting to define the natural history of periprosthetic osteolysis and the second is in the five and 10 years post surgery controls of high risk young active patients. Since osteolysis is often asymptomatic and not identified on radiographs, a CT at five and 10 years post surgery can identify and allow counseling for these patients.

Multislice CT scanning with metal artifact minimization is more sensitive for identifying and quantifying osteolysis around cemented and cementless cups than plain radiographs. Because CT scans can show the actual extent and location of osteolysis, they are useful adjuncts in planning cup revision, despite their relatively hip radioactive exposure (Fig. 2.3).

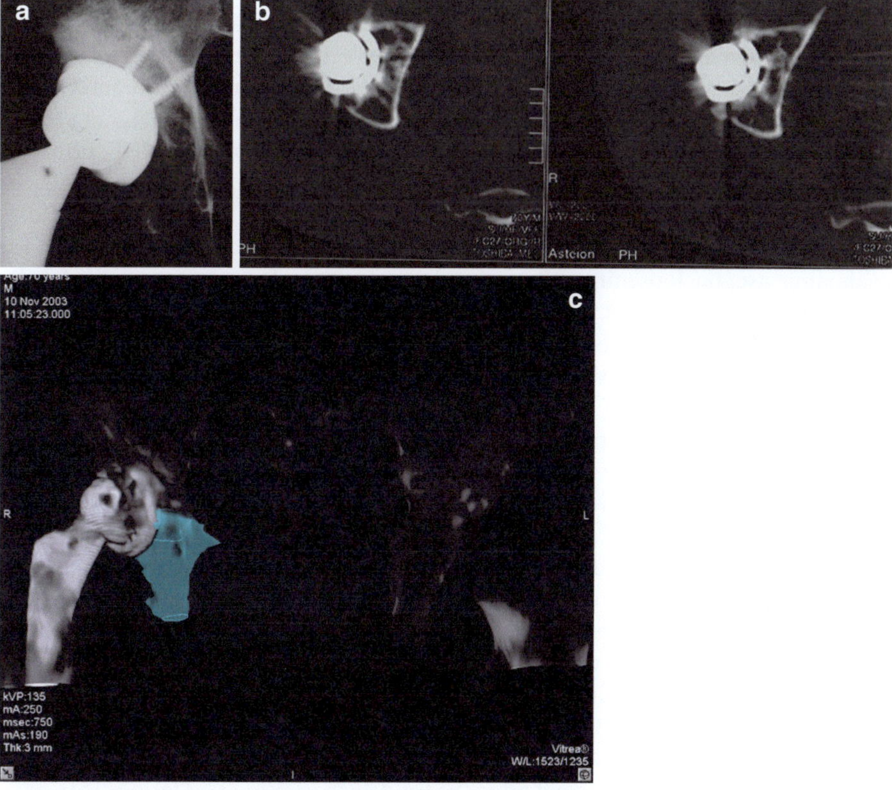


**Fig. 2.3** (**a**) An anteroposterior radiograph of a 70-year-old man seven years postsurgery shows an expansile and contained lytic cavity around a stable cementless cup. (**b**) A CT image shows a lytic cavity around the cup. (**c**) Multislice CT reconstruction shows a lytic cavity (in green) increasing the size of the radiographic preoperative bone defect

## *Magnetic Resonance Imaging*

MRI is another alternative to CT because there is no ionizing radiation exposure with MRI. However, metal, particularly chrome-cobalt, affects image quality on MRI because of artifacts. Factors that produce artifacts on MR images include the composition of the metallic implants, the orientation of the implants in relation to the direction of the main magnetic field, the strength of field, the pulse sequence type, and other imaging parameters (mainly voxel size, determined by the field of view, image matrix, section thickness, and echo train length) [5]. The use of lower field strength has been recommended to reduce metal artifacts. With high-field systems, increasing the band width can improve image. A small field of view with a high-resolution matrix, thin sections, and high gradient strength can also help to reduce metal-related artifacts [29].

Recently, specific metal suppression sequences have been developed, including multiacquisition with variable resonance image combination (MAVRIC) hybrid sequences [30, 31]. MAVRIC and fast spin-echo techniques can help visualize the hip after total hip arthrplasty, with fewer artifacts from the metallic hardware than traditional MRI and are useful in detecting periprosthetic osteolysis. MAVRIC can detect more damage from osteolysis than fast spin-echo sequences [31]. Wear debris after total hip arthroplasty will cause a soft-tissue sinovial reaction before it progresses to wear-induced osteolysis and an acetabular bone defect. Hayter et al. [32] showed that the presence of intermediate and low signal debris on MRI correlated with the debris characteristics found at the time of histologic analysis. MRI can be used for early osteolysis diagnosis and thus can allow earlier treatment. Cost, feasibility, and metal artifact remain as barriers to the clinical applicability of MRI for evaluating aseptic loosening. However, the superior soft-tissue imaging of MRI makes it quite likely that it will be increasingly used in imaging protocols.

MRI has been used to assess bone and soft tissue lesions after total hip replacement. It could reveal osteolysis, sinovitis, trochanteric bursitis, and loosening of components [33, 34] (Fig. 2.4). Walde et al. [26] compared the accuracy of radiography, CT, and MRI in assessing periacetabular osteolytic lesions in a cadaveric study and found that sensitivity for lesion detection was 22% with radiography, 75% with CT, and 95% with MRI. In lesions larger than 3 cm$^3$, which are of more concern clinically, their study found CT and MRI to be effective with detection rates greater than 80%. However, another study founds CT to be more accurate than MRI at measuring lesion volumen [6]. Metal-on-metal resurfacing or total hip arthroplasty can produce both osteolytic lesions in bone and so-called soft-issue pseudotumors. Pseudotumors, which has been associated with an adverse local reaction, can develop in soft tissue and are not well visualized in radiographs. The pseudotumors are filled with fluid and are well-visualized on MRI [35]. Ultrasound is also useful for detecting soft-tissue mass and can help to delinéate soft-tissue pseudotumors after placing a metal-on-metal prosthesis [36], but it is not effective for detecting osteolytic lesions [5].

Angiography of the iliac vessels is occasionally indicated when there is a concern that the external iliac vessels might have been damaged during extraction of a failed intrapelvic acetabular component. I it will detect if there is a close contact between the vessels and the implant (Fig. 2.5). If the angiograms confirm that the

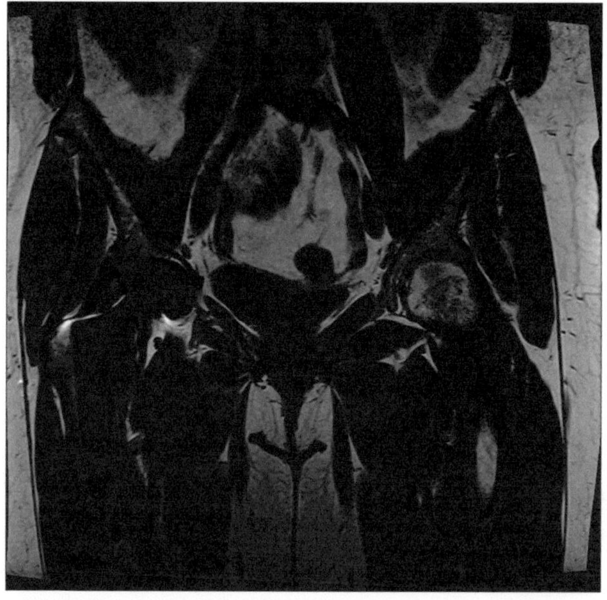

**Fig. 2.4** MRI used to assess bone and soft tissue lesions after total hip replacement. It can reveal osteolysis, synovitis, trochanteric bursitis, and component loosening

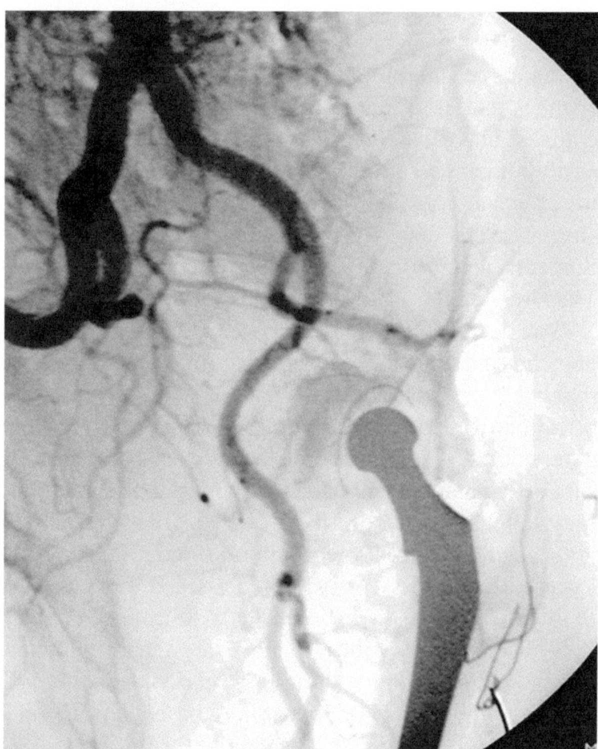

**Fig. 2.5** Angiography of the iliac vessels showing if there is any close contact between the vessels and the implant

vessels are sitting between the bony pelvis and the prosthesis, it may be wise to consider a retroperitoneal approach to extract the prosthesis [37].

## Classification of Acetabular Bone Defects

Because the complexity of acetabular revision surgery depends on the type, size and location of the bone loss, it is important to plan the surgery preoperatively, classifying the bone defects to prepare the appropriate surgical technique and avoid unexpected complications. However, the definitive bone defects are finally evaluated intraoperatively after removing the failed cup. A good bone defect classification system must be based on imaging findings and must include the following aspects [17].

1. The system must be based on plain radiographs. CT images and other modalities can be useful in complex cases or in resection-arthroplasty conversion in total hip replacement.
2. The classification must be validated by documented low rates of interobserver and intraobserver error prior to being accepted into routine usage [38].
3. The classification must be a guide to the surgeon that facilitates choosing the surgical technique.

A deficiency common to all classifications is the lack of information on how the radiographic interpretation of the degree of bone loss can be correlated with the changes that are found intraoperatively. The relative benefits of a simple versus a complex classification system are debatable. A simple system is likely to be more easily remembered and more widely used. However, it may not adequately define the exact nature of a given defect [17]. Several systems have been proposed for classifying acetabular bone defects, with the American Academy of Orthoaedic Surgeons (AAOS) and Paprosky systems being the most commonly used [39, 40]. The Gross et al. system is also very simple and useful for the surgeon [41].

**The AAOS classification** organizes the acetabular bone defects by pattern but does not quantify the size or location of the defect. Despite being the most commonly cited system, the AAOS defect classification system does not guide the identification of reconstruction options. The AAOS system distinguishes five types of defect: Type I, **segmental defects,** when bone loss involves any complete loss of supporting hemisphere of the acetabulum, including the medial wall; Type II, **cavitary defects**, which are those with a volumetric loss in the acetabular cavity but with an intact rim; Type III, c**ombined defects**; Type IV, **pelvic discontinuity**; Type V, **arthodesis**. Berry et al. classified the AAOS type IV defect, pelvic discontinuity, as type IVa, discontinuity with mild segmental or cavitary bone loss; type IVb, discontinuity with moderate or severe segmental or cavitary bone loss; and type IVc, discontinuity with prior pelvic irradiation [42].

**The Paprosky classification** is based on anatomic landmarks and uses four criteria to predict the location and severity of bone loss thus allowing appropriate planning [40]. The four criteria are: superior migration of the hip center, ischial osteolysis, acetabular teardrop osteolysis, and the position of the component relative to the Köhler line. Superior migration of the hip represents bone loss of the acetabular dome involving the anterior and posterior column. Ischial osteolysis indicates bone loss from the posterior column including the posterior wall. Teardrop osteolysis and migration beyond the Köhler line reflects medial acetabular bone loss. Paprosky distinguishes three types of bone loss: Type I is an intact, undistorted rim, no lysis or migration. Type II is intact, distorted rim with less than 3 mm of superomedial or superolateral migration. Type II can be subclassified into: Type IIA, superomedial; Type IIB, superolateral, no superior dome an less than 30% segmental rim defect; Type IIC, anterior column and medial defect, Köhler line violated, rim intact. Type III is superior migration greater than 3 mm with severe ischial and medial osteolysis. Type III can be differentiated into: Type IIIA, Köhler line intact, 30% to 60% of component supported by graft, bone loss between the 10- and 2-o'clock positions; Type IIIB, Köhler line is not intact, more than 60% component supported by graft, bone loss between the 9- and 5-o'clock positions.

**The Gross system** is based on the degree of bone loss seen on preoperative standard AP and lateral radiographs of the hip [43]. The degree of bone loss is classified as: Type I or cavitary, contained defects, with intact acetabular walls and column. A central defect, even if it involves more than 50% of the acetabulum, must be considered contained if the acetabular rim and column are intact and there is enough bone to fix a cup or ring. Type II or segmental defects that are uncontained, that involve structural bone loss. They can be classified in Type IIA, minor defects of the column that involve less than 50% of the structural wall, while Type IIB are major defects of the column involving at least 50% of the acetabulum [41]. Saleh et al. [43] developed another classification and distinguish: Type I, no substantial loss of bone stock; Type II contained loss of bone stock (columns and/or rim intact); Type III uncontained loss of bone stock (<50% acetabulum); Type IV, uncontained lose of bone acetabulum; Type V, Contained loss of bone stock with pelvic discontinuity.

## Planned Surgical Reconstruction

Because revision surgeries are long and complex operations, adequate preoperative planning of the reconstruction of the hip it is necessary to obtain as much as possible the original form and function of the hip joint. It is imperative to identify the component type and manufacturer before revision surgery to arrange for compatible implants to be available during the surgery.

Because each revision arthroplasty is unique, the surgeon must consider the previous approaches used, which components require revision and what defects need to be addressed. Despite the best preparation, unplanned events can occur. The surgeon should be prepared to enhance the surgical exposure with a combination of bony and soft-tissue procedures. Exposures must be more extensive than in primary or standard revision surgery. When another extensión is necessary to augment an old incision, it is safer to make this incision at right angles to the old one in order to leave flaps with wider base. Routinely, we prefer the postero lateral approach. It involves division of the short external rotators from their trochanteric attachment and excision of the posterior capsule. The hip is dislocated posteriorly in flexion, adduction and internal rotation, This approach allows good exposure of the posterior wall of the acetabulum but limited exposure of the superior rim. A retractor is placed in the obturator foramen to determine the level of the inferior border of the acetabulum. Aspiration of the hip should be done to obtain fluid for bacteriological studies. Removal of all scar tissue is essential to obtain a wide exposure of the entire cup. A circumferential capsulotomy is done an, if appropriate, the ilipsoas tendon is divided. After removing the cup, the fibrous interface is removed using curettes. At least three biopsy specimens are taken this fibrous membrane for histological and bacterial study.

Removing the components can be difficult and very time-consuming. The surgeon must be familiar with the basic techniques of implant removal [44]. Removal of a failed arthroplasty must be done efficiently and with every effort made to preserve host bone stock.

In cemented all-polyethylene components, the rim of the cup and the cement is easily seen in the majority of cases. If the component is grossly loose, the extraction will be easy with little force needed to drill ¼-in hole in the central aspect of the polyethylene cup and insert a threaded acetabular extractor into the hole. After cup removal, the remaining cement may be removed under direct line of sight with the use of osteotomes or curettes. Sectioning the remaining cement particles facilitates cement removal and decrease the amount of host bone injury. The presence of multiple cement anchoring holes increases the risk bone loss and fracture. Since intrapelvic cement fragments are larger than their respective acetabular defects they are frequently left in situ to avoid increasing the defect size. If necessary, the intrapelvic cement may be removed through a separate ilioinguinal incision [44].

The removal of a well-fixed cementless acetabular component begins with complete acetabular rim exposure and extraction of the polyethylene and screws. The entire perimeter of the metal shell must been clearly exposed before any attempt at extraction. Extraction of a well-fixed metal shell requires patience and caution to limit the amount of host bone destruction. The implant bone interface is disrupted with curve osteotomes used in a circumferential manner (Fig. 2.6). Peters et al. report that using curve osteotomes the revision component size was on average 6.5- mm wider than before [45]. The use of new cup extraction systems has been very useful in limiting bone destruction during cup removal. Mitchell et al. [46] report excellent results in a series of 31 hips with well-fixed cementless sockets using the Explant Acetabular Cup Removal System (Zimmer, Warsaw, Indiana) (Fig. 2.7). This system involves blades that closely match the outer diameter of the acetabular socket. The technique involves a centering head that matches the inner diameter of the socket to allow the stiff truncated blade to penetrate the dense peripheral bone and create channels while staying close to the shell. A second full radius blade, frees the dome of the cup from the iliac bone The time needed to remove the cup did not exceed 5 min in any hip. The mean difference between the

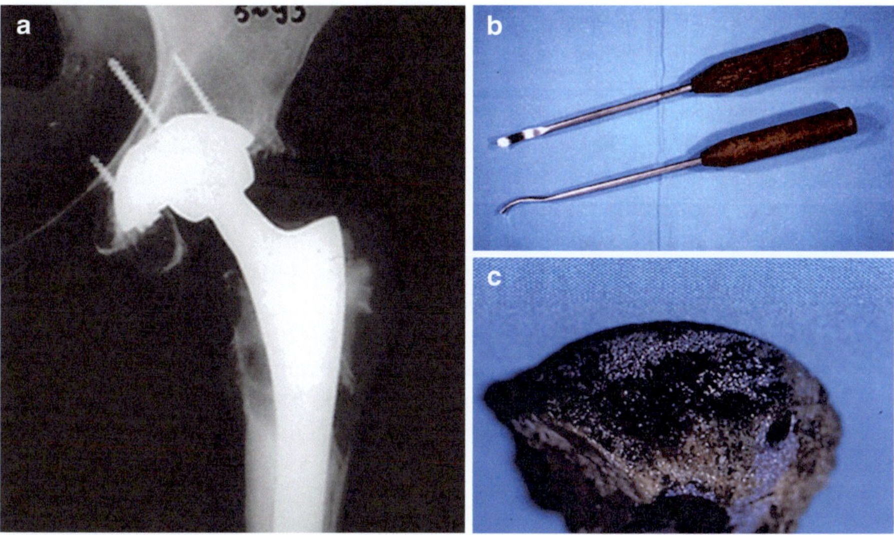

**Fig. 2.6** (**a**) Anteroposterior radiograph of a 74-year-old man twelve years postsurgery shows a stable cup with severe polyethylene wear. (**b**) Curve osteotomes were used in a circumferential manner to disrupt the bone-implant interface. (**c**) Photograph shows the removed host bone with the acetabular socket increasing the preoperative bone defect

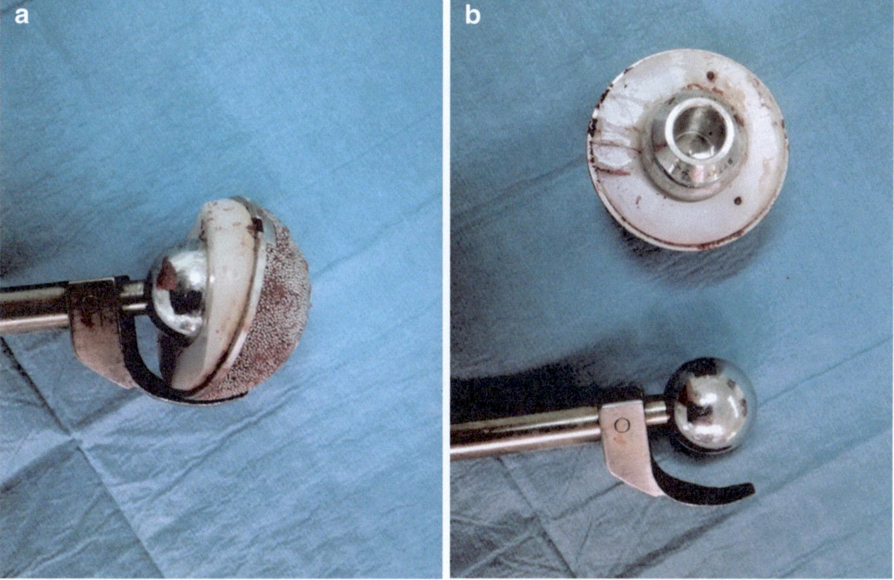

**Fig. 2.7** (**a**) System to remove an acetabular cup with ingrowth employs blades that closely match the outer diameter of the acetabular socket. (**b**) The resulting defect is no larger than the cup plus the thickness of the blades

size of extracted and the implanted cup 4 mm, indicating that no more host bone was removed than the thickness of the blades. The classification of the intraoperative bone defect did not change following removal of the implant in any hip [46].

Occasionally, an abdominal-retroperitoneal approach can be recommended to remove a prosthesis that has emigrated into the pelvis. The femoral prosthesis is removed using a posterolateral approach followed by removal of the acetabular componente via an abdominal retroperitoneal approach to permit exposure of the major intrapelvis structures and to ascertain their relationship to the acetabular component [37]. A vascular or general surgeon may need to be present to assist in the operative exposure and implant extraction.

After removing the implant, the resulting bone defect can be larger than preoperatively foreseen. The surgeon must meticulously examine the actual intraoperative bone defect, and it is who must then determine the necessary surgical technique to reconstruct the acetabulum and place the new socket in the anatomic center of hip rotation.

## References


1. Harris WH. Wear and periprosthetic osteolysis: the problem. Clin Orthop Relat Res. 2001;393:66–70.
2. Schmalzried TP, Guttman D, Grecula M, Amstutz HC. The relationship between the design, physician, and articular wear of acetabular components inserted without cement and the development of pelvic osteolysis. J Bone Joint Surg Am. 1994;76-A(5):677–88.
3. Schmalzried TP, Kwong OM, Jasty M, Sedlacek RC, Haire TC, O'Connor DO, Bragdon CR, Kabo JM, Malcolm AJ, Harris WH. The machanism of loosening and cemented acetabular components and total hip arthroplasty: analysis of specimens retrieved at autopsy. Clin Orthop Relat Res. 1991;274:60–78.
4. Schmalzried TP, Jasty M, Harris WH. Periprosthetic bone loss in total hip arthroplasty. Polyethylene wear debris and the concept of the effective joint space. J Bone Joint Surg Am. 1992;74-A(6):849–63.
5. Ries MD, Link TM. Monitoring and risk of progression of osteolysis after total hip arthroplasty. In: Pagnano MW, Hart RA, editors. AAOS instructional course lectures. 2013;62:207–14.
6. Stamenkov R, Howie D, Taylor J, Findlay D, McGee M, Kourlis G, Carbone A, Burwell M. Measurement of bone defects adjacent to acetabular components of hip replacement. Clin Orthop Relat Res. 2003;412:117–24.
7. Kitamura N, Naudie DD, Leung SB, Hooper RH Jr, Engh CA Sr. Diagnostic features of pelvic osteolysis associated with stable acetabulat component inserted without cement as part of a total hip replacement. J Bone Joint Surg Am. 2005;87-A(7):1542–50.
8. Maloney WJ, Paposky W, Engh CA, Rubash H. Surgical treatment of pelvic osteolysis. Clin Orthop Relat Res. 2001;393:78–84.
9. Kobayashi A, Freeman MAR, Bonfield W, Kadoya Y, Yamac T. Number of polyethylene particles and osteolysis in total joints replacements. A quantitative study using a tissue-digestion method. J Bone Joint Surg Br. 1997;79-B(5):844–8.
10. Maloney WJ, Smith RL. Periprosthetic osteolysis in total hip arthroplasty. The role of particulate wear debris. J Bone Joint Surg Am. 1995;77-A(9):1448–61.
11. Spangehl MJ, Masri BA, O'Connell JX, Duncan CP. Prospective analysis of preoperative and intraoperative investigation for the diagnosis of infection at the sites of two hundred and two revisión total hip arthroplasties. J Bone Joint Surg Am. 1999;81-A(5):672–83.

12. Alexander DP, Frew N. Preoperative optimisation of anaemia for primary total hip arthroplasty: a systemic review. Hip Int. 2017;27(6):515–22.
13. Gombotz H, Rehak PH, Shander A, Hofmann A. Blood use in elective surgery: the Austrian benchmark study. Transfusion. 2007;47(8):1468–80.
14. Dunne JR, Malone D, Tracy JK, Gannon C, Napolitano LM. Perioperative anemia: an independent risk factor for infection, mortality, and resource utilization in surgery. J Surg Res. 2002;102(2):237–44.
15. Bedair H, Yang J, Dwyer MK, McCarthy JC. Preoperative erytropoietin alpha reduces postoperative transfusions in THA and TKA by my not be cost-effective. Clin Orthop Relat Res. 2015;473(2):590–6.
16. Welton KL, Jesse MK, Kraeutler MJ, Garabekyan T, Mei-Dan O. The anteroposterior pelvic radiograph. Acetabular and femoral measurements and relation to hip pathologies. J Bone Joint Surg Am. 2018;100-A:76–85.
17. Masri BA, Masterson EL, Duncan CP. The classification and radiographic evaluation of bone loss in revision hip arthroplasty. Orthop Clin North Am. 1998;28(2):219–27.
18. Judet R, Judet J, Letournel E. Fractures of the acetabulum: classification and surgical approaches for open reduction, preliminary report. J Bone Joint Surg Am. 1964;46-A:1615–46.
19. Claus AM, Engh CA Jr, Sychterz CJ, Xenos JS, Orishimo KF, Engh CA Sr. Radiographic definition of pelvic osteolysis following total hip arthroplasty. J Bone Joint Surg Am. 2003;85-A(8):1519–26.
20. Shon WY, Gupta S, Biswal S, Han SH, Hong SJ, Moon JG. Pelvic osteolysis relationship to radiographs and polyethylene wear. J Arthroplasty. 2009;24(5):743–50.
21. Puri L, Wixson RL, Stern SH, Kohli J, Hendrix RW, Stulberg SD. Use of helical computed tomography for the assessment of acetabular osteolysis after total hip arthroplasty. J Bone Joint Surg Am. 2002;84-A(4):609–14.
22. Southwell DG, Bechtold JE, Lew WD, Schmidt AH. Improving the detection of acetabular osteolysis using oblique radiographs. J Bone Joint Surg Br. 1999;81-B(2):289–95.
23. Zimlich RH, Fehring TK. Underestimation of pelvic osteolysis: the value of the iliac oblique radiograph. J Arthroplasty. 2000;15(6):796–801.
24. Robertson DD, Magid D, Poss R, Fishman EK, Brooker AF, Sledge CB. Enhanced computed tomographic techniques for the evaluation of total hip arthroplasty. J Arthroplasty. 1989;4(3):271–6.
25. Claus AM, Totterman SM, Sychterz CJ, Tamez-Peña JG, Looney RJ, Engh CA Sr. Computed tomography to assess pelvic lysis after total hip replacement. Clin Orthop Relat Res. 2004;422:167–74.
26. Walde TA, Weiland DE, Leung SB, Kitamura N, Sychterz CJ, Engh CA Jr, Claus AM, Potter HG, Engh CA Sr. Comparison of CT, MRI, and radiographs in assessing pelvic osteolysis. A cadaveric study. Clin Orthop Relat Res. 2005;437:138–44.
27. Garcia-Cimbrelo E, Tapia M, Martin-Hervas C. Multislice computed tomography for evaluating acetabular defects in revision THA. Clin Orthop Relat Res. 2007;463(Oct):138–43.
28. Leung S, Naudie D, Kitamura N, Walde T, Engh CA. Computed tomography in the assessment of periacetabular osteolysis. J Bone Joint Surg Am. 2005;87(3):592–7.
29. Lee MJ, Kim S, Lee SA, Song HT, Huh YM, Kim DH, Han SH, Suh JS. Overcoming artifacts from metallic orthopedic implants at high-field-strength MR imaging and multi-detector CT. Radiographics. 2007;27(3):791–803.
30. Chen CA, Chen W, Goodman SB, Hargreaves BA, Koch KM, Lu W, Brau AC, Draper CE, Delp SL, Gold GE. New MR imaging methods for metallic implants in the knee: artifacts corection and clinical impact. J Magn Reson Imaging. 2011;33(5):1121–7.
31. Hayter CL, Koff MF, Shah KKM, Miller TT, Potter HG. MRI after arthroplasty: comparison of MAVRiC and conventional fast spin-echo techniques. AJR Am J Roentgenol. 2011;197(3):W405–11.
32. Hayter CL, Koff MF, Porter HG. Magnetic resonance imaging of the postoperative hip. J Magn Reson Imaging. 2012;35(5):1013–25.

33. Potter HG, Nestor BJ, Sofka CM, Ho ST, Peters SL, Salvati EA. Magnetic resonance imaging after total hip arthroplasty: evaluation of periprosthetic soft tissue. J Bone Joint Surg Am. 2004;86-A(9):1947–54.
34. Cooper HJ, Ranawat AS, HGF P, Foo LF, Jawetz ST, Ranawat CS. Magnetic resonance imaging in diagnosis and management of hip pain after total hip arthroplasty. J Arthroplasty. 2009;24(5):661–7.
35. Hayter CL, Potter HG, Su EP. Imaging of metal-on-metal resurfacing. Orthop Clin North Am. 2011;42(2):195–205.
36. Williams DH, Greidanus NV, Masri BA, Duncan CP, Garbuz DS. Prevalence of pseudotumor in asymptomatic patients after metal-on-metal hip arthroplasty. J Bone Joint Surg Am. 2011;93-A(23):2164–71.
37. Eftekhar NS, Nercessian O. Intrapelvic migration of total hip prostheses: operative treatment. J Bone Joint Surg. 1989;71-A(10):1480–6.
38. Frandsen PA, Andersen E, Madsen F, Skjodt T. Garden's classification of femoral neck fractures: an assessment of inter-observer variation. J Bone Joint Surg Br. 1988;70-B(4):588–90.
39. D'Antonio JA, Capello WN, Borden LS, Bargar WL, Bierbaum BF, Boettcher WG, Steinberg ME, Stulberg SH, Wedge JH. Classification and management of acetabular abnormalities in total hip arthroplasty. Clin Orthop Relat Res. 1989;243:126–37.
40. Paprosky WG, Perona PG, Lawrence JM. Acetabular defect classification and surgical reconstruction in revision arthroplasty: a 6-year follow-up evaluation. J Arthroplasty. 1994;9(1):33–44.
41. Gross AE, Duncan CP, Garbuz D, Mohamed EMZ. Revision arthroplasty of the acetabulum in association with loss of bone stock. J Bone Joint Surg Am. 1998;80-A(3):440–51.
42. Berry DJ, Lewallen DG, Hanssen AD, Cabanela ME. Pelvic discontinuity in revision total hip arthroplasty. J Bone Joint Surg Am. 1999;81-A(12):1692–702.
43. Saleh KJ, Holtzman J, Gafni A, Saleh L, Jaroszynski G, Wong P, Woodgate I, Davis A, Gross AE. Development, test reliability and validation of a classification for revision hip arthroplasty. J Orthop Res. 2001;19(1):50–6.
44. Paprosky WG, Weeden SH, Howling JW Jr. Component removal in revision total hip arthroplasty. Clin Orthop Relat Res. 2001;393:181–93.
45. Peters CL, Erickson JA, Dunn HK. Revision of well-fixed cementless acetabular components for polyethylene failure. Clin Orthop Relat Res. 2003;414:129–35.
46. Mitchell PA, Masri BA, Garbuz DS, , Greidanus NV, Wilson D, Duncan CP. Removal of well-fixed, ccementless, acetabular components in revisión hip arthroplasty. J Bone Joint Surg Br 2000;85-B(7):949–952.

# Chapter 3
# Prosthetic Component Fixation and Bone Defect Determine Acetabular Revision Surgery

**Eduardo García-Cimbrelo and Eduardo García-Rey**

## Introduction

Acetabular revision surgery can present a considerable technical challenge to surgeons depending on the type of cup fixation and the intraoperative bone defect. The decision surgically to treat osteolytic lesions around well-fixed acetabular components or to observe them is made on the basis of the presence or absence of symptoms, as well as the size, location, and rate of progression of the lesion. The relative urgency of surgical treatment is based on the potential adverse consequences of waiting. Catastrophic consequences are loss of superior supporting bone resulting in a segmental bone defect that would convert a cavitary-contained defect into an uncontained segmental defect. Another very difficult-to-solve consequence is the loss of anterior and posterior column support, which results in a pelvic discontinuity. While a superior defect can be visualised on an anteroposterior (AP) radiographs, pelvic discontinuity can require oblique radiographs and computed tomography (CT) scans to assess the integrity of the posterior and anterior columns. For patients at risk of developing these complications, surgical treatment is indicated [1].

## Osteolytic Lesions Around Well-Fixed Acetabular Components. Timing of Surgery

The natural history of osteolysis and the timing of surgical intervention is not clearly defined. Timing of surgical intervention for polyethylene wear and asymptomatic osteolysis is complicated by different factors: (1) osteolysis is difficult to quantify

E. García-Cimbrelo (✉) · E. García-Rey
Orthopaedic Surgery Department, Hospital Universitario La Paz-IdiPaz, Madrid, Spain



E. García-Rey, E. García-Cimbrelo (eds.), *Acetabular Revision Surgery in Major Bone Defects*, https://doi.org/10.1007/978-3-319-98596-1_3

only using two-dimensional radiographs; and (2) it is difficult to predict when complete wear-through of the poletyhelene liner or catastrophic loosening of the socket due to bone less will finally occur [2]. Asymptomatic patients with radiographically wear but no evidence of ostelysis should be advised of this and undergo yearly evaluations. Although most patients develop symptoms and associated osteolysis, osteolysis can be radiographically diagnosed without symptoms, but, and as soon as osteolysis is seen, socket should be revised regardless of symptoms. The development of radiographic lysis means a higher degree of technical difficulty for the reconstruction. From the perspective of the revisiön surgery, there is great value in an early intervention in the face of polyethylene wear and pelvic osteolysis [3]. Mehin et al. advise that osteolysis affecting 50% of the cup contour is more predictive of loosening than the amount of affected area [4]. Changing the polyethylene liner while possible should be considered before allowing the osteolysis to affect cup fixation.

While bone destruction in the acetabulum is associated with loosening in cemented total hip arthroplasties, the surgeon is not faced with removing a well-fixed socket during revision surgery. In contrast, the surgeon frequently must decide whether to remove a well-fixed porous-coated cup when reoperating for osteolysis and polyethylene wear. The first strategy is to remove the well-fixed cup, graft defects, and revise the cup. A second strategy involves doing a liner exchange with debriding and grafting of osteolysis lesions. According to the cup fixation type of fixation, Maloney et al. [5] classified patients with acetabular osteolysis in three types:

1. **Type I**. The porous-coated cup is radiographically stable. in addition, the polyethylene is replaceable. For the liner to be replaceable different criteria must be met: (1) The cup is not malpositioned. If the cup is malpositioned, cup must be removed to avoid recurrent postoperative dislocation; (2) The locking mechanism for the modular component must be intact so the replacement of the liner is stable; (3) The metal shell must not be damaged secondary to head penetration; (4) The polyethylene liner must be of adequate thickness, a mínimum of 6–8 mm.
2. **Type II**. The metal shell is radiographically stable, however, because of factors noted previously (malpositioned cup, a damaged metal shell, locking mechanism failure, poor cup design, impossibility of providing a liner with adequate thickness), the well-fixed cup is removed.
3. **Type III**. The cup is loosened. The only treatment is to revise the cup.

## *Type I. Treatment When the Cementless Cup Is Radiographically Stable and the Polyethylene Is Replaceable*

When a preoperative evaluation determines that a case is potentially Type I, it is necessary to confirm at the time of the revision surgery (Fig. 3.1). After dislocating the hip, the acetabular line and screws are removed. The stability of the

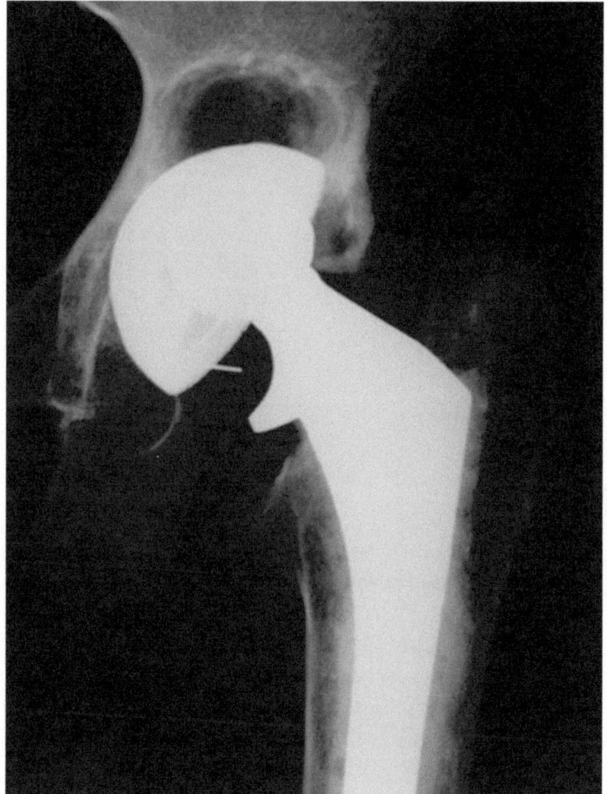

**Fig. 3.1** Anteroposterior radiograph of a hip shows a stable cup with significant polyethylene wear and a rounded and well-limited osteolytic cavity

metal-backed shell is also confirmed manually. If Type I classification continues, accessible osteolytic lesions are debrided and grafted with particulate graft material. A new polyethylene liner is inserted and it should be as thick as possible (Fig. 3.2) [5].

Maloney et al. [5], in a series of 40 hips with a mean follow-up of 3.5 years (Type I cases), exchanged the polyethylene liner and debrided the ostolytic lesion. Allograft bone chips were packed into the lytic defect in 29 patients. In the remaining 11 patients, the lesion was debrided but not grafted. At final follow-up all acetabular cups were stable and no new lesions were identified. One third of the lesions had resolved completely regardless of whether they received graft material. The remaining two thirds of the lesions had decreased in size. Maloney et al. [6] suggest that the replacement of the liner and elimination of the source of the high particle load is more important than removing all of the granulation tissue. Leaving the metal shell prevented complete debridement of the granuloma because it made it more difficult to access the entire lesion [6].

Several techniques can be used to graft bone in osteolytic defects when there is a well-fixed acetabular component. The technique depends on the accessability of the lesions. Lesions in the anterior column and pubic symphysis are difficult to assess

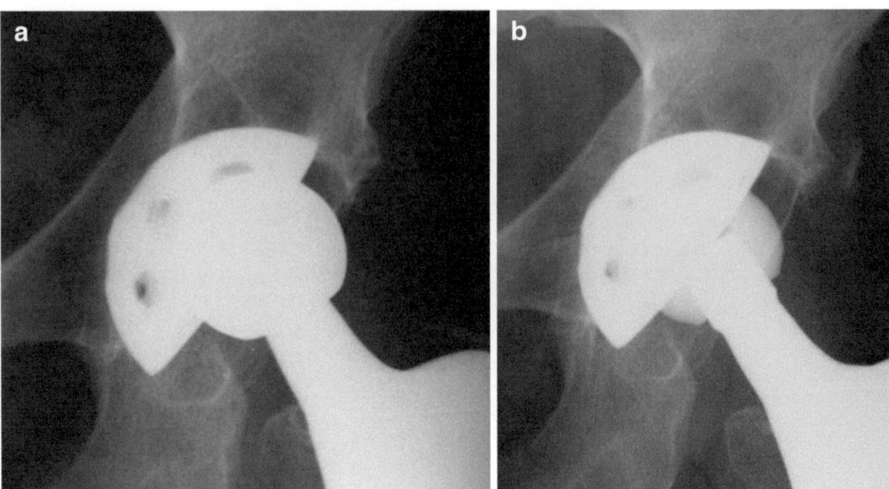


**Fig. 3.2** (**a**) Anteroposterior radiograph of hip a shows a radiographically stable cementless cup and replaceable polyethylene. (**b**) Osteolytic lesions were debrided and grafted and a new polyethylene liner was inserted with a ceramic femoral head

with a stable socket [7]. Therefore only a liner change is done and these lesions are not grafted. In a well-fixed socket with screw holes, the osteolytic lesions can be grafted through the holes. The process of placing graft through such a small area is labor-intensive and usually results in less than optimum grafting. Different series report good results using simple devices to facilitate the accessing and debriding of the granulomata and grafting of dome lesions, such as special cones made in different diameters and a long cylindrical body with a funneled top, or chondrotome shaver blades [7, 8].

Modular component exchange surgery is considered more benign for the treatment of polyethylene wear and osteolysis than full actabular revisión and has induced no significant intraoperative complications [9, 10]. However, Boucher et al. [11] report in a series of 24 patients who had an isolated polyethylene liner exchange for wear or osteolysis, at a mean of 56-months follow-up time, six hips (25%) had dislocation. Griffin et al. in a series of 55 patients treated with modular exchange, reported 18% of patients experienced postoperative dislocation, three of which required re-revision surgery. One additional patient required re-revision due to catastrophic failure of the socket after 5 years [9]. Hip instability is the problem associated to this procedure, so more stable constructs should be emphasized. Alberton et al. using a 32-mm-diameter femoral head, report a significantly lower clinical risk of dislocation [12]. However, the necessity for a fairly thick polyethylene component did not permit the use of a larger femoral head with modular exchange surgery. The new highly cross-linked polyethylene may allow the use of larger femoral heads and thinner liners [13]. Talmo et al. also report that 14 hips (25%) with acetabular revision used this technique, and of these in eight were revised due to liner dislodgment [14].

## *Type II. Treatment When the Cementless Cup is Radiographically Stable But the Polyethylene Is Not Replaceable*

When the preoperative or intraoperative evaluation determines that the clssification should be Type II, the surgeon has to be prepared to remove a stable cup. This has the potential to result in major bone destruction producing segmental defects in the medial wall of the acetabulum, the posterior or anterior columns, and even pelvic discontinuity [5]. Carefull attention to the preoperative radiographs is necessary and helps the surgeon to plan the optimal technique for removing a stable shell (Fig. 3.3). An ingrown cup that is abutting the medial wall should not be removed with space occupying tools (curved osteotomes). Peters et al. found that the revision component size was an average 6.5-mm larger due to the increase in the acetabular cavitary diameter when curve osteotomes were used [15].

The cementation of a new polyethylene liner into damaged shells has been done and may enable retention of old cups when there is a deficient locking mechanism or matching liners are unvailable for patients classified as Type II [16]. Cementing a liner into a stable socket is a good alternative for suitable patients who have a well-fixed cementless cup with an inner diameter that is larger than the outer diameter of the cemented liner. Biomechanical testing of cemented polyethylene liners has shown initial fixation strengths that exceed conventional locking mechanisms [17]. Clinical reports with follow-ups of as many as 6 years have shown survival in 90% of cases [17, 18]. This technique requires the proper patient selection, accurate sizing of the new liner, careful preparation of the substrate of the liner and the shell, and good cementing technique. The potential advantages of this technique are less surgical morbidity, more rapid surgery and patient recovery.

The use of new cup extraction systems has been very useful to limit bone destruction during cup removal. Mitchell et al. report excellent results in a series of 31 hips with well-fixed cementless sockets using the Explant Acetabular Cup Removal System (Zimmer, Warsaw, Indiana). The time taken to remove the cup did not

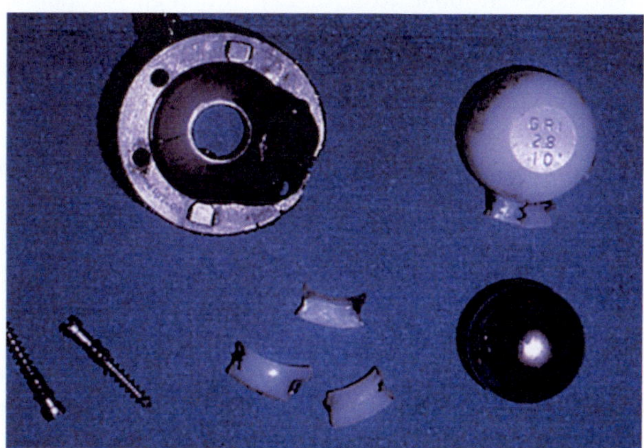


**Fig. 3.3** Photograph shows an explanted cementless cup due to a liner rupture, the polyethylene is not replaceable

exceed 5 min in any hip. The median difference between the size of the removed component the size of the new cup was 4 mm, indicating that no more host bone was removed than the thickness of the blades. The classification of the intraoperative bone defect did not change in any hip following implant removal [19].

After removing the metal shell, granulomatous tissue and osteolytic defects are debrided. Depending on the intraoperative bone defect after removing the stable shell, the surgeon must be prepared to solve possible major bone defects using the necessary graft material and tools to reconstruct the defects.

Talmo et al. [14] in a series 128 revisions involving a well-fixed Harris-Galante Porous (HGP-I) or HGP-II acetabular component found that, of the hips that underwent modular liner exchange at revision, 14 hips (25%) required re-revision of the socket., 8 for liner dislodgement, 3 for osteolysis, 2 for dislocation and 1 for aseptic loosening. Of the hips that underwent liner cementing, six (27%) were re-revised: four for dislocation and two for loosening. Of the hips that underwent revision of a well-fixed shell, four (15%) required re-revision, two for dislocation and two for loosening. For these authors using new acetabular cup removal systems, complete revision of the socket is more reliable than liner exchange or liner cementation.

## *Type III. Revision Surgery in Loosened Acetabular Cups*

Cup loosening produces bone defects and cup migration. The bone defect determines the technique used in acetabular cup revision [20]. Cup migration also make it necessary to reconstruct the centre of rotation of the hip to place the cup in the anatomic rotation centre of the hip to obtain a good clinical result [21]. Restoration of the bone stock and the hip rotation centre of the hip remain a problem in acetabular revision surgery.

As yet there is little consensus on acetabular revision surgery because there is a wide variety of available implants and techniques and questions regarding the possible use of morselised and structural bone-allograft that can be necessary when there is severe bone loss [6, 22]. Although preoperative planning is necessary in order to forestall potential difficulties, the intraoperative findings determine what intervention will be performed. The cup requires appropriate acetabular bone stock support. There must be enough medial bone stock and supportive rims to obtain a long-term result. A pelvic discontinuity that may be very difficult to diagnose, makes it necessary to stabilise the acetabular columns before implanting the cup [23].

## Classification of Acetabular Defects

The use of an adequate system to classify the acetabular defects helps plan the operation. However, the different classifications have not been universally validated. The Paprosky et al. system [24] is based on the extent of the bone defect, and allows the surgeon to choose the most adequate technique in every case. According to Paprosky, types 1 and 2 represent a bone loss of less than 30% of the acetabular surface, type 3A represents a bone loss of between 30% and 50%, and type 3B is a defect affecting more than 50% of the acetabular surface.

## *Minor Acetabular Bone Defects Paprosky Types 1 and 2*

### Cemented Techniques in Acetabular Revision Surgery

Conventional cemented techniques without additional bone grafting were widely used in acetabular revision surgery in the seventies and early eighties. The long-term results of revision surgey using early cementing techniques were inferior to those of primary surgery [25–28]. The use of a cemented socket alone requires healthy bone and an intact acetabular rim to be effective. Radiolucent lines around the socket are frequent in revision surgery, increase in width progressively over time, and must be considered a sign of prosthetic loosening [27]. This lack of initial fixation in revision surgery may be due to residual tissue debris or an inadequate bone-cement interlock on the smooth sclerotic bed. The use of contemporary cementing techniques seems to have improved the results [29]. Currently, cement alone techniques in acetabular revision surgery should be used in non complicated cases with an adequate bone bed, for old and less active patients (Fig. 3.4). The early clinical results in revision surgery can be similar to those obtained in primary surgery, but the radiographic signs must be assessed, even in asymptomatic patients,

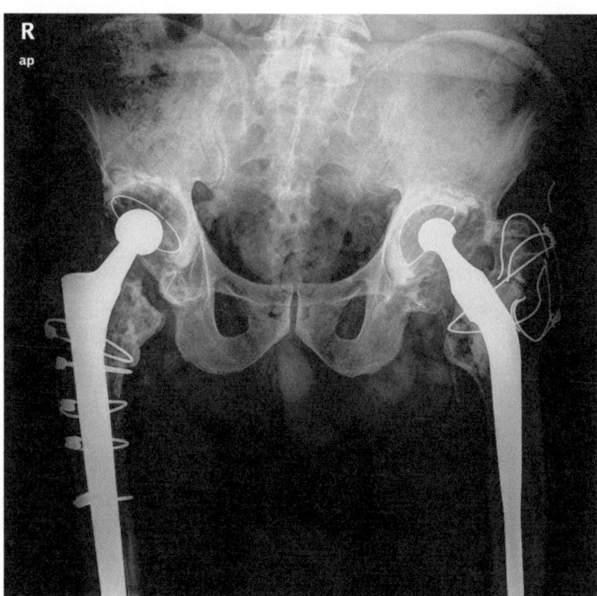


**Fig. 3.4** Anteroposterior radiograph of pelvis shows bilateral revised cemented total hip arthroplasties. Radiolucent lines around both components are clearly visible in both prostheses

to check for progressive widening of radiolucent lines, which indicate poor bone-cement fixation that causes late failures. Any major bone defect counter indicates the use of cement alone techniques [27].

## Cementless Porous-Coated Cup in Revision Surgery

A hemispherical titanium porous cementles cup supplemented with screws and frequently associated with morsellised allografts is currently used in most institutions for revision surgery and shows excellent results [30–34]. Supplemental fixation with multiple screws is advised in revision surgery to minimise micromotion and promote bone ingrowth. Screws should be placed not only posterosuperiorly into the dome of the acetabulum but also inferiorly into the ischium [34]. Good results should be expected in cases with a bone defect less than 30% and poor results in cases with a bone defect greater than 50% [33]. A major bone defect rarely reproduces the geometry of the implant, in these cases, contact between the cup and the healthy bone is very poor, and osseointegration is not obtained. Intimate apposition of the acetabular component against intact viable host is necessary to obtain a good result, and if the only viable host-bone is high on the acetabulum, the cementless cup must be placed here. When the cup is implanted in a vascularised bone bed, cup fixation should be similar to that obtained in primary surgery. Morsellized graft associated with a porous cementless cup is only useful in small cavitary defects. Biologic fixation of a cementless porous-coated cup is not to be expected in regions supported by solid allograft [35, 36].

The use of new biomaterials, such as porous tantalum trabecular metal, have afforded a superior capacity for bone ingrowth that make the use of hemispherical cementless cups feasible for acetabular revision despite marked bone loss. Tantalum has excellent mechanical and biological compatibility with host bone and induces bone ingrowth with complete osseointegration of the scaffoldat 4–6 months. Different series report encouraging results in revision surgery [37–41]. The incidence of radiolucent lines observed around the tantalum trabecular metal acetabular components is lower than that displayed around the conventional porous-coated components [37]. The excellent osteoconductive properties of porous tantalum trabecular metal may enable stronger biologic fixation even when limited viable bone host is available [42]. The properties of tantalum trabecular metal promote bone formation even across periacetabular defects up to 5 mm in width [43]. Ingrowth is easily obtained if the component is initially stable. In Paprosky types 1 and 2 acetabular defects, excellent stability can be achieved by the tight press-fit of the tantalum trabecular metal components (Fig. 3.5) [37]. Although the use of tantalum trabecular metal cups improves the press-fit of the cups in revision surgery, we do not yet know yet the minimum bone bed necessary to obtain an adequate and reliable osseointegration [44].

Newer porous titanium trabecular cups have a similar architecture to the porous tantalum trabecular metal cups, with 60–70% porosity and pore diameter ranging from 250 to 650 μm. Basic science studies have validated both porous metals by demonstrating excellent bony ingrowth potential as well as mechanical strength

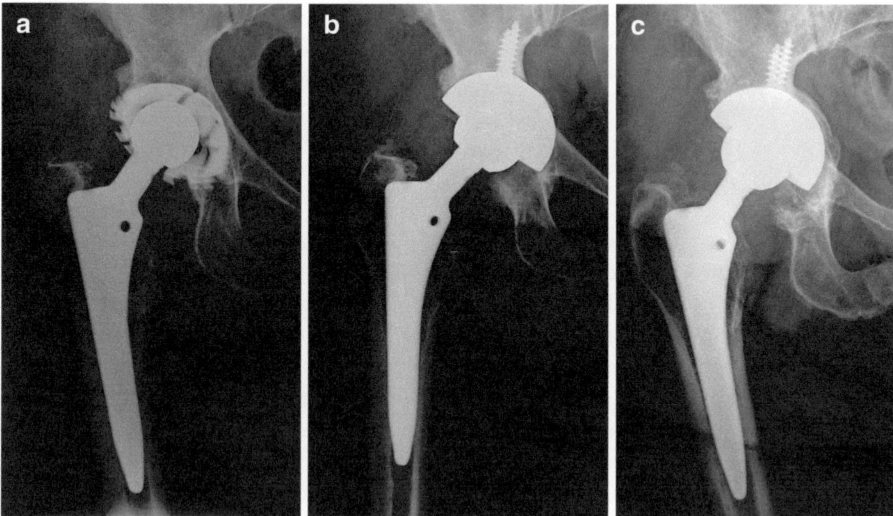


**Fig. 3.5** (**a**) Preoperative radiograph shows a loosened cementless cup. (**b**) A porous tantalum cup was used in revision surgery. (**c**) Two years later medial wall remodelling was observed and the clinical outcome is good

[45, 46]. Gallart et al. reported a series of 67 revisions using trabecular titanium cups with a mean follow-up of 30.5 months, eight patients underwent cup re-revision: two for loosening, three for infection, and three for hip dislocation. The remaining cases did not present radiological signs of loosening [47]. None of the cases with Paprosky type I classifications needed revision, while four with type II and four with type III needed revision. Ayers et al. in a series using RSA, found no significant difference in proximal migration between tantalum and titanium acetabular cups over a 5-year follow-up period [48].

Laaksonen et al. in a large registry approach compare the clinical outcome of porous-tantalum cups with other cementless designs [49]. Authors found similar results for implant survival in both groups for first-time revision. They were also unable to identify a "protective effect" by porous tantalum cups against re-revision for infection. Severe defects treated with tantalum augments were excluded from this study. Although trabecular metal could be slightly superior to cups with porous coating, more evidence is still needed before any definitive statements [50].

## Major Acetabular Bone Defects (Paprosky Types 3A and 3B)

Uncemented hemispherical cups are the treatment of choice in small acetabular defects, but it is accepted that they will provide poor results when acetabular bone defects are greater than 50% [33]. Another limitation for these implants in revision hip surgery is bone resection. Although extra-large uncemented components have achieved good results [51], the extensive reaming required to obtain good bone contact with the host bone, which is more important in the antero-posterior diameter of the acetabulum, can ultimately affect implant stability [52]. In these difficult cases, we use metallic rings, oblong cups, tantalum cementles porous cup associated with tantalum augments, and the bone impacting grafting technique.

## Metallic Rings

During the 1970s, Müller developed a metallic ring to increase a deficient acetabular bone bed. Burch and Schneider also developed an anti-protrusio cage. There are several similar designs today. These rings try to provide a greater contact between the implant and the acetabular bone bed in the hope of distributing the stresses over a greater area. In the early period only cement was used in conjunction with the ring to secure cup fixation. The Müller ring was used in segmental defects, and the Burch and Schneider cage was used in major defects [53].The advantages of antoprotrusio cages are that the reinforcement device seems to protect grafts from overstress, helps to restore the appropriate centre of rotation of the hip and support the polyethylene cemented cup. The best results obtained with the Müller ring are seen in cavitary and anterior segmental defects, while the Burch-Schneider antiprotrusio cage is indicated in major bone defects, but its use requires experience and good exposure, since the screws must be placed in zones with good bone stock [54]. Most series reporting poor long-term results have cases with only a cemented cup associated with a metallic ring. Allografts are currently associated with these devices and have improved those poor results. Grafts are protected from forces that might contribute to graft failure and allograft remodelling is frequently seen (Fig. 3.6). All series described the best results when metal rings were used in association with graft [53–56]. Coscujuela et al. [57], in a series of 96 acetabular revisions using a Burch-Schneider antiprotrusio cage with a mean follow-up of 8.1 years (range, from 5 to 13 years), found three re-revisions, one because of aseptical loosening and two because of deep infection. The Kaplan-Meier survivorship rate, with aseptic component loosening as the criterion of failure, was 92.4% (95% confidence interval, 85.1–99.8%) at 13 years. Radiographic evaluation determined that three cages were considered definitely loose. The distance from the prosthetic femoral head to the approximate anatomic rotation centre of the hip was lowered an average of 4.3 mm and lateralised an average of 1.3 mm.

Metal ring and cemented cup alone could be used for salvage surgery in elderly patients and in low-demand patients [58]. The Burch-Schneider antiprotrusio cage long-term survival rate compares favourably with that for other devices.

## Oblong Cups

The purpose of an oblong cup is to obtain sufficient stability in both the anterior and posterior column of the acetabulum without sacrificing the longitudinal axis [59, 60]. This should allow the reconstruction of the anatomic centre of hip rotation and is desirable in order to obtain good results in acetabular revision surgery. Using these cups, different authors have reported excellent clinical and radiological results

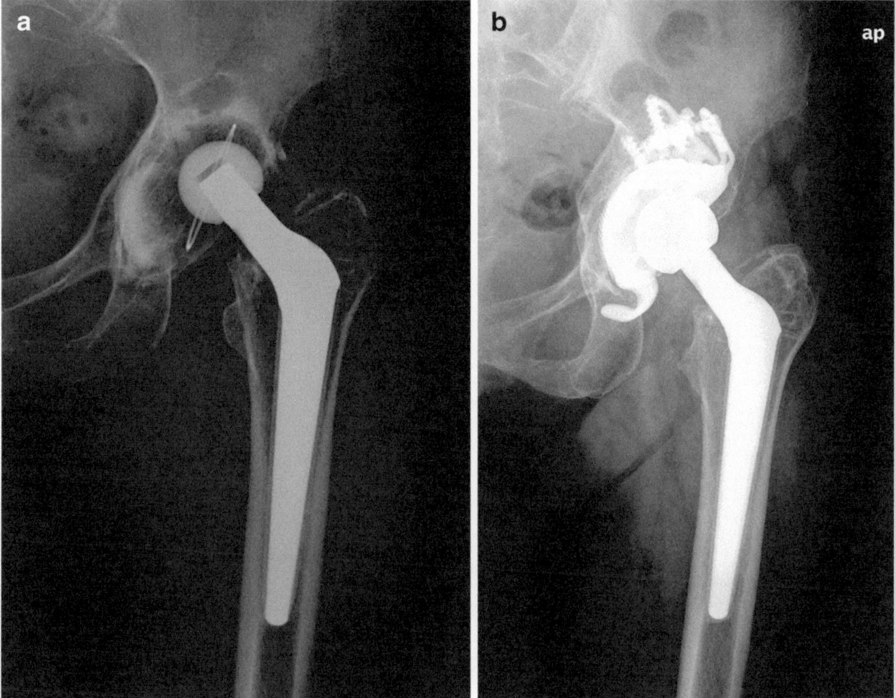


**Fig. 3.6** (**a**) Preoperative radiograph shows a loosened cemented cup. (**b**) A metallic cage was used in revision surgery with a good clinical outcome

[60]. Herrera et al. reported a 14.2% migration rate that was greater in vertical cups and in major bone defects with an incomplete cup contact at the acetabular rim [61]. Landor et al. reported a survival rate for aseptic loosening of 90% at 12 years without deep infection in patients with different bone defects; they do not recommend these implants for large bone defects and also emphasize a need of correct cup positioning [62]. Garcia-Rey et al. report in a series of 46 hips with a mean follow-up of 7.2 years, four re-revisions (three due to aseptic loosening); the survival rate for re-revision due to aseptic loosening was 60.1% at 7 years, but the survival rate for radiological loosening at 7 years was 40.54% [63] (Fig. 3.7). Chen et al. reported an early rate of probable or definite loosening of 24% in a follow-up that ranged from 24 to 41 months; failure was greater with major bone defects and undersized components and they did not recommend the routine use of these types of implants [64]. Abeyta et al. reported the long term results of 15 hips using S-ROM (DePuy Johnson and Johnson, Leeds, UK) oblong bi-hemispherical cups; three cups were revised due to aseptic loosening and one showed complete radiolucencies around the cup [65]. On the other hand, Moskal et al. assessed 11 bilobed components in combined acetabular defects that did not require revision over a 5 year follow-up [66]. Although most series observe good results for oblong or bilobed cups, Babis et al. have reported poor results with the Procotyl E cup (Wright Medical Technology, Arlington, TN) in Paprosky defect type 3A and do not recommend this

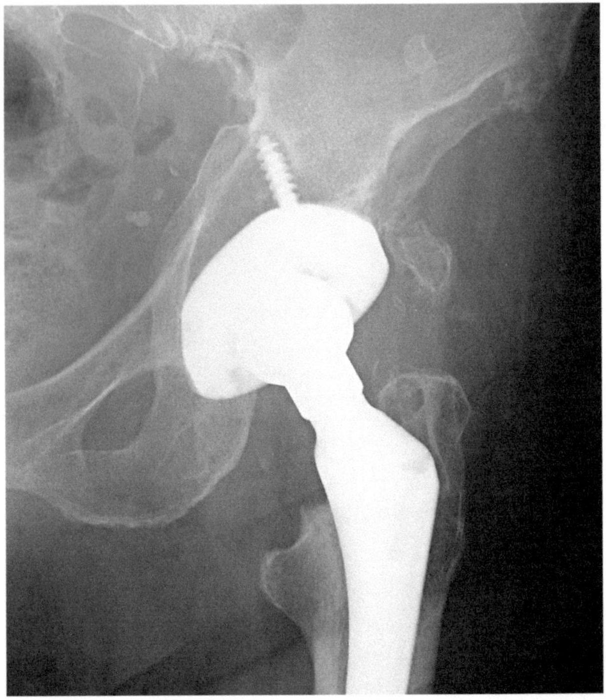

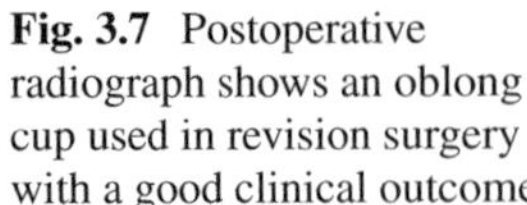

**Fig. 3.7** Postoperative radiograph shows an oblong cup used in revision surgery with a good clinical outcome

technique [67]. Many factors may be responsible for the acetabular cup loosening. A shorter horizontal distance was related to the appearance of radiological cup loosening in the Babis et al. study. Similarly, Surace et al. correlated the clinical results of the LOR cup to its proper postoperative positioning [68]. Bone defect is considered to be the most important factor in obtaining a good result in hip revision surgery. Several authors have reported worse results in major bone defects when oblong cups were used [60, 61]. Currently, clinical and radiological results for these oblong cup designs are not encouraging in medium term follow-ups. The high rate of radiological loosening is a concern since this failure was observed regardless of the grade of the bone defect. Although a good reconstruction of the center of rotation of the hip is frequently achieved, and the postoperative position is frequently correct, this was not enough to achieve an acceptable rate of radiological loosening with these cups. We recommend careful evaluation of the patient before using these types of devices in revision hip surgery.

## Porous Trabecular Metal Cementles Cup Associated with Trabecular Metal Augments

The use of porous trabecular metal cementless cups is currently more and more associated with the use of trabecular metal augments [40, 69, 70]. The theoretical advantages are that, as augments are not oblong cups, there is not allograft risks such as disease and bone graft resorption, and well as the simplicity of their use. Different series report excellent results using this technique [71–74].

Acetabular component augments are added to reduce a large acetabular bone defect volume and restore the acetabular rim to aid in the support of the revision cup. A trabecular metal modular augment shaped like a partial hemisphere with rim screw holes is indicated when less than 50% host acetabular bone is present [75]. The acetabulum is reamed in the anatomic position for the eventual reconstruction until two points of fixation are achieved and this will determine the size of acetabulum. Once the desired cup position is identified, the augment is positioned to optimize the filling and fit to the bone defect and provide primary support for the acetabular component [37]. In cases presenting Paprosky type 3 defects, augment can be used to fill the large defect and allow for direct apposition of the tantalum surface to host bone (Fig. 3.8). Location and orientation of augments depends on the pattern of bone loss. It is more common to use augments with the wide base placed laterally and the apex medially. The revision acetabular cup directly contacts the augments, and the augments are necessary to achieve press-fit by the acetabular cup. Particulate bone graft is placd into any remaining cavity before implanting the cup in place. The interface between the revision shell and the augment is cemented to minimize micromotion and subsequent fretting. Multiple screws into both the ilium and ischium are used for fixation. In cases where augments may not provide adequate defect repair and component stability, an acetabular cage may be used [75–77]. Ballester and Sueiro also reported excellent results in a series of 35 patients with severe bone defects using buttress tantalum augments [71].

## Impacting Morsellized Allograft and Cemented Cup

In the light of the good results with impacting autografts taken from the femoral head and a cemented cup in acetabular protrusio, Slooff et al. used a similar technique in acetabular revision surgery [78]. Impacted morselized bone allograft and cement in the acetabulum used in revision surgery have given good clinical results [79–81]. The use of metallic meshes converts segmental defects into cavitary defects, making it possible to the fill the cavity with bone-bank impacted morsellized allografts. After this, the cup is cemented onto the graft. In the impacting graft technique, open cancellous bone allows rapid revascularisation of the graft, and bone formation preceeds resorption, thus avoiding the loss of mechanical properties of the bone. What is more, the morsellized allograft can fill in an irregular bone defect [80].

We commonly use this technique in acetabular defects greater than 30%, where our porous cementless cups results have been poor [33]. In a series of 181 hips with either a Paprosky grade 3A (98 hips) or grade 3B defect (83 hips) [82], 12 hips were re-revised and 17 hips showed bone resorption. The total cumulative probability of not having a probable or definite radiographic loosening after 8 years was 94.6% in Paprosky grade 3A hips and 85.9%in grade 3B hips ($p = 0.0453$) (Fig. 3.9). Placing the acetabulum in the anatomic position is important for good long-term results

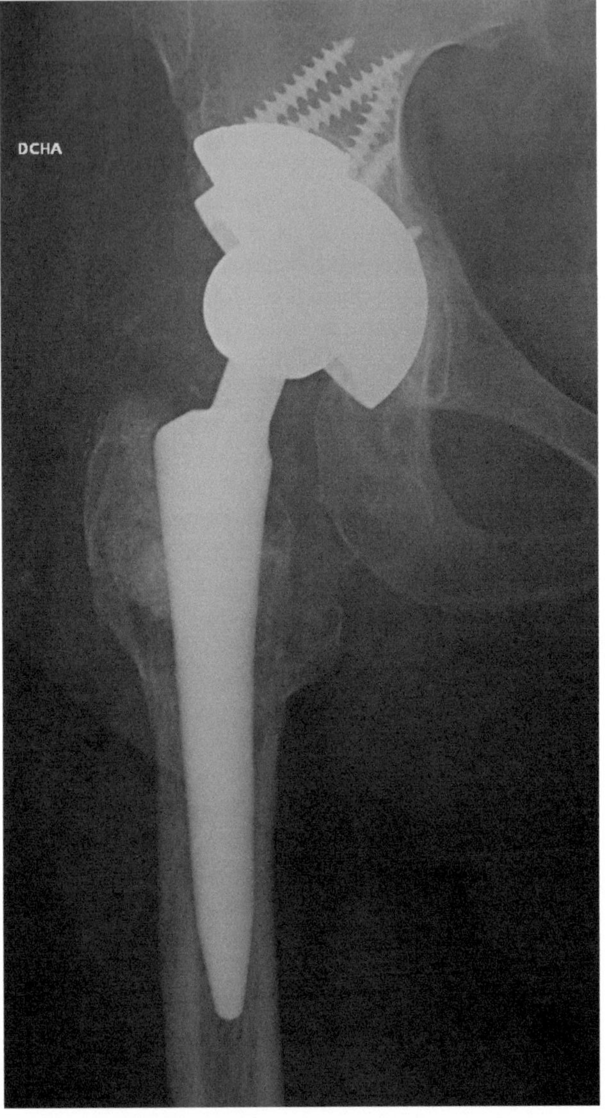


**Fig. 3.8** Postoperative radiograph shows a porous tantalum cup associated with a tantalum augment, with a good clinical outcome

[83, 84]. The mid-term results for impacted bone allograft and cemented all-polyethylene cups are more favorable in Paprosky grade 3A than in Paprosky grade 3B hips and acetabular reconstruction allows anatomic positioning of the cups and promotes good final results. Van Haaren et al. [85] report a high rate of failure with impaction bone grafting in large acetabular defects, including those with pelvic discontinuities. Our series excluded cases with pelvic discontinuity because major bone defects associated with pelvic discontinuity usually require complex acetabular reconstructive techniques using cages or plates, which effectively excluded them from the series [23]. Buttaro et al. suggested considering metal mesh, impaction

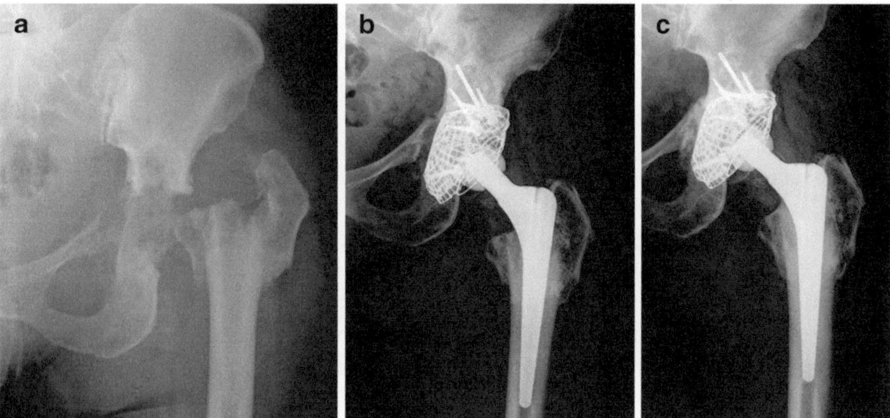


**Fig. 3.9** (**a**) Preoperative radiograph of the hip after removal of a metal-metal total hip arthroplasty that developed a pseudotumor and a bone defect at the acetabular medial wall. (**b**) Postoperative radiograph shows impacting bone grafting in the acetabulum and a cementless femoral stem than were used in revision surgery. (**c**) The bone defect is remodeled at 7 years. The clinical result is excellent

bone grafting, and a cemented acetabular component when reconstructing acetabular defects of medium severity, but advised treating severe combined deficiencies with an acetabular ring [86]. Waddell et al. report their American experience in 21 patients with Paprosky 3B acetabular defect who underwent total hip arthroplasty revision using impacting bone grafting [87]. After an average follow-up of 47 months for the entire series, one patient has had radiographic loosening without symptoms at 120 months postoperatively. No patients have been revised for a related reason. Authors concluded that impacting bone grafting is a reliable technique for the treatment of Paprosky 3B acetabular defects. As in other series [80], the impression at re-revision was that the original bone graft had been incorporated, and a new bone impacting grafting was performed because part of the existing graft looked viable and well incorporated to the host-bone. Radiological assessment of bone graft resorption is difficult when impacted bone allograft has been used with cement in an acetabular revision, but the cup and remodeled graft is clearly stable. Most hips presented uniform graft and host bone radiodensity. Histologic studies of cup loosening in humans report bone substitution, but at a slower rate than in animal models [88–91]. The open structure of the cancellous bone graft, associated with cement, permits good vascularization, and thus bone substitution takes place without mechanical loosening [79]. Board et al. report in an in vitro study that strain, as from vigorous graft impaction and postoperative loading, can transform bone allograft from osteoconductive to osteoinductive, since BMP-7 was found to be released from the graft in proportion to the strain imposed on it [92]. Clinical studies using PET to evaluate the spatial and temporal development of bone formation after acetabular revision surgery report that the impacted bone allograft had transformed to living bone [93].

Cup migration and bone graft resorption are some of the limitations after acetabular impaction bone grafting in revision surgery when used for large segmental defects. Garcia-Rey et al. have reported in a series of 204 hips that the survival rate for loosening at 15 years was 83.2 ± 12% for Paprosky Type defect 3A and 72.5 ± 12% for group 3B defects (Mantel-Cox, p = 0.04) [94]. The survival rate for loosening was lesser when using rim meshes (Mantel Cox, p = 0.008). Patients with a bone defect 3B and a metallic mesh rim had a higher risk for loosening (p = 0.047; Hazard Ratio: 2.36, Confidence Interval 95% (IC) 1.01–5.5, and, p = 0.026; OR: 3.7, CI 95%: 1.13–12.4, respectively). Rigby et al. explain that the mechanism of failure of these cups consisted of movement and rotation of the cup/cement composite within the graft [95]. This was followed, eventually, by the mesh being pulled off the reconstructed rim. Failure of the metalwork did not initiate the rotation and migration process. Another possible explanation for the high failure rate in this series could be that in large segmental defects the absence of superior bony support leads to a large amount of bone graft placed at the most loaded area above the acetabular component. Owing to insufficient support for the bone graft, it is likely that micromovement of the prosthesis results in implant failure [85]. RSA studies have shown that almost all impacted sockets migrate in the postoperative period, although the rate of migration decreases with time. Ornstein et al. report that 41% of the sockets were still found to be migrating 18–24 months after surgery [96]. Mohaddes et al. conducted a randomised study with 17 years follow-up, including RSA, and concluded that cemented fixation with bone grafting in acetabular revision surgery results in higher proximal migration [97]. Better results for cemented fixation would probably have been obtained if bigger graft particles and a more consistent impaction technique had been used. It could also be argued that the increased proximal migration of the cemented acetabular components is due to a different pattern of bone remodelling when cemented fixation is used in conjunction with bone impaction grafting. Garcia-Rey et al. also concluded that impacting bone grafting improves the reconstruction of the rotation of the hip center in acetabular revision surgery [94]. Although results are good for large contained or medial defects, hips with a large segmental rim defect may need other options for reconstruction in these challenging surgeries. A large metal mesh does not avoid cranial femoral head migration when there is a large segmental defect of the acetabular roof. Porous trabecular metal augments associated with impacting grafting technique have obtained good early results in this situation (Fig. 3.10). The combination of biological fixation offered by tantalum and impaction grafting seems to generate an adequate cranial support for the cemented cup [98–100]. We must perform more prospective comparative and ideally, randomized studies examining impacting bone grafting versus metal augments as well as the results of impacting bone grafting with and without the augments.

## Pelvic Discontinuity

Pelvic discontinuity (acetabular disassociation) is one of the more challenging situations for the hip arthroplasty surgeon to manage. Pelvic discontinuity is a distinct form of bone loss. Occurring in association with total hip arthroplasty, in which

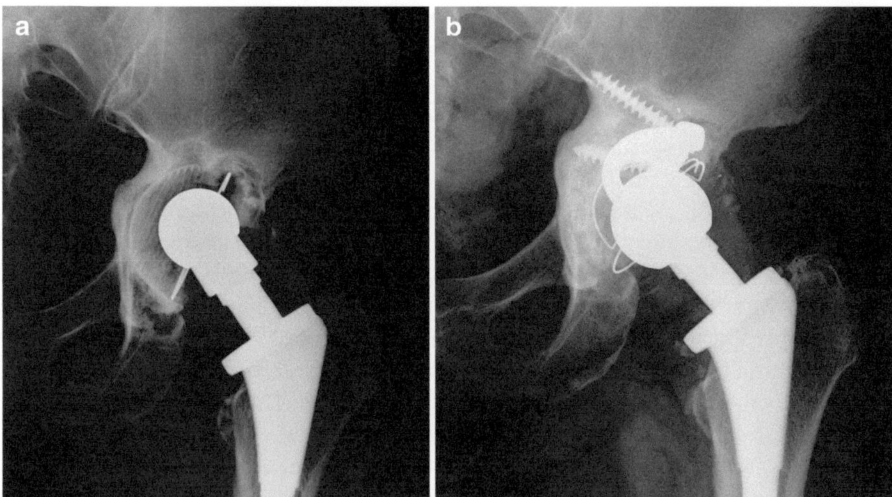


**Fig. 3.10** (**a**) Anteroposterior radiograph of a hip shows a failed impacting bone grafting of a revised cup. (**b**) A new impacting bone graft associated with tantalum augments were used in re-revision surgery

there is loss of structural bone between the superior and inferior part of the pelvis resulting from bone loss or fracture through the acetabulum [23, 38]. Its incidence is rare, around 0.9%, and several surgical techniques including ilioisquial cages, or acetabular plates have been recommended [23]. Preoperative diagnosis is important to avoid surgical complications. The radiographic findings include a visible fracture line through the anterior and posterior columns, medial translation of the inferior aspect of the hemipelvis relative to the superior aspect (seen as a break in Köhler's line), and rotation of the inferior aspect of the hemipelvis relative to the superior aspect (seen as asymmetry of the obturator rings) on a true anterioposterior radiograph [23]. However, the diagnosis of pelvic discontinuity using standard imaging views (i.e., anteroposterior, pelvic inlet and outlet views) is challenging because the prosthetic implant can obstruct full visualisation of the defect, especially if the posterior column is involved. Multiple reports support the superiority of the computed tomography (CT) over traditional radiographs in monitoring periprosthetic osteolysis [101, 102]. Massive acetabular bone loss is the most common cause of pelvic discontinuity, making a reliable means of monitoring osteolysis in the hip arthroplasty patient important. Leung et al. found that while radiographs were able to detect at most 52% of osteolytic lesions, CT scans were able to detect 87% [102].

Intraoperative diagnosis of pelvic discontinuity can be made by placing stress on the inferior hemipelvis in the anteroposterior direction and observing any disassociated movement between the superior and inferior portions of the acetabulum. This approach can be limited by the fracture line not being very mobile. Furthermore, visual assessment also presents challenges because the fracture line may pass through areas of bone loss or be filled with fibrous tissue [23].

Berry et al. [23] subclassified the AAOS Type IV defect (pelvic discontinuity) into three subgroups: Type IVa, if the pelvic discontinuity is associated only with cavitary defect and or mild-moderate segmental bone loss; as Type IVb if the discontinuity is associated with more severe segmental or combined bone loss; and as Type IVc if it was associated with previous irradiation of the pelvis with or without cavitary or segmental bone loss. Rogers et al. distinguish acute and chronic pelvic discontiniutes [38]. Acute pelvis discontinuity is secondary to a blunt trauma or iatrogenic intraoperative trauma to impact the uncemented componenet into the acetabulum. A "T "pattern or transverse acetabular fracture is frequent in these cases, and the resulting bone loss is moderate and the acetabular reconstruction relatively simple, however, the posterior column must be stabilized with a reconstruction plate initially in addition to revising the acetabulum. Chronic pelvis discontinuity is secondary to septic or aseptic periprosthetic bone loss. The bone loss is frequently severe and reconstruction requires the use of an ischial cage or a cup-cage. The diagnosis is frequently not obvious before surgery, despite the use of CT and oblique x-Ray. Therefore, a high-level of suspicion should be maintained during surgery, with the possibility of a pelvic discontinuity specifically being checked after any initial gente reaming [38].

## Reconstruction Techniques

**Porous Metal Components** The implantation of the acetabular component is complex and complications and poor results are frequent. A hemispheric acetabular component alone does not provide adequate implant stability in patients with pelvic discontinuity and a number of different methods have been used for reconstruction depending on the degree of severity. The best results are obtained in patients who do not have severe segmental acetabular bone loss (Type IVa) and are worse in those with severe segmental or combined defects (Type IVb) or those who have previously been treated with irradiation in the pelvis (Type IVc) [23].

**Internal Fixation with Acetabular Reconstruction** In cases of acute pelvic discontinuity with moderate segmentl bone-loss, the use of a compression posterior column plating supplementing a trabecular metal acetabular revision shell can solve the problem depending on the size and nature of the cavitary defect that is the result of stabilizing the posterior column. Plates are used in conjunction with acetabular reconstruction to stabilize the pelvic discontinuity (Fig. 3.11). Dual plating of posterior and anterior columns and plating of just the posterior or anterior column have been described in the literature [38, 103, 104]. Dual plating requires combined ilio-inguinal pelvic and posterior surgical approaches to the hip. Berry et al. found unfavorable results using plating with a cemented cup, and none of the five cases had good long term survivorship [23]. Better results were found in the eight cases in whom a cementless cup and dual or single plating was used: four (three type IVA and one type IVB) had satisfactory results, while the other four (all type IVB) did not. Stiehl et al. used structural allografts with dual plating or single column plating.

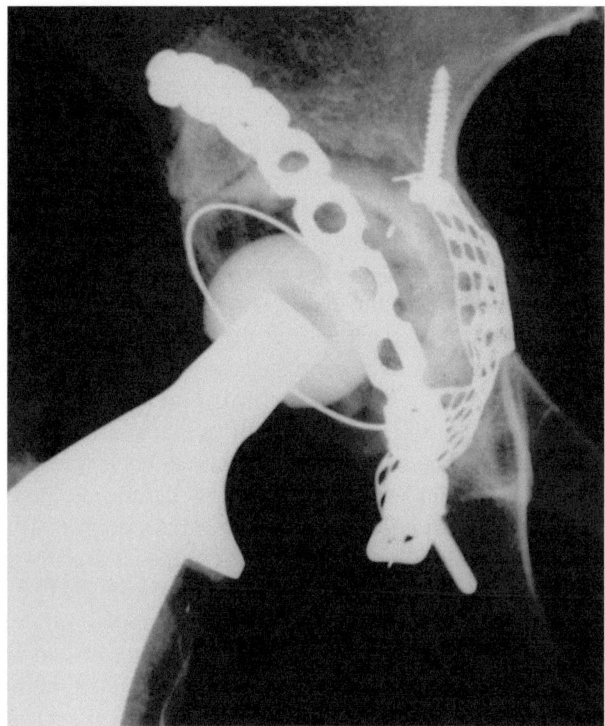

**Fig. 3.11** Anteroposterior radiograph of the hip shows a pelvis discontinuity after an acetabular fracture that was treated using an acetabular plate recontruction to stabilize the posterior column and total hip arthroplasty

Of the 10 pelvic discontinuities, seven out of the nine Type IVB and the single Type IVC pelvic discontinuities shaved actual healing of the discontinuity. The utility of fixation was called into question in these cases by the high complication rate of 60%. Eggli et al. used plating of either the posterior or anterior column along with reconstruction using allograft chips covered by autograft [104], and at a mean follow-up of 8 years, reported reoperation had occurred in two of the seven cases but at their last follow-up, all cases demonstrated a stable and healed pelvic discontinuity. Rogers et al. used compression plating of the posterior column, revision cup, and screw supplementation in eight of their patients with acute pelvic discontinuity and, at a mean follow-up of 34 months, there were no further revisions in any of those eight cases [38].

**Metallic Rings** The Kerboull plate was developed in 1974 to address pelvic discontinuity [105]. The vertical plate is proximally fixed to the ilium via screw fixation and distally via a hooked end that inserts under the inferior acetabular margin. It has traditionally been used with bone grafts, providing the grafts with mechanical support, to address areas of acetabular bone loss. The failure rate during the period analyzed was only 5% (three hips) and these were due to partial or complete resorption of allograft. However, in their study only 12 of the 60 hips had Type IV acetabular bone loss (AAOS) and the remainder (48 hips) had Type III loss [105]. The study did not specify how the Type IV hips fared with this reconstruction technique. The promising results in the above study need validation with further studies focusing on Type IV acetabular defects.

**Acetabular Distraction with Porous Acetabular Cup** The acetabular distraction technique is another novel approach to managing pelvic discontinuities. Paprosky et al. [106] recommend the use of metal acetabular augments to distract across the pelvic discontinuity, since the amount of bone loss along the posterior column is often too severe to provide direct bone apposition during compression plating. The goal of the distraction technique is to address the acetabular nonunion with distraction by expanding the defect and creating elastic recoil forces that should compress the porous metal construct and provide a stable construct. Intraoperatively, a Cobb elevator is used to delineate the fracture line and debride the granulation tissue followed by acetabular reaming that is performed to better define the acetabular bone that is suitable for fixation using augmentation [107]. The location and severity of bone loss determine the type and position of the acetabular augments used to enhance initial component stability. Augments are frequently used to reconstruct portions of the anterosuperior aspect of the acetabulum as well as the posteroinferior aspect; they provide two secure points of fixation for the acetabular component. A porous acetabular cup, which is 6–8 mm larger than the hemisferic reamer that engaged the anterior and posterior columns, is used to distract the superior hemipelvis from the inferior hemipelvis. Multiple screws are placed in ilium and ischium, and the augment is secured to the cup with polymethylmethacrylate [107]. Sporer et al. reported good mid-term results using acetabular distraction and only one case (1/20) required revision for aseptic loosening at 9 months, at the 4 year follow-up, four hips showed migration of the acetabular component but they were clinically stable [107]. The acetabular distraction technique is a reasonable option for many patients but the long-term data is limited in this regard.

**Cup-Cage Construct** In cases with chronic pelvic discontinuity or major column defects, different aurthors recommend the use of a cup-cage acetabular reconstruction owing to the inherent beneficial biological and biomechanical properties of porous tantalum metal [23, 38, 56, 71, 108, 109]. The cup-cage construct is a well-described technique to correct large acetabular defects and pelvic discontinuity. Using this technique, a porous metal cup is secured to host bone and allograft, if used. An acetabular cage is subsequently anchored to the pelvis. Placing a screw through both the cage and the cup adds a level of unity and stability to the construct. The rationale behind the cup and cage is that it removes loading forces on the cup and allows time to optimize ingrowth of new bone into the cup [74]. Cup-cage reconstruction has yielded encouraging short-term outcomes, including one study that demonstrated no clinical or radiological evidence of loosening in 23 out of 26 (88.5%) hips with an average follow-up of 44.6 months (range, 24–68) [110]. Another study with a mean follow-up of 82 months reported a survival rate of 87.2% for cup-cage reconstructions as opposed to just 49.9% for the group treated with only a cage [74]. Despite the use of new biomaterials, Rogers et al. report only an 8-year survivorship of 86.3% using cup-cage reconstructions [38]. Ballester and Sueiro [71] reported excellent results in a series of 35 patients with severe bone defects including five cases of chronic pelvic discontinuity using buttress tantalum augments with cup-cage construct; no mechanical failure had occurred in any hip and all patients had a radiographically stable cup. Radiographic assessment showed an improvement in the position of the rotation centre of the hip. Konan et al. [108] in a series of 24 patients with pelvic discontinuity treated using a cup-cage construct, at median 6-year (minimum 2 year, maximum 10 years) follow-up reported that one patient was converted to excision arthroplasty for infection. A further three patients required revision for instability but the cup-cage construct was not revised. The cup-cage construct is a viable method of dealing with a complex pelvic discontinuity. However, the failure rate due to loosening in most reports does prompt the need for further refinement of the technique and technology in this very challenging group of patients, as well as continued evaluation at the mid- and long-term so as to confirm the ongoing success of this method of reconstruction [111].

The cup-cage technique is technically challenging, and forceful impaction of the ischial flange of the cage into the ischium risks producing an iatrogenic pelvic dissociation [112]. Furthermore, the increased dissection required for placement of the ischial flange may increase the risk of sciatic nerve injury [113]. Sculco et al. report good results using the half cup-cage modification, designed to simplify cage insertion [112]. The half-cup cage involves removal of the ischial flange to create a single-flanged cup-cage construct. Sculco et al. found both full and half cup-cage constructs gave successful clinical outcomes in the treatment of major acetabular defects and pelvic discontinuities. Each method should be used on the basis of individual intraoperative findings, including the extent of bone loss, the quality of the remaining bone stock, and the presence of pelvic discontinuity.

**Custom Triflange Implants** Triflange implants are custom-made, porous-coated titanium alloy components considered to be a final therapeutic salvage option in patients with pelvic discontinuity and/or large acetabular defects. A triflange construct is designed and manufactured based on pelvic CT scans with metal subtraction software converted into a 3-D representation of the patient's hemipelvis. The manufacturer generates personalized implants from the corresponding images. Triflange components have had produced wide-ranging clinical results. DeBoer et al. reported zero cases (0/20) requiring revision of the triflange construct and average Harris Hip Score (HHS) of 80 at 10 years follow-up [114]. Taunton et al. reported a revision rate of 30% (20/57) at 5.4 years and a 21% dislocation rate most likely attributable to instability generated from he preoperative trochanteric escape performed in 51% of patients, as well as possible traction injury to the superior gluteal nerve during exposure leading to abductor muscle weakness [115]. When comparing manufacturing cost, triflange components are priced similar to other constructs used to treat pelvic discontinuity, including the cup-cage construct. The major drawback of the triflange construct is that it may take up to several weeks or longer to prepare the implant for surgery. However, custom triflange components may be the only viable reconstructive option for discontinuity with massive segmental bone loss [111].

The outcome for reconstruction of pelvic a discontinuity is dependent on many factors including the extent of bone loss associated with the discontinuity, severity of osteopenia, vascularity of the pelvic bone, chronicity of discontinuity and reconstruction technique. Healing of the discontinuity can be achieved more effectively for defects associated with cavitary or mild to moderate segmental bone loss (AAOS type IVa) than those with more severe bone loss or poor vascularity (AAOS types IVb and IVc). However, stable fixation of the revision component to the iliac portion of the pelvis may still be feasible with a cup cage or custom triflange reconstruction without union of the discontinuity.

## Conclusion

The type of cup fixation and the degree of pelvic osteolysis determines the surgical technique to reconstruct the acetabulum and implantation of a stable acetabular component. Table 3.1 shows recommendations according to this variables. Table 3.2 shows results of different surgical techniques depending on the acetabular bone defect.

**Table 3.1** Surgical techniques recommended depending on type of cup fixation and the degree of pelvic osteolysis in acetabular revision surfery

| Socket fixation | Surgical technique |
|---|---|
| Type I: cementless cup stable and polyethylene replaceable | Retain shell, exchange liner, ± grafting |
| Type II: cementless cup stable but the polyethylene not replaceable | Revise socket ± bone grafting |
| Type III. Loosened socket | Revise component |
| Paprosky bone defect types 1 and 2 | Porous cup± bone grafting |
| Paprosky bone defect type 3 A | Trabecular porous augment and cups/ impacting bone grafting |
| Paprosky bone defect type 3B | Impacting bone grafting ± porous augments |
| Pelvic discontinuity | |
| Acute pelvic discontinuity | Acetabular plates to stabilize the posterior column |
| Chronic pelvic discontinuity | Cup-cages/distraction technique |

**Table 3.2** Results of differents techniques used according to the acetabular bone defect in revision surgery

| Author | Surgical technique | Year | Bone defect according to Paprosky | Number of cases | Follow-up (years) | Revised cups | Loosened cups |
|---|---|---|---|---|---|---|---|
| Garcia-Cimbrelo et al. [27] | Cemented cup | 1995 | 1–3 | 180 | 11.5 | 19 | 29 |
| Garcia-Cimbrelo [33] | Cementless cup | 1999 | 1–3 | 65 | 8.3 | 7 | 18 (grade 3) |
| Fernandez-Fairen et al. [37] | Porous-tantalum | 2010 | 1–3 | 253 | 6.1 | 2 (infections) | 0 |
| Coscujuela-Maña et al. [57] | Antiprotrusio-cage | 2010 | 2–3 | 68 | 8.1 | 3 (2 infections) | ° |
| Garcia-Rey et al. [64] | Oblong cups | 2013 | 2-3A | 45 | 7.2 | 2 | 8 |
| Ballester-Alfaro et al. [72] | Tantalum augments | 2010 | 3A-3B | 19 | 2.2 | 0 | 0 |
| Garcia-Cimbrelo et al. [82] | Impacting bone grafting | 2010 | 3A-3B | 181 | 7.7 | 12 | 14 |
| Garcia-Rey et al. [94] | Impacting bone grafting | 2015 | 3A-3B | 204 | 10.4 | 14 | 24 |
| Gallart et al. [47] | Trabecular titanium | 2016 | 1–3 | 67 | 2.5 | 8 | 2 |

# References


1. Ries MD, Link TM. Monitoring and risk of progression of osteolysis after total hip arthroplasty. In: Pagnano MW, Hart RA, editors. AAOS instructional course lectures, 62. 2013. p. 207–14.
2. Dumbleton JH, Manley MT, Edidin AA. A literatura review of the association between wear rate and osteolysis following total hip arthroplasty. J Arthroplasty. 2002;17(5):649–61.
3. Hozack WJ, Mesa JJ, Carey C, Rothman RH. Relationship between polyethylene wear, pelvic osteolysis, and clinical symptomatology in patients with cementless acetabular components. A framework for decisión making. J Arthroplasty. 1996;11(7):769–72.
4. Mehin R, Yuan X, Haydon C, Rorabeck CH, Bourne RB, McCalden RW, MacDonald SJ. Retroacetabular osteolysis. When to operate? Clin Orthop Relat Res. 2004;428:247–55.
5. Maloney WJ, Paposky W, Engh CA, Rubash H. Surgical treatment of pelvic osteolysis. Clin Orthop Relat Res. 2001;393:78–84.
6. Maloney WJ, Herzwurm PW, Rubash HE, Engh CA. Treatment of pelvic osteolysis associated with a stable acetabular component inserted without cement as part of a total hip replacement. J Bone Joint Surg Am. 1997;79(11):1628–34.

7. Chiang PP, Burke DW, Freiberg AA, Rubash HE. Osteolysis of the pelvis. Evaluation and treatment. Clin Orthop Relat Res. 2003;417:164–74.
8. Jeer PJS, Oakeshott RD. Debridement of wear granulomata in revision total hip arthroplasty. Use of a chondrotome saber blade. J Arthroplasty. 2004;19(8):1042–4.
9. Griffin WL, FehringTK MJB, TH MC, Odum S, Sychterz Terefenko C. Early morbidity of modular exchange for polyethylene wear and osteolysis. J Arthroplasty. 2004;19(Suppl 2):61–6.
10. Beaulé PE, LeDuff MJ, Dorey FJ, Amstutz HC. Fate of cementless acetabular components retained during revision total hip arthroplsty. J Bone Joint Surg Am. 2003;85(12):2288–93.
11. Boucher HR, Lynch C, Young AM, Engh CA Jr, Engh C Sr. Dislocation after polyethylene liner exchange in total hip arthroplasty. J Arthroplasty 2003;18(5):654–7.
12. Alberton GM, High WA, Morrey BF. Dislocation after revisión total hip arthroplasty: an analysis of risk factors and treatment options. J Bone Joint Surg Am. 2002;84(10):1788–92.
13. Burroughs BR, Rubash HE, Harris WH. Femoral head sizes with larger than 32 against highly-cross-linked polyethylene. Clin Orthop Relat Res. 2002;405:150–7.
14. Peters CL, Erickson JA, Dunn HK. Revision of well-fixed cementless acetabular components for polyethylene failure. Clin Orthp Relat Res. 2003;414:129–35.
15. Beaulé PE, Ebramzadeh E, LeDuff M, Prasad R, Amstutz HC. Cementing a liner into a stable cementless acetabular shell: the double-socket tecnique. J Bone Joint Surg Am. 2004;86-A(5):929–34.
16. Jiranek WA. Acetabular liner fixation by cement. Clin Orthop Relat Res. 2003;417:217–23.
17. Haft GF, Heiner AD, Callaghan JJ, et al. Polyethylene liner cementation into fixed acetabular shells. J Arthroplasty. 2002;17(4 Suppl 1):167–70.
18. Mitchell PA, Masri BA, Garbuz DS, Greidanus NV, Wilson D, Duncan CP. Removal of well-fixed, ccementless, acetabular components in revisión hip arthroplasty. J Bone Joint Surg (Br). 2003;85-B(7):949–52.
19. Talmo CT, Kwon Y-M, Freiberg AA, Rubash HE, Malchau H. Management of polyethylene wear associated with a well-fixed modular cemented shell during revisión total hip arthroplasty. J Arthroplasty. 2011;26(4):576–81.
20. García-Cimbrelo E, García-Rey E. Bone defect determines acetabular revisión surgery. Hip Int. 2014;24(Suppl 10):S33–6.
21. Pagnano MW, Hanssen AD, Lewallen DG, Shaughnessy WJ. The effect of superior placement of the acetabular component on the rate of loosening after total hip arthroplasty: long-term results in patients who have Crowe type-II congenital dysplasia of the hip. J Bone Joint Surg Am. 1996;78(7):1004–14.
22. Gross AE, Duncan CP, Garbuz D, Mohamed EMZ. Revision arthroplasty of the acetabulum in association with loss of bone stock. J Bone Joint Surg Am. 1998;80(3):440–51.
23. Berry DJ, Lewallen DG, Hanssen AD, Cabanela ME. Pelvic discontinuity in revision total hip arthroplasty. J Bone Joint Surg Am. 1999;81(12):1692–702.
24. Paprosky WG, Perona PG, Lawrence JM. Acetabular defect classification and surgical reconstruction in revision arthroplasty. A 6-year follow-up evaluation. J Arthroplasty. 1994;9(1):33–44.
25. Katz RP, Callaghan JJ, Sullivan PM, Johnston RC. Long-term results of revision total hip arthroplasty with improved cementing technique. J Bone Joint Surg (Br). 1997;79(2):322–6.
26. Retpen JB, Varmarken JE, Röck ND, Jensen S. Unsatisfactory results after repeated revision of hip arthroplasty: 61 cases followed for 5 (1–10) years. Acta Orthop Scand. 1992;63:120–7.
27. Garcia-Cimbrelo E, Munuera L, Diez-Vazquez V. Long-term results of aseptic cemented Charnley revisions. J Arthroplasty. 1995;10(2):121–31.
28. Hultmark P, Hötsner J, Herberts P, Kärrholm J. Radiographic evaluation of Charnley cups used in first-time revision: repeated observations for 7-15 years. J Arthroplasty. 2003;18(8):1005–15.
29. Estok DM II, Harris WH. Long-term results of cemented femoral revision surgery using second-generation techniques: an average 11–7-year follow-up evaluation. Clin Orthop Relat Res. 1994;299:190–202.

30. Deaborn JT, Harris WH. Acetabular revision arthroplasty using so-called jumbo cementless component: an average 7-year follow-up study. J Arthroplasty. 2000;15(1):8–15.
31. Della Valle CJ, Shuaipaj T, Berger RA, Rosenberg AG, Shott S, Jacobs JJ, Galante JO. Revision of the acetabular component without cement after total hip arthroplasty. A concise follow-up, at fifteen to nineteen years, of a previous report. J Bone Joint Surg Am. 2005;87(8):1795–800.
32. Hallstrom BR, Golladay GJ, Vittetoe DA, Harris WH. Cementless acetabular revision with the Harris-Galante prosthesis. Results after a minimum of ten years of follow-up. JBone Joint Surg Am. 2004;86(5):1007–11.
33. Garcia-Cimbrelo E. Porous-coated cementless acetabular cups in revision surgery. A 6- to 11-year follow-up study. J Arthroplasty. 1999;14(4):397–406.
34. Weeden SH, Paprosky WG. Porous-ingrowth revision acetabular implants secured with peripheral screws. A minimum twelve-year follow-up. J Bone Joint Surg Am. 2006;88(6):1266–71.
35. Hooten JP Jr, Engh CA Jr, Engh CA. Failure of structural acetabular allografts in cementless revision hip arthroplasty. J Bone Joint Surg (Br). 1994;76:419–22.
36. Hooten JP Jr, Engh CA, Heekin RD, Vinh TN. Structural bulk allografts in acetabular reconstruction. Analysis of two grafts retrieved at post-morten. J Bone Joint Surg (Br). 1996;78-B(2):270–5.
37. Fernandez-Fairen M, Murcia A, Blanco A, Meroño A, Murcia A Jr, Ballester J. Revision of failed total hip arthroplasty acetabular cups to porous tantalum components. A 5-year follow-up study. J Arthroplasty. 2010;25(6):865–72.
38. Rogers BA, Whittingham-Jones PM, Mitchell PA, Safir OA, Bircher MD, Gross AE. The reconstruction of periprosthetic pelvic discontinuity. J Arthroplasty. 2012;27(8):1499–506.
39. Jafari AM, Bender B, Coyle C, Parvizi J, Sharkey PF, Hozack WJ. Do tantalum and titanium cups show similar results in revision hip arthroplasty? Clin Orthop Relat Res. 2010;468:459–65.
40. Lachiewicz PF, O'Dell JA. Tantalum components in difficult acetabular revisions have good survival at 5 to 10 years: longer term follow-up of a previous report. Clin Orthop Relat Res. 2018;476:336–42.
41. Lakstein D, Backstein D, Safir O, Kosashvili, Gross AE. Trabecular metal TM cups for acetabular defects with 50% or less host bone contact. Clin Orthop Relat Res. 2009;467(9):2318–24.
42. Gross AE, Goodman SB. Rebuilding the skeleton: the intraoperative use of trabecular metal in revision total hip arthroplasty. J Arthroplasty. 2005;20(4 Suppl 2):91–3.
43. Macheras GA, Papagelopoulos PJ, Kateros K, Kostakos AT, Baltas D, Karachalios TS. Radiological evaluation of the metal-bone interface of a porous tantalum monoblock acetabular component. J Bone Jojnt Surg Br. 2006;88-B(3):304–9.
44. Sternheim A, Backstein D, Kuzyk PRT, Goshua G, Berkovich Y, Safir O, Gross AE. Porous metal revision shells for management of contained acetabular bone defects at a mean follow-up of six years. A comparison between up to 50% bleeding host bone contact and more than 50% contact. J Bone Joint Surg (Br). 2012;94(2):158–62.
45. Bobyn JD, Stackpool GJ, Hacking SA, Tanzer M, Krygier JJ. Characteristics of bone ingrowth and interface mechanics of a new porous tantalum biomaterial. J Bone Joint Surg (Br). 1999;81(5):907–14.
46. Frenkel SR, Jaffe WL, Dimaano F, Iesaka K, Hua T. Bone response to a novel highly porous surface in a canine implantable chamber. J Biomed Mater Res B Appl Biomater. 2004;71(2):387–91.
47. Gallart X, Fernández-Valencia JA, Riba J, Bori G, García S, Tornero E, Combalía A. Trabecular titanium™ cups and augments in revision total hip arthroplasty: clinical results, radiology and survival outcomes. Hip Int. 2016;26(5):486–91.
48. Ayers DC, Greene M, Snyder B, Aubin M, Drew J, Bragdon C. Radiostereometric analysis study of tantalum compared with titanium acetabular cups and highly cross-linked compared with conventional liners in young patients undergoing total hip replacement. J Bone Joint Surg Am. 2015;97(8):627–34.
49. Laaksonen I, Lorimer M, Grosmov K, Rolfson O, Mäkelä KT, Graves SE, Malchau H, Mohaddes M. Does the risk of rerevision vary between porous tantalum cups and other cementless designs after revision hip arthroplasty? Clin Orthop Relat Res. 2017;475(12):3015–22.

50. Kärrholm J. CORR insights: does the risk of rerevision vary between porous tantalum cups and other cementless designs after revision hip arthroplasty? Clin Orthop Relat Res. 2017;475(12):3023–5.
51. Patel JV, Masonis JL, Bourne RB, Rorabeck CH. The fate of cementless jumbo cups in revision hip arthroplasty. J Arthroplasty. 2003;18(2):129–33.
52. Whaley AL, Berry DJ, Harmsen WS. Extra-large uncemented hemispherical acetabular components for revision total hip arthroplasty. J Bone Joint Surg Am. 2001;83(9):1352–7.
53. Berry DJ, Müller ME. Revision arthroplasty using an anti-protrusio cage for massive acetabular bone deficiency. J Bone Joint Surg (Br). 1992;74-B(5):711–5.
54. Roson J, Schatzker J. the use of reinforcement rings to reconstruct deficient acetabula. J Bone Joint Surg (Br). 1992;74-B(5):716–20.
55. Zehntner MK, Ganz R. Midterm results (5.5–10 years) of acetabular allograft reconstruction with the acetabular reinforcement ring during total hip revision. J Arthroplasty. 1994;9(5):469–79.
56. Regis D, Sandri A, Bonetti I, Bortolami O, Bartolozzi P. A minimum of 10-year follow-up pf the Burch-Schneider cage an bulk allografts for the revision of pelvic discontinuity. J Arthroplasty. 2012;27(6):1057–63.
57. Coscujuela Maña A, Angles F, Tramunt C, Casanova X. Burch-Schneider antiprotrusio cage for acetabular revision: a 5- to 13-year follow-up study. Hip Int. 2010;20(Suppl 7):S112–8.
58. Garcia-Cimbrelo E, Alonso-Biarge J, Cordero-Ampuero J. Reinforcement rings for deficient acetabular bone in revision surgery: long-term results. Hip Int. 1999;7(2):57–64.
59. DK DB, Christie MJ. Reconstruction of the deficient acetabulum with an oblong prosthesis: three- to seven-year results. J Arthroplasty. 1998;13(6):674–80.
60. Köster G, Willert HG, Kohler HP, Dopkens K. An oblong revision cup for large acetabular defects: design rationale and two- to seven-year follow-up. J Arthroplasty. 1998;13(5):559–69.
61. Koster, Surace MF, Zatti G, De Pietri M, Cherubino P. Acetabular revision surgery with the LOR cup: three to 8 years' follow-up. J Arthroplasty. 2006;21(1):114–21.
62. Herrera A, Martinez AA, Cuenca J, Canales V. Management of types III and IV acetabular deficiencies with the longitudinal oblong revision cup. J Arthroplasty. 2006;21(6):857–64.
63. Landor I, Vavrik P, Jahoda D, Pokorny, Tawa, Sosna A. The long oblique revision component in revision arhtoplasty of the hip. J Bone Joint Surg (Br). 2009;91(1):24–30.
64. Garcia-Rey E, Fernández-Fernández R, Duran D, Madero R. Reconstruction of the rotation center of the hip after oblong cups in revision total hip arthroplasty. J Orthopaed Traumatol. 2013;14:39–49.
65. Chen WM, Engh CA Jr, Hopper RH Jr, McAuley JP, Engh CA. Acetabular revision with use of a bilobed component inserted without cement in patients who have acetabular bone-stock deficiency. J Bone Joint Surg Am. 2000;82(2):197–206.
66. Abeyta PN, Namba RS, Janku GV, Murray WR, Kim HT. Reconstruction of major segmental acetabular defects with an oblong-shaped cementless prosthesis: a long-term outcomes study. J Arthroplasty. 2008;23(2):247–53.
67. Moskal JT, Higgins ME, Shen J. Type III acetabular defect revision with bilobed components: five years results. Clin Orthop Relat Res. 2008;466:691–5.
68. Babis GC, Sakellariou VI, Chatziantoniou AN, Soucacos PN, Megas P. High complication rate in reconstruction of Paprosky IIIa acetabular defects using an oblong implant with modular side plates and a hook. J Bone Joint Surg (Br). 2011;93(12):1592–6.
69. Surace MF, Zatti G, De Pietri M, Cherubino P. Acetabular revision surgery with the LOR cup: three to 8 years' follow-up. J Arthroplasty. 2006;21(1):114–21.
70. Sporer SM. How to do a revision total hip arthroplasty: revision of the acetabulum. J Bone Joint Surg Am. 2011;93(14):1359–66.
71. Flecher X, Sporer S, Paprosky W. Management of severe bone loss in acetabular using a trabecular metal shell. J Arthroplasty. 2008;23(7):949–55.
72. Ballester Alfaro JJ, Sueiro FJ. Trabecular metal buttress augment and the trabecular metal cup-cage construct in revision hip arthroplasty for severe acetabular bone loss and pelvic discontinuity. Hip Int. 2010;20(Suppl 7):S119–27.

73. Del Gaizo DJ, Kancherla V, Sporer SM, Paprosky WG. Tantalum augments for Paprosky IIIA defects remain stable at midterm followup. Clin Orthop Relat Res. 2012;470:395–401.
74. Unger AS, Lewis RJ, Gruen T. Evaluation of a porous tantalum uncemented acetabular cup in revision total hip arthroplasty. Clinical and radiological results of 60 hips. J Arthroplasty. 2005;20(8):1002–9.
75. Abolghasemian M, Tangsataporn S, Sternheim A, Backstein D, Safir O, Gross AE. Combined trabecular metal acetabular shell augment for acetabular revision with substantial bone loss. Bone Joint J. 2013;95-B(2):166–72.
76. Weeden SH, Schmidt RH. The use of tantalum porous metal implants for Paprosky 3A and 3B defects. J Arthroplasty. 2007;22(6 Suppl 2):151–5.
77. Nehme A, Lewallen DG, Hanssen AD. Modular porous metal augments for treatment of severe acetabular bone loss during revision hip arhroplasty. Clin Orthop Relat Res. 2004;429:201–8.
78. Slooff TJJH, Van Horn J, Lemmens A, Huiskes R. Bone grafting in total hip replacement for acetabular protrusion. Acta Orthop Scand. 1984;55:593–6.
79. Slooff TJ, Schimmel JW, Buma P. Cemented fixation with bone grafts. Orthop Clin North Am. 1993;24:667–77.
80. Schreurs BW, Keurentjes JC, Gardeniers JWM, Verdonschot N, Slooff TJJH, Veth RPH. Acetabular revision with impacted morselised cancellous bone grafting and a cemented acetabular component. A 20- to 25-year follow-up. J Bone Joint Surg (Br). 2009;91(9):1148–53.
81. Schmitz MWJL, Hannink G, Gardeniers JWM, Verdonschot N, Slooff TJJH, Schreurs BW. Acetabular reconstructions with impaction bone-grafting and a cemented cup in patients younger than 50 years of age. A concise follow-up, at 27 to 35 years of a previous report. J Bone Joint Surg Am. 2017;99(19):1640–6.
82. Garcia-Cimbrelo E, Cruz-Pardos A, Garcia-Rey E, Ortega-Chamarro J. The survival and fate of acetabular reconstruction with impaction grafting for large defects. Clin Orthop Relat Res. 2010;468:3304–13.
83. Crowninshield RD, Brand RA, Pedersen DR. A stress analysis of acetabular reconstruction in protrusion acetabuli. J Bone Joint Surg Am. 1983;65:495–9.
84. Garcia-Cimbrelo E, Diaz-Martin A, Madero R, Munuera L. Loosening of the cup after low-friction arthroplasty in patients with acetabular protrusion. The importance of the position of the cup. J Bone Joint Surg (Br). 2000;82-B(1):108–15.
85. van Haaren EH, Heyligers IC, Alexander FG, et al. High rate of failure of impaction grafting in large acetabular defects. J Bone Joint Surg (Br). 2007;89(3):296–300.
86. Buttaro MA, Comba F, Pusso R, Piccaluga F. Acetabular revision with metal mesh, impaction grafting, and a cemented cup. Clin Orthop Relat Res. 2008;466:2482–90.
87. Waddell BS, Boettner F, Gonzalez Della Valle A. Favorable early results of impaction bone grafting with reinforcement mesh for the treatment of Paprosky 3B acetabular defects. J Arthroplasty. 2017;32:919–23.
88. Buma P, Lamerigts N, Schreurs BW, et al. Impacted graft incorporation after cemented acetabular revision. Histological evaluation in 8 patients. Acta Orthop Scand. 1996;67:536–40.
89. Schimmel JW, Buma P, Versleyen D, Huiskes R, Slooff TJJH. Acetabular reconstruction with impacted morcellized cancellous allografts in cemented hip arthroplasty: a histologic and biomechanical study on the goat. J Arthroplasty. 1998;13(4):438–48.
90. Schreurs BW, Buma P, Huiskes R, Slagter JL, Slooff TJ. Morselized allografts for fixation of the hip prosthesis femoral component: a mechanical and histological study in the goat. Acta Orthop Scand. 1994;65:267–75.
91. Singer GC, Muirhead-Allwood SK. The histology of impacted cancellous allograft in acetabular reconstruction. Hip Int. 1999;9(1):20–4.
92. Board TN, Rooney P, Kay PR. Strain imparted during impaction grafting may contribute to bony incorporation; an in vitro study of the release of BMP-7 from allograft. J Bone Joint Surg (Br). 2008;90(6):821–4.

93. Ullmark G, Sörensen J, Nilsson O. Bone healing of severe acetabular defects after revision arthroplasty. A clinical positron emission tomography study of 7 cases. Acta Orthop. 2009;80:179–83.
94. Garcia-Rey E, Madero R, Garcia-Cimbrelo E. THA revision using impacting grafting allografting with mesh is durable for medial but not lateral acetabular defect. Clin Orthop Relat Res. 2015;473:3882–91.
95. Rigby M, Kenny PJ, Sharp R, Whitehouse SL, Gie GA, Timperley JA. Acetabular impaction grafting in total hip replacement. Hip Int. 2011;21(4):399–408.
96. Ornstein E, Franzen H, Johnsson R, Stefansdottir A, Sundberg M, Tagil M. Hip revision with impacted morselized allograft: unrestricted weight-bearing and restricted weight-bearing have similar effect on migration. A radiostereometry analysis. Arch Orthop Trauma Surg. 2003;123:261–7.
97. Mohaddes M, Herberts P, Malchau JP-E, Kärrholm J. High proximal migration in cemented acetabular revisions operated with bone impaction grafting; 47 revision cups followed with RSA for 17 years. Hip Int. 2017;27(3):251–8.
98. Borland WS, Bhattacharya R, Holland JP, Brewster NT. Use of porous trabecular metal augments with impaction bone grafting in management of acetabular bone loss. Early to medium-trem results. Acta Orthop. 2012;83(4):347–52.
99. Gehrke T, Bangert Y, Schwantes B, Gebauer M, Kendoff D. Acetabular revision in THA using tantalum augments combined with impaction bone grafting. Hip Int. 2013;23(4):359–65.
100. Gill K, Wilson MJ, Whitehouse SL, Timperley AJ. Results using trabecular metal augments in combination with acetabular impaction bone grafting in deficient acetabula. Hip Int. 2013;23(6):522–8.
101. Puri L, Wixson RL, Stern SH, Kohli J, Hendrix RW, Stulberg SD. Use of helical computed tomography for the assessment of acetabular osteolysis after total hip arthroplasty. J Bone Joint Surg Am. 2002;84(4):609–14.
102. Leung S, Naudie D, Kitamura N, Walde T, Engh CA. Computed tomography in the assessment of periacetabular osteolysis. J Bone Joint Surg Am. 2005;87(3):592–7.
103. Stiehl JB, Saluja R, Diener T. Reconstruction of major column defects and pelvic discontinuity in revision total hip arthroplasty. J Arthroplasty. 2000;15:849–57.
104. Eggli S, Müller C, Ganz R. Revision surgery in pelvic discontinuity. An analysis of seven patients. Clin Orthop Relat Res. 2002;398:136–45.
105. Kerboull M, Hamadouche M, Kerboull L. The Kerboull acetabular reinforcement device in major acetabular reconstructions. Clin Orthop Relat Res. 2000;378:155–68.
106. Paprosky WG, O'Rourke M, Sporer SM. The treatment of acetabular bone defects with an associated pelvic discontinuity. Clin Orthop Relat Res. 2005;441:216–20.
107. Sporer SM, Bottros JJ, Hulst JB, Kancherla VK, Moric M, Paprosky WG. Acetabular distraction: an alternative for severe defects with chronic pelvic discontinuity? Clin Orthop Relat Res. 2012;470(11):3156–63.
108. Konan S, Duncan CP, Masri BA, Garbuz DS. The cup-cage reconstruction for pelvic discontinuity has encouraging patient satisfaction and functional outcome at median 6-year follow-up. Hip Int. 2017;27(5):509–13.
109. Abolghasemian M, Tangsaraporn S, Drexler M, Barbuto R, Backstein D, Safir O, Kuzyk P, Gross A. The challenge of pelvic discontinuity: cup-cage reconstruction does better than conventional cages in mid-term. J Bone Joint Surg (Br). 2014;96-B(2):195–200.
110. Kosashvili Y, Backstein D, Safir O, Lakstein D, Gross AE. Acetabular revision using an anti-protrusion (ilio-ischial) cage and trabecular metal acetabular component for severe acetabular bone loss associated with pelvic discontinuity. J Bone Joint Surg (Br). 2009;91(7):870–6.
111. Schwarzkop R, Ihn HE, Ries MD. Pelvic discontinuity: modern techniques and outcomes for treating pelvic disassociation. Hip Int. 2015;25(4):368–74.
112. Sculco PK, Ledford CK, Hanssen AD, Abdel MP, Lewallen DG. The evolution of the cup-cage technique for major acetabular defects. Full and half-cup reconstructions. J Bone Joint Surg Am. 2017;99(13):1104–10.

113. Goodman S, Saastamoinen H, Shasha N, Gross A. Complications of iliischial reconstruction rings in revision total hip arthroplasty. J Arthroplasty. 2004;19(4):436–46.
114. DeBoer DK, Christie MJ, Brinson MF, Morrison JC. Revision total hip arthroplasty for pelvic discontinuity. J Bone Joint Surg Am. 2007;89(4):835–40.
115. Taunton MJ, Fehring TK, Edwards P, Bernasek T, Holt GE, Christie MJ. Pelvic discontinuity treated with custom triflange component: a reliable option. Clin Orthop Relat Res. 2012;470(2):428–34.

# Chapter 4
# Biology of Bone Grafting

**Eduardo García-Rey and Enrique Gómez-Barrena**

## Introduction

Bone defects due to trauma or pathological bone resorption represent a major challenge for surgeons. The need for bone regeneration is one of the central clinical issues in regenerative medicine. Autografts have always been considered the "gold standard of bone transplantation". Bone autografts were originally used to unite fractures, and in this situation the quantity of graft material that can be harvested from the host is usually sufficient. Posteriorly, with improved techniques for limb salvage surgery in orthopedic oncology, allograft bone has been more and more used [1]. In total hip arthroplasty (THA), at revision surgery, the magnitude of bone loss around the implant can make reconstruction of the hip using conventional methods impossible, and bone allograft must be used on both the acetabular and femoral sides.

On the acetabular side, allografts have been used as morselised pieces to fill cavitary defects [2] or as structural grafts to support acetabular components in more severe defects [3, 4]. Kwong et al. have questioned the longevity of hip reconstructions using structural allografts [5]. Reconstructive oncologic surgery with structural allografts has been associated with a high complication rate including infection, fracture of the allograft, and nonunion of the graft-host junction [6, 7]. However, in revision surgery using morselised allografts, even structural allografts, complication rates have been low [3, 4, 8–10]. Currently, the overall clinical experience with the use of allografts in acetabular revision surgery has been positive and its use is a major part of the armamentarium in orthopedic reconstructive surgery [1].

Bone repair is a special process in which sequential cellular and molecular events take place to generate new bone, rather than causing a fibrous scar as in other

E. García-Rey (✉) · E. Gómez-Barrena
Orthopaedic Surgery Department, Hospital Universitario La Paz-IdiPaz,
Madrid, Spain



E. García-Rey, E. García-Cimbrelo (eds.), *Acetabular Revision Surgery in Major Bone Defects*, https://doi.org/10.1007/978-3-319-98596-1_4

connective tissues. The precise serial, ordered events required to produce the new bone are modulated by systemic and local factors, and disruption of these events or their organisation may cause healing problems.

## Bone Healing Process

The general pattern of bone healing, based on endochondral ossification, includes chronological phases of haematoma, inflammation, angiogenesis, chondrogenesis to osteogenesis, and bone remodeling [11]. Membranous ossification, with no periosteal reaction or visible callus formation, is seldom obtained. The well-established characteristics of the mentioned phases require different processes of cell migration and differentiation, extracellular matrix formation and organization towards calcification, as well as both local and systemic modulation.

Formation of a hematoma related to blood vessel damage is accompanied by an inflammatory response [12] where pro-inflammatory cytokines such as Interleukin (IL-1), −6, and particularly Tumor necrosis factor (TNF), initiate the bone healing cascade towards endochondral bone formation and remodeling [13]. Secondarily, growth and differentiation factors, particularly the Transforming growth factor (TGF), superfamily including Bone morphogenetics proteins (BMP), as well as platelet derived growth factor (PDGF), fibroblast growth factor (FGF), and insulin-like growth factors (IGF), orchestrate crucial events for chondro-osteogenesis, including chemotaxis, mesenchymal and osteoprogenitor cell proliferation and differentiation, continuing into the extracellular matrix ossification [14]. Finally, angiogenesis is also regulated at the molecular level, and an angiopoietin pathway has been described in the early days of the healing process [15], but a Vascular endothelial growth factor (VEGF) dependent pathway related to endochondral bone formation, with BMPs stimulating the expression of VEGF by osteoblasts and osteoblast-like cells has also been described [16]. Inhibitory molecules are needed to control growth factors and various BMP antagonists are released with this purpose to the extracellular compartment (sclerostatin, follistatin, etc.). Other inhibitory mechanisms include receptor inhibition of some members of the TGF-b superfamily, which has been related to a pseudo-receptor called BAMBI (BMP and activin membrane bound inhibitor) [17], but also intracellular inhibition by the activation of I-SMADs [18, 19], among other mechanisms. Many aspects are known in this bone healing cascade of molecules, cells, and events, yet the complex interactions and processes, with simultaneous sequences, are still only partially understood.

Besides the triad controlling bone healing, with the participation of cells, extracellular matrix, and osteoinductive factors, a fourth major controller has been stressed by different authors [20, 21]; and it is related to the biomechanics of the callus. Mechanical influence on biological processes significantly affects all the phases of bone formation. Major external forces are not the only influences to disrupt the healing process, mechanical loading influences endochondral ossification since compression enhances bone apposition [20]. The earlier phases of osteogenesis show increased cell proliferation if cyclic motion with associated shear stresses occurs, while intramembranous ossification may occur in areas with low stress and strain. Mechanical signaling at the cellular level may modulate molecular changes in cytoskeleton, integrins, and ion channel activities with consequences in the differentiation and gene expression of cells involved in the healing process. Transduction mechanisms range from direct mechanical stimulation of cells [22], to fluid shear stresses and various matrix effects that indirectly affect cells [23]. Clinical studies showed the beneficial influence of interfragmentary motion (of about 0.6 mm) in the early stages of the healing process [24], and the role of mechanical stimulus in general to influence the rate of healing.

Despite this mechanism of bone healing, alteration of local and systemic factors may impair healing. While systemic factors are recognised to influence the outcome of bone healing, nonsteroidal anti-inflammatory drugs (that inhibit the Cox-2 required in the inflammation phase), age (with decreased expression of mediators, hormonal changes, impaired osteoblast function), or smoking [25], local factors and the mechanical environment are determinant for bone healing.

## Biology of Bone Grafting

The properties of the bone tissue that are critical for successful healing and incorporation of bone grafts. These include osteogenesis, osteoclastic resorption, osteoinduction, and osteoconduction. Osteogenesis refers to the ability of bone to regenerate itself by production of new bone. This function is accomplished by osteoblasts. Osteoclastic resorption is the ability to remove bone mineral and is mediated by osteoclasts. Osteoinduction is the ability to stimulate new bone formation by recruitment of pluripotential mesenchymal cells from the surrounding host bed. This unique property of bone is mediated by several bone matrix-derived soluble proteins of which the best characterized group is the family of BMP. BMP function does not require living cells and its activity is triggered by removing bone mineral [26]. Osteoconduction refers to the bone graft's ability to function as a scaffold for the ingrowth of capillaries, perivascular tissue, and osteoprogenitor cells from the host bed. This scaffold is critical to the remodeling of bone and allows gradual replacement of the bone graft over time by resorption of old bone trabeculae and formation of new bone, a process known as creeping substitution.

Autograft bone possesses all of the four unique properties lasted above. Processed allograft bone only possesses the property of osteconduction. This explains why autograft heals and incorporates faster than allograft bone. From a clinical point of view, bone graft success of a bone graft is defined as the point in time when the host-graft interface unites and the graft-host bone construct tolerates physiologic weight bearing without fracture or pain [1]. Clinical success will vary depending on the type of bone graft procedure. In cancellous grafting to a defect in spongious bone, the graft needs to be remodeled and incorporated before the construct can sustain physiologic loads. In cases in which a massive cortical graft has to join to host bone for a successful clinical result, it does not have to and will not incorporate or remodel completely. Despite this lack of biologic incorporation an allograft construct can be a clinical success when united and supported by internal fixation. Complete incorporation may mask success from a biological view point; however, it may not be necessary for clinical function [1].

## *Autogenous Bone Graft*

Healing and incorporation of autogenous grafts is an orderly sequential process whose histologic sequence is similar to that seen in fracture healing. The early phase after transplantation is predominated by inflammation. Surface osteoblasts and osteocytes from the graft survive and are capable of producing early new bone [27]. During this early phase, vascular invasion from the host bed occurs. Along with these new blood vessels come pluripotential mesenchymal cells that can differentiate into osteoblasts through the mechanism known as osteoinduction. These newly-formed osteoblasts will secrete seams of osteoid around the central core of necrotic bone [1]. Both the donor and the recipient contribute osteogenic cells. The early phase following transplantation is similar for cancellous and cortical autografts. The late phase after autogenous bone grafting differs significantly between cancellous and cortical bone. In cancellous grafting bone formation occurs concomitantly with bone resorption. Osteoblasts secrete seams of osteoid on the surface of the necrotic bone while the osteoclasts gradually resorb the dead trabeculae. This process, known as creeping substitution, characterises the late phase of autogenous cancellous bone grafting. This remodeling phase eventually results in complete replacement of the graft by host bone and marrow. In cortical grafting, bone formation occurs only after complete resorption of dead lamellar bone. Thus, haversians systems have to be gradually broken down by osteoclasts before any bone formation can occur. This is a very slow process and is reflected in the slow revascularisation. Unlike cancellous grafts, resorption predominates for long periods of time in cortical grafts. Widespread graft resorption can be seen as early as 2 weeks after transplantation and can last for many months or years [28] with the consequence that the cortical graft will be weaker than normal bone. Another major difference between cancellous and cortical autografts is that the cancellous grafts are completely remodeled and replaced by host bone, whereas cortical grafts are never completely remodeled and will always be a combination of necrotic and live bone. Autograft taken from the femoral head have been frequently used for reconstructing the acetabular medial wall in acetabular protrusio (Fig. 4.1) and for acetabular roof in severe developmental dysplasia of the hip (Fig. 4.2).

Awareness of the biology of autogenous bone grafts is important to understanding events related to healing and incorporation of allograft bone. Although autogenous bone grafts possess all the unique features required for successful healing and incorporation, they are limitations to their derived from the lack of suitable quantity and donor site morbidity. These difficulties have lead to the increasing clinical use of allograft bone.

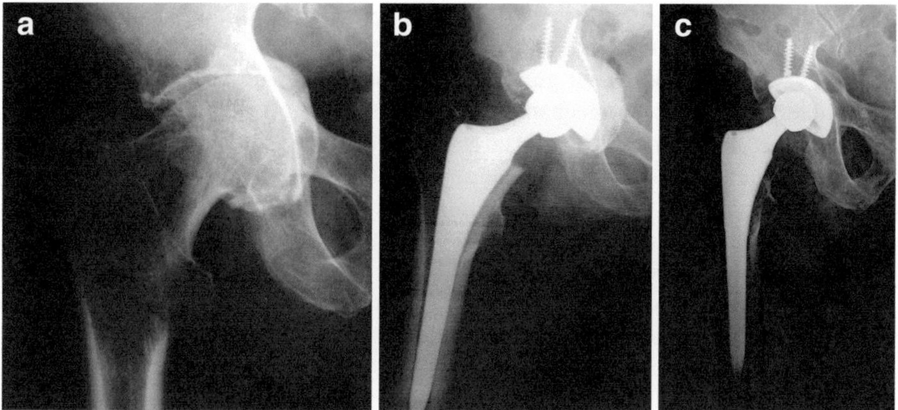

**Fig. 4.1** (**a**) Anteroposterior radiograph of a hip shows acetabular protrusio. (**b**) Postoperative radiograph, a cancellous autograft taken from the femoral head was used to reconstruct the acetabular protrusio. (**c**) Postoperative radiograph at 10 years shows good trabecular remodelling of the autograft

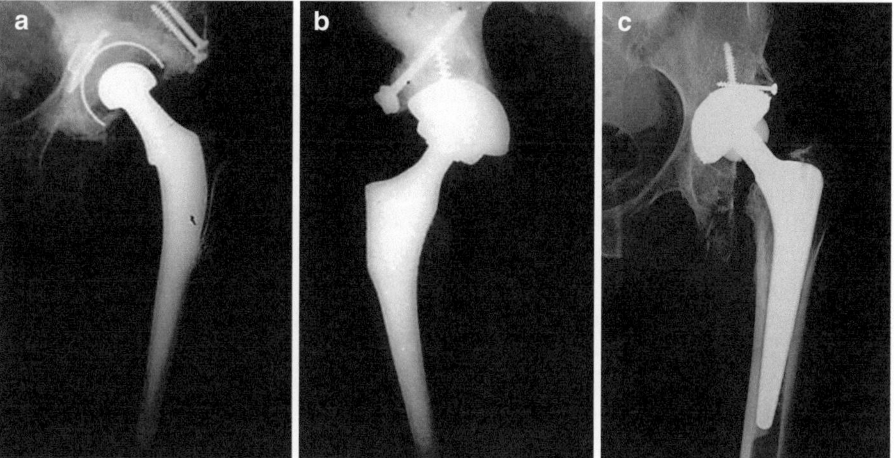

**Fig. 4.2** (**a**–**c**) Radiographs show structural autograft taken from the femoral head to reconstruct the acetabular roof in developmental dysplasia of the hip in cemented and cementless total hip arthroplasties. We can see good trabecular remodelling in all hips

## *Allograft Bone Graft*

Allograft bone is an attractive alternative to autogenous bone. Its advantages are that it is available in unlimited quantities and various shapes that can be tailored to the defect encountered at surgery and it avoids donor site morbidity. These characteristics make it a very useful alternative in revision surgery with severe bone defects. The biology of allograft bone healing and incorporation is very similar to the biology of autografts with the main difference being the lack of donor cells that can contribute to healing. One of the problems with allograft is the low level of osteoprogenitor cells but the use of growth factors, scaffolds, mesenchymal stem cells, and achieving proper biomechanics are known to promote bone healing [21]. However, the incorporation of cancellous bone and the healing (union) of cortical allografts is generally slower than that of equivalent autograft [1].

Understanding the biology of allograft incorporation and the mechanisms that can alter the biology is critical to the successful application of allografts in revision surgery. Bone loss in revision surgery can be cavitary or segmental [29, 30], and the process of allograft incorporation will vary with the clinical situation in which it is used. The most critical factor in allograft incorporation is the recipient host bed. Morselised allograft has been successfully used as a filler in acetabular revision surgery where there is a cavitary defect [8, 10]. From a biological point of view this is the ideal environment-consisting of a well-vascularised bed. This recipient bed results in incorporation of the allograft through a combination of revascularisation, osteoconduction, and remodeling. The contrasting situation is one in which a segmental allograft must be used to replace a segmental bone loss. In this situation the junction between graft and host is cortex to cortex, although most of the allograft is in contact with soft tissue. The allograft can unite to the host in these circumstances but there will be very limited internal remodeling of the allograft [28].

Allograft incorporation has been studied extensively in animals to help us understand the biology of allografting. Fresh allografts are rejected by the host immune system. The initial response in fresh allografts is inflammation followed by complete graft resorption or marked delay in graft incorporation [1]. Because of the immune response to fresh allografts, bone allografts for use in clinical surgery are processed. The most common methods of processing are freezing or freeze-drying. These techniques allow the long-term preservation of the graft. Bone frozen at −70 °C has a shelf life of 5 years. These techniques have been shown to decrease or eliminate the immunogeneity of the bone allografts although it does decease graft biological activity by removing all live cells.

Allograft in the form of morselised chips to fill cavitary defects in revision surgery has had good clinical results [2] (Fig. 4.3). These grafts biologically lack osteogenesis but they do possess osteoconductive properties and remodel like cancellous autografts, although at a slower rate. Despite their slower incorporation, cancellous allografts are widely accepted as a reconstructive alternative in cavitary well-vascularised host defects [2, 8–10, 31, 32]. Sclerotic bone is frequently observed on the acetabulum. This condition will affect the osteogenia and osteoinductive properties, but it will still usually have more preserved cells and growth factors than femoral bone. The fact that the pelvis is mostly made up of cancellous bone with bone marrow and blood together with the morphology of the acetabular bone defects (often cavitary and suitable for containing bone grafts), have contributed to the use of bone allograft on the acetabular side [33] (Fig. 4.4).

The use of structural allografts in revision surgery is controversial with contradictory reports of long-term results. Complications such as infection, nonunion, and fracture have been reported in approximately 30% of cases [7]. Structural grafts can

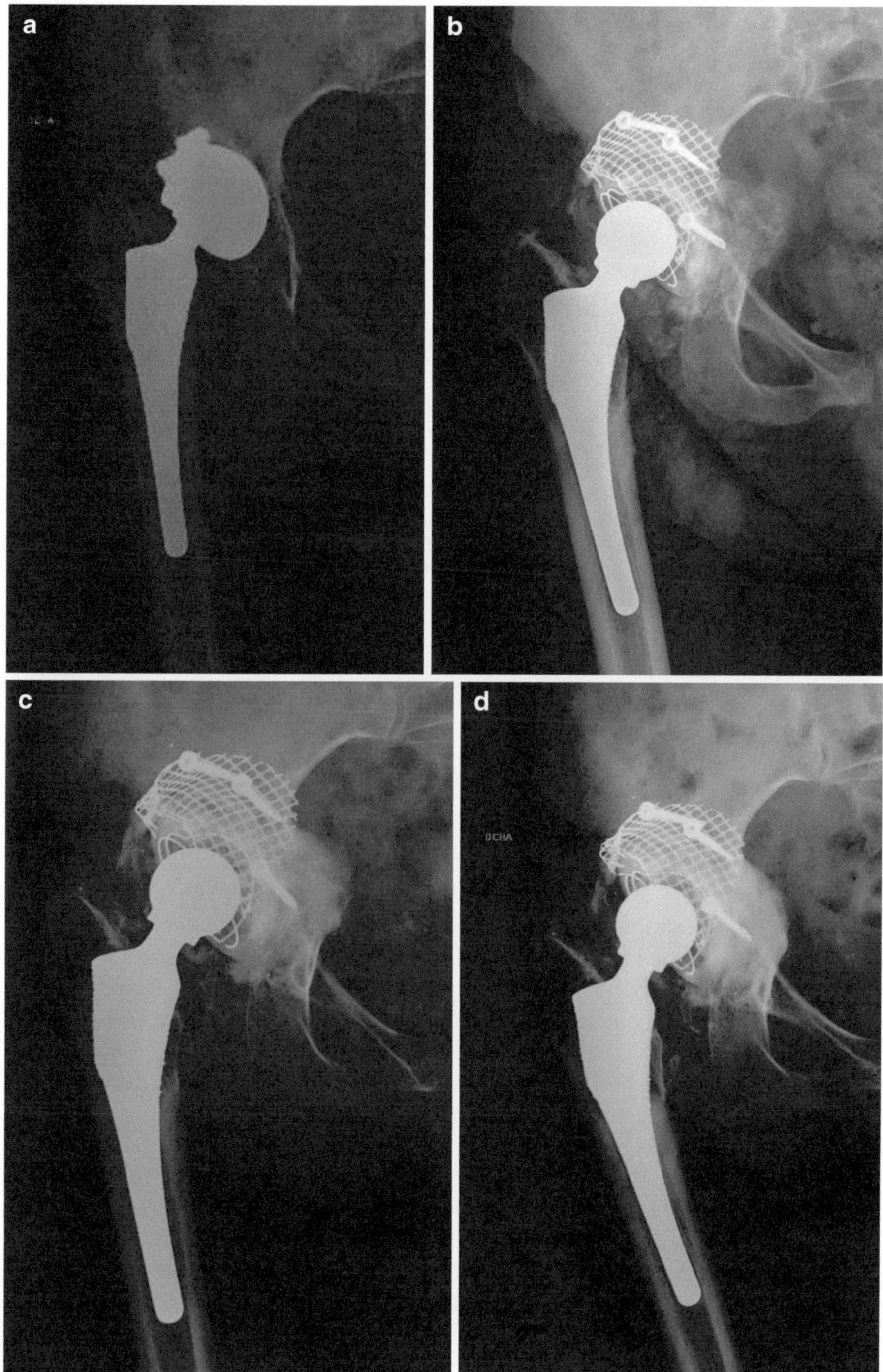


**Fig. 4.3** (**a**) Anteroposterior radiograph of a hip shows a cementless loosened cup. (**b**) Postoperative radiograph 3 months after impacting allograft bone grafting with a cemented cup used in revision surgery. (**c**) Radiograph 6 months post-surgery. (**c**) Radiograph 1 year post-surgery. (**d**) Radiograph at 5 years post surgery. Observe the progression of allograft remodelling

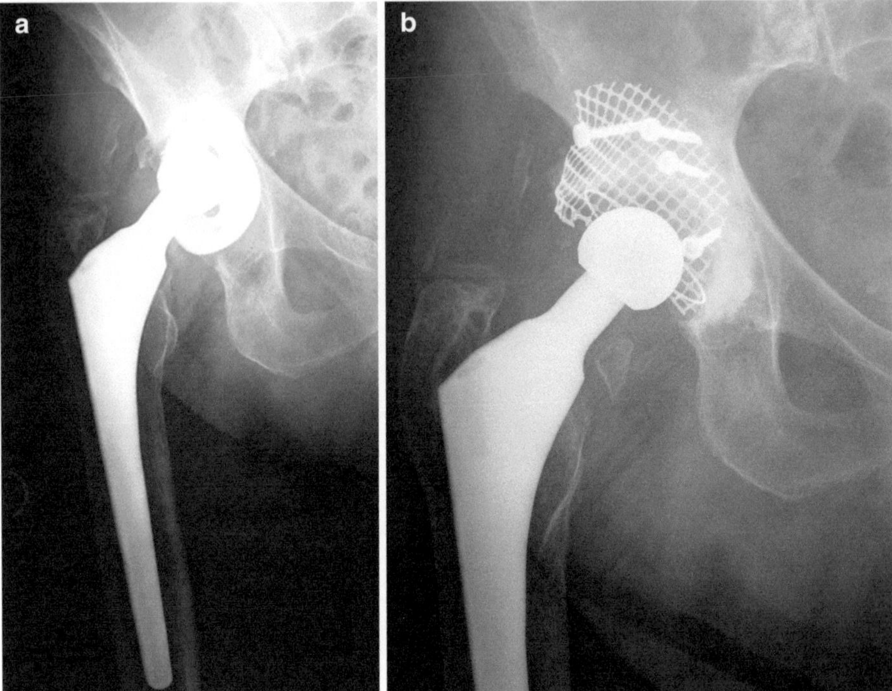


**Fig. 4.4** (**a**) Anteroposterior radiograph of a hip shows a cementless loosened cup. (**b**) Postoperative radiograph 10 years after impacting allograft bone grafting with a cemented cup in a revision surgery

be cortical, as in proximal femoral replacement, or cortico-cancellous as in acetabular reconstruction. These structural allografts have limited biologic activity. The first step in the healing of structural allografts is the inflammatory response. This response brings in the pluripotential cells required for new bone formation. In most cases union will then occur at the allograft host junction (Fig. 4.5). The success of union is highly dependent on the host. Revascularisation, creeping substitution and remodeling occur to a very limited degree in processed allografts [33]. Many factors have been implicated as having an effect on structural allograft incorporation, including immune response, mechanical response, and graft host stability [1]. Despite these multiple confounding factors, experiments that have controlled for them [34] have shown that processed structural allograft bone unites to the host but lacks the ability to remodel, and the arthroplasty relies on internal fixation devices for clinical function.

Although controlled animal experiments have provided insight into the basic science of allograft incorporation, ultimately the clinical fate and the biologic response to these allografts in humans are what matters. Human retrieval studies [28, 35, 36] have provided great insights into the biological behavior of frozen allografts in humans. Enneking et al. [28] found that union in massive allografts occurs at the

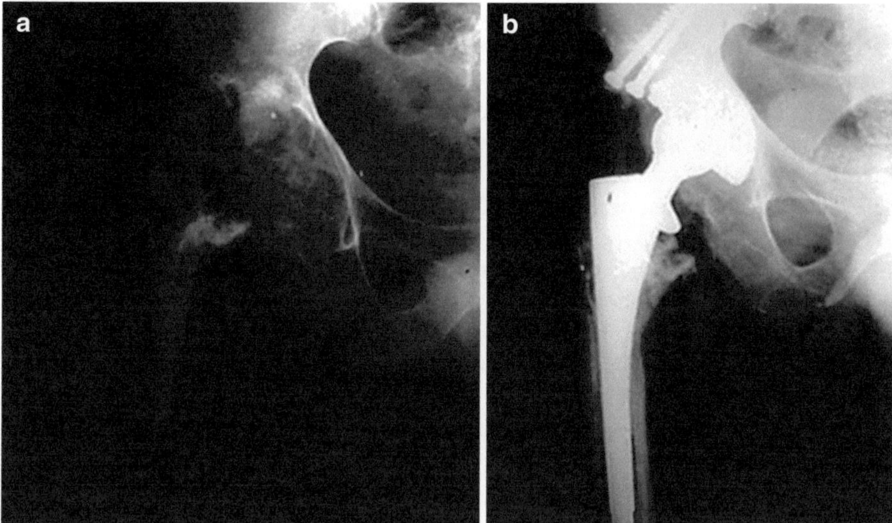


**Fig. 4.5** (**a**) preoperative radiograph of a hip shows a resection-arthroplasty. (**b**) Radiographs show structural allograft taken from the femoral head to reconstruct the acetabular roof. The bone allograft provided mechanical support for the skeleton with a good clinical outcome

host graft junction slowly at cortical junctions, by formation of external callus from the host. In addition, they found that internal repair (remodeling) took place on the superficial ends of the graft and involved less than 20% of the graft. An important clinical finding was that soft tissues become firmly attached to the graft by a seam of new bone. Human retrieval has confirmed previous results in animal experiments. Frozen structural allografts are biologically inert and only possess the osteoconductive property of bone grafts, and therefore function as implants. This has important biological and biomechanic consequences.

In terms of structural function, acellular dead allograft supported by internal fixation is biomechanically as strong as live bone because it is the mineralised bone matrix of bone that serves this structural function. Therefore, once union occurs at the graft-host junction, an allograft prosthesis composite, such as would be used in the reconstruction of a massive proximal femoral deficiency, can be considered a clinical success. Achieving union can be difficult because allograft is only osteoconductive. To improve union rates, autograft should be placed at the graft-host junction because autograft possesses cells capable of osteogenesis and proteins capable of osteoinduction.

Once union has been achieved at the graft-host junction, allograft composites can continue to function well clinically in spite of the fact that they are incapable of remodeling. This lack of remodeling ability has important clinical implications in terms of the methods to fix allograft to host bone. It is also this remodeling ability that may be responsable for the fractures seen in these large weight-bearing allografts. It has been shown that holes in allografts and the use of plates lead to an increased fracture risk fractures that are a common and serious complications in allograft. Being biologically inert allograft is also susceptible to fatigue fracture.

Regarding the increasingly-used impacting bone grafting technique, the main question regarding the biology of impacting grafting is whether cancellous allograft incorporates when combined with cement. Clinical studies on impacting bone grafting on both the femoral and acetabular sides have been encouraging [2, 8, 37]. Radiographic follow-up indicates that the impacted allograft does incorporate [37]. In biopsies of cases that have previously undergone impacting bone grafting, allograft incorporation was seen on histology in all patients. The grafts were revascularised, remodeled, and had experienced creeping substitution [38, 39]. Because these were limited biopsies, we do not know whether incorporation was complete. Animal experiments support the fact that allograft that has been impact-grafted does at least partially incorporate [40]. Schreurs et al. using goats, found partial graft incorporation very similar to when morselized allograft is used in cavitary defects without cement [41]. In a vitro study, Board et al. [42] report that strain, as from vigorous graft impaction and postoperative loading, can transform bone allograft from osteoconductive to osteoinductive, since BMP-7 was found to be released from the graft in proportion to the strain imposed on it. Clinical studies using positron emission tomography (PET) to evaluate the spatial and temporal development of bone formation after acetabular revision surgery report that the impacted bone allograft had transformed to living bone [43]. It seems that cement does not interfere with the incorporation process.

Complete allograft incorporation may not be the goal in all clinical situations. Clinical success ultimately depends on the bone graft providing mechanical support for the skeleton.

## *Immunology of Allografting*

Fresh allografts will provoke an immune response in the host that can result in graft resorption or a marked delay in graft incorporation. For this reason techniques were developed to decrease the immunogenicity of transplanted allograft bone. The most common clinical techniques used today are deep-freezing and freeze-drying. These methods allow for long-term preservation and storage of allograft bone. Originally these techniques were also shown to eliminate the host immune response. It was clear that because these preserved allografts had no living cells they would not elicit a strong alloreactive immune response when transplanted. With the advent of modern immunologic assay techniques it became apparent that fresh and processed allograft bone can invoke immune responses. Although processed allograft bone can elicit ahost immune response, the exact role of immunology in the biological incorporation is unclear [1].

The evidence from experimental studies indicates that processed allograft bone is definitely immunogenic. However, the role of this immune response in the fate of allograft bone incorporation is not clearly defined. The immune response seems to delay revascularization and incorporation but whether this mechanism actually plays a role in humans has not yet been examined.

## Bone Extenders and Enhancers

Different materials have been used to enhance graft incorporation, including bioceramics, DBM or mesenchymal cells.

So-called bioactive bioceramics can act as a scaffold for bone regeneration. These bioinert biomaterials are osteoconductive, and may have some osteoinductive properties in certain environments [44]. The use of different mostly synthetic composites of biphasic calcium phosphates (BCP) or hydroxyapatite (HA as powder, granules, pellets or cement)mixed with bone allograft has been assessed in acetabular revision surgery. Different authors report good clinical results using both cemented or cementless cups [45, 46].

Used as a demineralised freez-dried allograft, the DBM has some properties such as inducing growth factor release, which may it to act as a osteoinductive substitute. When mixed with bone allograft, DBM can serve for bone reconstruction in the acetabulum [47].

For their part, mesenchymal stem cells are probably the best osteogenic progenitors given their potential capacity to differentiate into osteoblasts. Harvested from crest iliac bone and centrifugated, afterwards, good clinical data have been reported when mixing with structural frozen-irradiated allograft in severe bone defects [48].

## References

1. Garbuz DS, Masri BA, Czitrom AA. Biology of allografting. Orthop Clin North Am. 1998;28(2):199–204.
2. Schmitz MWJL, Hannink G, Gardeniers JWM, Verdonschot N, Slooff TJJH, Schreurs BW. Acetabular reconstruction with impaction bone-greafting and a cemented cup in patients younger than 50 years of age. A concise follo-up, at 27 to 35 years, of a previous report. J Bone Joint Surg Am. 2017;99(19):1440–6.
3. Garbuz D, Morsi E, Gross AE. Revision of the acetabular component of a total hip arthroplasty with a massive structural allograft. J Bone Joint Surg Am. 1996;78-A:693–7.
4. Paprosky WC, Perona PG, Lawrence JM. Acetabular defect classification and surgical reconstruction in revision arthroplasty. A 6-year follow-up evaluation. J Arthroplasty. 1994;9(1):33–44.
5. Kwong LM, Jasty M, Harris WH. High failure rate of bulk femoral head allografts in total hip acetabular reconstructions at 10 years. J Arthroplasty. 1993;8:341–6.
6. Berrey BH Jr, Lord CF, Gebhardt MC. MankinHJ. Fractures of allografts. Frequency, treatment and results. J Bone Joint Surg Am. 1990;72(6):825–33.
7. Lord CF, Gebhardt MC, Tomford WW, Mankin HJ. Infection of bone allografts: Incidence, nature and treatment. J Bone Joint Surg Am. 1988;70(3):369–76.

8. Schreurs BW, Keurentjes JC, Gardeniers JW, Verdonschot N, Slooff TJ, Veth RP. Acetabular revision with impacted morsellised cancellous bone grafting and a cemented acetabular component: a 20- to 25-year follow-up. J Bone Joint Surg (Br). 2009;91(9):1148–53.
9. Buttaro MA, Comba F, Pusso R, Piccaluga F. Acetabular revision with metal mesh, impaction bone grafting, and a cemented cup. Clin Orthop Relat Res. 2008;466(10):2482–90.
10. Garcia-Cimbrelo E, Cruz-Pardos A, Garcia-Rey E, Ortega CJ. The survival and fate of acetabular reconstruction with impaction grafting for large defects. Clin Orthop Relat Res. 2010;468(12):3304–13.
11. Phillips AM. Overview of the fracture healing cascade. Injury. 2005;36(Suppl 3):S5–7.
12. Einhorn TA, Majeska RJ, Rush EB, Levine PM, Horowitz MC. The expression of cytokine activity by fracture callus. J Bone Miner Res. 1995;10(8):1272–81.
13. Gerstenfeld LC, Cho TJ, Kon T, Aizawa T, Tsay A, Fitch J, Barnes GL, Graves DT, Einhorn TA. Impaired fracture healing in the absence of TNF-alpha signaling: the role of TNF-alpha in endochondral cartilage resorption. J Bone Miner Res. 2003;18(9):1584–92.
14. Tsiridis E, Upadhyay N, Giannoudis P. Molecular aspects of fracture healing: which are the important molecules? Injury. 2007;38(Suppl 1):S11–25.
15. Gerstenfeld LC, Cullinane DM, Barnes GL, Graves DT, Einhorn TA. Fracture healing as a post-natal developmental process: molecular, spatial, and temporal aspects of its regulation. J Cell Biochem. 2003;88(5):873–84.
16. Deckers MM, van Bezooijen RL, van der Horst G, Hoogendam J, van Der Bent C, Papapoulos SE, et al. Bone morphogenetic proteins stimulate angiogenesis through osteoblast-derived vascular endothelial growth factor A. Endocrinology. 2002;143(4):1545–53.
17. Onichtchouk D, Chen YG, Dosch R, Gawantka V, Delius H, Massagué J, Niehrs C. Silencing of TGF-beta signalling by the pseudoreceptor BAMBI. Nature. 1999;401(6752):480–5.
18. Nakao A, Afrakhte M, Morén A, Nakayama T, Christian JL, Heuchel R, Itoh S, Kawabata M, Heldin NE, Heldin CH, ten Dijke P. Identification of Smad7, a TGFbeta-inducible antagonist of TGF-beta signalling. Nature. 1997;389(6651):631–5.
19. Bai S, Shi X, Yang X, Cao X. Smad6 as a transcriptional corepressor. J Biol Chem. 2000;275(12):8267–70.
20. Carter DR, Beaupre GS, Giori NJ, Helms JA. Mechanobiology of skeletal regeneration. Clin Orthop Relat Res. 1998;355:S41–55.
21. Giannoudis PV, Einhorn TA, Marsh D. Fracture healing: the diamond concept. Injury. 2007;38(Suppl 4):S3–6.
22. Zhuang H, Wang W, Tahernia AD, Levitz CL, Luchetti WT, Brighton CT. Mechanical strain-induced proliferation of osteoblastic cells parallels increased TGF-beta 1 mRNA. Biochem Biophys Res Commun. 1996;229(2):449–53.
23. Chiquet M. Regulation of extracellular matrix gene expression by mechanical stress. Matrix Biol. 1999;18(5):417–26.
24. Kershaw CJ, Cunningham JL, Kenwright J. Tibial external fixation, weight bearing, and fracture movement. Clin Orthop Relat Res. 1993;293:28–36.
25. Kwong FN, Harris MB. Recent developments in the biology of fracture repair. J Am Acad Orthop Surg. 2008;16(11):619–25.
26. Reddi AH, Wientroub S, Muthukumaran. Biologic principles of bone induction. Orthop Clin North Am. 1987;18:207–12.
27. Chalmers J. Transplantation immunity in bone homografting. J Bone Joint Surg (Br). 1959;41:160–78.
28. D'Antonio JA, Capello WN, Borden LS, Bargar WL, Bierbaum BF, Boettcher WG, Steinberg ME, Stulberg SH, Wedge JH. Classification and management of acetabular abnormalities in total hip arthroplasty. Clin Orthop Relat Res. 1989;243:126–37.
29. Gross AE, Duncan CP, Garbuz D, Mohamed EMZ. Revision arthroplasty of the acetabulum in association with loss of bone stock. J Bone Joint Surg Am. 1998;80(3):440–51.
30. Enneking WF, Mindell E. Observations on massive retrieved human allografts. J Bone Joint Surg Am. 1991;73:1123–42.

31. Waddell BS, Boettner F, Gonzalez Della Valle A. Favorable early results of impaction bone grafting with reinforcement mesh for the treatment of Paprosky 3B acetabular defects. J Arthroplasty. 2017;32:919–23.
32. Colo E, Rijnen WHC, Schreurs BW. The biological approach in acetabular revision surgery: impaction bone grafting and a cemented cup. Hip Int. 2015;25(4):361–7.
33. Pierannunzii L, Zagra L. Bone grafts, bone graft extenders, substitutes and enhancers for acetabular reconstruction revision total hip arthroplasty. EFORT Open Rev. 2017;1(12):431–9.
34. Stevenson S, Li XQ, Martin B. The fate of cancellous and corticl bone after transplantation of fresh and frozen tissue-antigen-matched and mismatched osteocondral allograft in dogs. J Bone Joint Surg Am. 1991;73:1143–56.
35. Hooten JP Jr, Engh CA Jr, Engh CA. Failure of structural acetabular allografts in cementless revision hip arthroplasty. J Bone Joint Surg (Br). 1994;76(3):419–22.
36. Heekin RD, Engh CA, Vinh T. Morselized allograft in acetabular reconstruction. A postmortem retrieval analysis. Clin Orthop Relat Res. 1995;319:184–90.
37. Gie GA, Linder L, Ling RSM, Simon J-P, Slooff TJJH, Timperley AJ. Impacted cancellous allografts and cement for revision total hip arthroplasty. J Bone Joint Surg (Br). 1993;75:14–21.
38. Buma P, Lamerigts N, Schreurs BW, Gardeniers J, Versleyen D, Slooff TJ. Impacted graft incorporation after cemented acetabular revision. Histological evaluation in 8 patients. Acta Orthop Scand. 1996;67(6):536–40.
39. Schimmel JW, Buma P, Versleyen D, Huiskes R, Slooff TJ. Acetabular reconstruction with impacted morselized cancellous allografts in cemented hip arthroplasty: a histological and biomechanical study on the goat. J Arthroplasty. 1998;13(4):438–48.
40. van der Donk S, Buma P, Slooff TJ, Gardeniers JW, Schreurs BW. Incorporation of morselized bone grafts: a study of 24 acetabular biopsy specimens. Clin Orthop Relat Res. 2002;396:131–41.
41. Schreurs BW, Buma P, Huiskes R, Slagter JL, Slooff TJ. Morselized allografts for fixation of the hip prosthesis femoral component: a mechanical and histological study in the goat. Acta Orthop Scand. 1994;65:267–75.
42. Board TN, Rooney P, Kay PR. Strain imparted during impaction grafting may contribute to bony incorporation; An in vitro study of the release of BMP-7 from allograft. J Bone Joint Surg (Br). 2008;90:821–4.
43. Ullmark G, Sörensen J, Nilsson O. Bone healing of severe acetabular defects after revision arthroplasty. A clinical positron emission tomography study of 7 cases. Acta Orthop. 2009;80:179–83.
44. Le Nihouannen D, Daculsi G, Saffarzadeh A, Gauthier O, Delplace S, Pilet P, Layrolle P. Ectopic bone formation by microporous calcium phosphate ceramic particles in sheep muscles. Bone. 2005;36:1086–93.
45. Bolder SB, Verdonschot N, Schreurs BW, Buma P. The initial stability of cemented acetabular cups can be augmented by mixing morsellized bone grafts with tricalciumphosphate/hydroxyapatite particles in bone impaction grafting. J Arthroplasty. 2003;18(8):1056–63.
46. Whitehouse MR, Dacombe PJ, Webb JC, Blom AW. Impaction grafting of the acetabulum with ceramic bone graft substitute mixed with femoral head allograft: high survivorship in 43 patients with a median follow-up of 7 years: a follow-up report. Acta Orthop. 2013;84:365–70.
47. Hamadouche M, Karoubi M, Dumaine V, Courpied JP. The use of fibrebased demineralised bone matrix in major acetabular reconstruction: surgical technique and preliminary results. Int Orthop. 2011;35:283–8.
48. Hernigou P, Pariat J, Queinnec S, Homma Y, Flouzat Lachaniette CH, Chevallier N, Rouard H. Supercharging irradiated allografts with mesenchymal stem cells improves acetabular bone grafting in revision arthroplasty. Int Orthop. 2014;38:1913–21.

# Chapter 5
# Acetabular Revision with Impaction Bone Grafting

**Berend Willem Schreurs and Wim Rijnen**

## Introduction

Impaction bone grafting was started at end of the 1970s by Tom Slooff at the Radboud University Medical Centre in Nijmegen [1]. He started this technique by modifying bone reconstruction methods that were introduced by Hastings and Parker [2] and McCollum et al. [3] (1980) in acetabular protrusion. He started to use the technique in primary total hips with acetabular protrusion and in revision hip surgery in patients with contained bone defects [1]. The difference with the previous described techniques was that he used larger bone chips produced by hand with a rongeur and that he impacted the bone grafts using a metal hammer and the trial cup as impactor. He used the technique only in combination with a cemented cup, at that time the Mueller 32 mm cup. Initially, all patients had a long time recovery period with 6 weeks bed rest. After the initial favourable results, the technique was extended to more complex primaries like reconstructions in developmental dysplasia of the hip (DDH) and more demanding revisions. For medial wall defects he used metal titanium perforated meshes to strengthen the medial wall to prevent a blowout during impaction. At that time there was a lot of concerns about this new technique and suggestions were made that too much contact between the reconstructed bone layer and bone cement would harm the incorporation of the bone graft [4]. By using the same metal meshes as he used for reconstructing of the medial wall mesh directly on top of these reconstruction, he was able to limit the bone cement contact. However, in retrospect the suggestion that bone cement would hamper bone incorporation was wrong, as was shown in many experiments. About 10 years after the start of this technique at our institution, we quit stopping these meshes on top of the

B. W. Schreurs (✉) · W. Rijnen
Radboud university medical center, Nijmegen, The Netherlands
e-mail: wim.schreurs@radboudumc.nl



E. García-Rey, E. García-Cimbrelo (eds.), *Acetabular Revision Surgery in Major Bone Defects*, https://doi.org/10.1007/978-3-319-98596-1_5

bone graft. Also during the years we learned that early mobilisation of the patients was possible after these reconstructions, and we followed the trend to start early mobilisation after revision.

After our initial experience we started many experiments to underpin the science around this technique. We performed mechanical experiments in vitro using human cadaveric pelvic bone as well as an artificial developed acetabular model to study the mechanical effects of bone impaction grafting [5]. We found that after a technically proper impaction using a metal hammer and a metal impactor, and after pressurizing of the cement on top of these reconstructions a very nice cement bone graft interface was obtained, and that the cement did only slightly protrude into the impacted bone reconstruction. We also found out that it is important to use larger bone chips to obtain a better stability. For acetabular impaction bone grafting bone chips with a diameter of 8–12 mm seems to be the most attractive [5]. There have been studies from other centres suggesting that mixes of larger and smaller bone chips are also attractive [6]. However, there is certainly agreement that small sized bone chips (2–4 mm) are not attractive, as they will lead to more migration and less cup stability. We also learned that washing of the bone grafts may be attractive and hence reducing the fat in the bone chips is also attractive to improve cup stability [7], as was earlier confirmed by Dunlop et al. [6]. However, all our long-term clinical data are based on non-washed bone chips. We also performed animal experiments in goats use bone chambers to investigate the incorporation process of the bone graft [8]. In other animal experiments in goats, we did realistic hip surgery implanting cemented total hips in combination with acetabular bone impaction grafting [9]. These experiments showed that the impacted bone grafts do effectively incorporate. This was confirmed in human biopsy data and retrievals [10]. In our center we published two papers studying bone biopsies taken during re-opertions after previous reconstructions with bone impaction grafting [10]. Overall, the bone chips were nicely incorporated with few remnants of the original bone chips. There was also a retrieval study by Heekin [11] that showed that these bone chips really incorporate into normal bone.

## Indications and Guidelines for Use

Acetabular bone impaction grafting can be considered in all cases with acetabular bone stock loss in revision hip surgery. However, infection should be ruled out before the reconstruction is performed. In septic loosening, we advise two stage surgery if acetabular bone impaction grafting is considered. There is some information about using this technique also in one stage revisions in infective cases, however this is scientifically not sufficiently underpinned yet. There is a tendency to start using bone impaction grafting in the more extensive defects, when the surgeons primary choice of revision technique is not suitable anymore. This is a potential drawback for the technique of impaction bone grafting. Like in all techniques, it is important to start the experience with a technique in the less demanding and hence forgiving cases. Once familiar with a technique one can start to use it in the more demanding cases. This is of course the same with impaction bone grafting. And as with all other techniques, the outcome in the more extensive defects is less favourable. However, this bone reconstruction technique is one of the few techniques that can make a future revision, despite a failure, less demanding as more bone can be present at the re-revision.

## Technique

The posterolateral approach is our favourable exposure, because of the excellent view on the acetabulum. This exposure also facilitates the insertion of a superolateral mesh. Especially the fixation of these meshes on the posterior wall is difficult when using other approaches. If only a medial wall mesh is needed, other surgical approaches can certainly be considered. Identifying the major landmarks is helpful for orientation purposes because in many cases the anatomy is disturbed extensively by the loosening process itself or by methods to remove the cup. The important landmarks guiding the reconstruction are the tip of the greater trochanter, the tendinous part of the gluteus maximus, the lower border of the gluteus medius and minimus, the transverse ligament and the tuber ischiadicum, if needed. Be aware of the position of the sciatic nerve, although exposure of this structure is not advised. After exposure of the joint, three biopsies of the capsule are taken for cultures. Three other biopsies are taken of the interface behind the cup or of the femur.

Releasing the gluteus maximus tendon on the femoral side can be helpful to mobilize the femur anteriorly. A circumferential exposure of the entire acetabulum is achieved by removing all scar tissue anterior, superior and posterior at the acetabular rim, and perform a circumferential capsulotomy and or even capsulectomy. Sometimes a release of the tendinous part of the iliopsoas attachment is helpful for exposure, however one should consider that this will hamper the future activity level of the patient. In case of a noncemented cup in most cases a modern device that facilitates explantation is helpful using curved chisel mounted on a head that is central in the inner diameter of the cup. In cases of a still well fixed cemented cup the technique of reaming out the polyethylene cup using acetabulum reamers and subsequently splitting the cement with osteotomes is a technique that will prevent unnecessary bone stock loss. After removing the component, and is applicable the cement, the fibrous interface is removed completely from the irregular acetabular wall using sharp spoons and curettes. Care is taken to locate and trim the transverse ligament at the inferior part of the acetabulum. The acetabular walls are reconstructed from this level upwards. After taking of the biopsy samples, systemic antibiotic therapy is started although some evidence suggests that a shot of antibiotics at the beginning of the procedure will not hamper the outcome of the cultures and may prevent superimposed infections from the revision procedure itself.

The acetabular floor and walls are examined meticulously for any segmental defects. Often these defects can only be detected by manual examination of the walls. Check carefully is there is a dissociation of the pelvis, in these cases additional plating is necessary to prevent failure of the revised reconstruction. Meshes are not strong enough to stabilize these defects. The plates can be used on the outside of the acetabulum but also inserted on the inner side of the acetabulum, depending on the case and the preference of the surgeon. Special care is given to the transverse ligament, this is still often available at revision surgery. This ligament can be used for especially estimating the extent of the superolateral wall defect. By placing a suitable sized trial prosthesis on this ligament in the correct position, the extent of the superolateral defect can be visualized. The defects are now reconstructed using wire meshes being able to contain the bone grafts. If one want to use a reamer to optimize the bone bed for bone impacting grafting and to remove more debris, this has to be done before fixation of the meshes. If there is a medial wall defect or a weak medial wall that maybe will not resist the forces during bone impaction grafting, a medial wall mesh should be used. There are several options available that can be performed, we prefer titanium meshes. Often, these do not need any screw fixation and will snap in nicely, however screw fixation is an option. For segmental defects, using scissors and pliers, a flexible stainless steel or titanium preformed wire mesh is trimmed and adapted to fit the acetabular rim defects. The superolateral pelvic bone can be exposed by lifting up the abductors, there are no major structures that will be damaged by this exposure. The wire mesh is fixed to the remaining acetabular wall with at least three small fragment screws to ensure rigid fixation. In most cases 6 screws are used, one can use standard 3.5 mm small fragment screws or selftapping screws. Screws are placed on the most anterior and posterior positions in the mesh an on the superolateral position in the pelvis. If the posterior wall is weak or there is a significant bone defect of the posterior wall, bony support can be found by exposing the tuber ischiadicum. In these cases one can choose to support the often quite extensive mesh by a plate that is bowed flat over the mesh and extents from the tuber area to the anterior side of the acetabulum. Both pelvic reconstruction plates as well as one-third tubular plates can be used.

After closing of the defects on the rim and medial wall the acetabulum is now contained and transformed into a cavitary defect. If a sclerotic acetabular wall exists despite previous reaming, many small holes must be drilled into the sclerotic host bone to enhance surface contact and promote vascular invasion into the graft. Allograft bone chips are then ordered, some bone banks offer washed deep frozen trabecular bone chips of 8–12 mm. If not, deep-fresh-frozen femoral heads from the a bone bank are first cleaned after thawing in saline. These heads can then be divided in four parts and using rongeurs with a large beak bone chip of the suitable size can be produced by hand. Alternatively, one can use a bone mill in the operation theatre. All fibrous tissues and cartilage is removed. An option is to use a specially designed head reamer to remove the cartilage. Next, the remaining bone is divided into four equal parts. Substantial chips of at least 8–12 mm are by a specially designed Noviomagus Bone Mill (A One Medical, Oss, The Netherlands). Most commercial bone mill produce bone chips that are small (2–5 mm).

After cleaning and washing the acetabulum, any small cavity is packed tightly with chips and subsequently impacted using the small round, half moon and large round impactors. Next, the entire socket is filled, layer-by-layer with cancellous chips. Acetabular shaped large metal impactors hammer the chips in situ, starting with the smallest-possible-size impactor and ending with the largest-size-impactor suitable for a new acetabular wall of preferable at least 5 mm thick. Consequently, the whole acetabular hemisphere is covered with an impacted and stable layer of allograft chips. It is evident that after impaction this bone layer is not circumferentially equal in thickness. The thickness of the bone graft layer depends of course on the variety of depth of the acetabular defect. After impaction, the pre-existing enlarged acetabular diameter has been reduced to a normal size. Next the size of the suitable cup is planned, this planning should allow a cement mantle of 2–4 mm around the cup. While the antibiotic-loaded cement is being prepared, pressure on the graft is maintained using the last impactor. After inserting and pressurizing the cement, the cup is placed and held in position with the pusher until the cement has been polymerized. The advantage of impaction bone grafting is clearly that within certain limits the surgeon decides during surgery the size and shape of the new acetabulum and subsequently the size and position of the new implant. It is important to reconstruct the anatomy of the hip in such a way that the cup is placed at the level of the transverse ligament, the anatomical centre of rotation that guarantees the best mechanical properties.

Postoperative management includes anticoagulation therapy for 4–6 weeks using subcutaneous low molecular weight heparins, and if one prefers systemic antibiotics for 24 h. Indomethacin is administered for 7 days to prevent the development of heterotopic ossification. Mobilization of the patient is nowadays like in the primary total hip replacement, out of bed the day of surgery or the next day and walking with two crutches and but only touch weight bearing for the first 6 weeks. In the second period of 6 weeks 50% weight bearing is allowed. In smaller defects we start loading with 50% in the first 6 weeks and after 6 weeks full weight bearing. In cases of pelvic discontinuity the protocol is individualized according to the different circumstances of the revision arthroplasty. A period of two to maximum of 6 weeks bed rest is not used anymore, only after rare cases with very extensive acetabular reconstructions.

## Results

Two recent reviews of the literature on outcomes of bone impaction grafting on the acetabular side were published in 2013 and 2018 [12].

The first paper on the outcome of bone impaction grating from our institution was a mixed series of both primary and revision case and was published by Slooff et al. [1]. This was only short to medium follow-up. However, we published our long term experience in several subsequential publications focussing on a group of 62 consecutive revisions all done at our center [13, 14]. Between 1979 and 1986, four surgeons performed 62 acetabular reconstructions in 58 consecutive patients (13 men, 43 women) for the management of failed hip arthroplasty.

The indication for the revision surgery was aseptic or septic loosening in 58 hip and 4 hips respectively. The mean age of the patients at the time of the procedure was 59 years. Defects were cavitary in 39 hips and in 23 hips the defects were combined segmental cavitary according to the AAOS classification. All patients could be followed and no hip was lost to follow-up during this long term review. At the last publication in 2015 the follow-up was between 25 and 30 years, the Kaplan-Meier survivorship of the cup with the end point of revision for any reason was 52% at 25 years postoperatively (95% CI, 45–99%). Excluding two revisions that were performed for the management of septic loosening at 3 and 6 years postoperatively, survivorship with the end point of aseptic loosening was 58% at 25 years postoperatively (95% CI, 38–73%). Most hips had a stable radiologic appearance. In this last study we evaluated also the outcome of the re-revisions performed for the management of the acetabular reconstruction to prove that reconstructions with bone impaction grafting facilitates future revisions. In this part of the study we evaluated the clinical and radiographic outcomes of 11 consecutive repeat acetabular revisions in 10 patients with all repeat bone impaction grafting again and a cemented polyethylene cup. The mean follow-up was 10 years after repeat revision and 28 years after the primary revision. Data of all re-revisions were available. Using again a Kaplan-Meier survival analysis the survival with further revision of the cup for any reason as the end point was 91% (95% CI, 51–99%) at 10 years postoperatively. On the basis of the results of this study long-term follow-up, including the data of the re-revisions bone impaction grafting was considered to be a safe and adequate biological reconstruction technique of acetabular bone defects in revision surgery.

In patients with revision of the cup and diagnosis rheumatoid arthritis, the best results in the literature have been achieved using simple repeat cementation or bone impaction grafting with a cemented cup. In one of our studies, 35 consecutive acetabular revisions were performed in 28 patients with rheumatoid arthritis using acetabular bone impaction grafting and a cemented cup. At 8–19 years postoperatively, no patient was lost to follow-up, but outcomes were included for eight patients (ten hips) who died during the follow-up period. Acetabular bone stock defects were cavitary (11 hips) or combined segmental and cavitary (24 hips). At minimum 8-year follow-up, eight hips had a re-revision. With septic loosening excluded, Kaplan-Meier analysis demonstrated a survival rate with aseptic loosening as the end point of 85% (95% CI, 71–99%) at 11-year follow-up [15]. The literature on revisions with a noncemented cup in rheumatoid arthritis has been very disappointing [16]. In a recent study we showed that the bone impaction grafting techniques also works in revisions in young patients [17]. We studied the outcome of 34 hips (33 patients) who had a revision by performing both a femoral and acetabular bone impaction grafting in one revision procedure. All patients were under 55 years, the average age at surgery was 46 years. At a mean follow-up of more than 11 years, survival rate with the endpoint of re-revision for any component for any reason was 87% (95% confidence interval [CI], 67%–95%) and with the endpoint of re-revision for aseptic loosening, the survival rate was 97% (95% CI, 80%–100%). This is in striking contrast with the only study on the outcome on uncemented revisions in young patients by Gross and Lee [18] who reported only a survival of less than 70% with also a lot of patients lost to follow-up.

Several studies from other centres have confirmed the data from our original studies. Certainly in the less extensive defects results outcomes overall are very satisfying. Comba et al. [19] stated that the survival rate for the reconstruction was 95.8% (95% confidence interval 92.3–99.1) overall, and 98%, excluding revision due to sepsis. They concluded that their study from an independent center has reproduced the results of the originators of the method. Garcia-Cimbrelo and Cordero [20] concluded that the mid-term results with impacted allograft and cemented all-polyethylene cups were favourable in acetabular revision surgery. Other studies had the same conclusion, bone impaction grafting works well and most patients are satisfied, however in some cases there is radiological loosening of the cup with radiolucent lines, but patients have few complaints [21, 22].

However, the outcome in the larger defects type Paproski 3A and 3B the outcomes are less favourable and as in all techniques, the more extensive the defect the less favourable the long term outcomes. Buttaro et al. [23] stated that metal mesh, impaction grafting, and a cemented cup should be considered for reconstruction of medium uncontained acetabular defects, but not for severe combined deficiencies. Garcia-Rey et al. [24] reported in their paper the outcome of 226 of these cases with a lateral rim reconstruction with a metal mesh. In the more extensive defects at 15 years follow-up, the outcome for endpoint aseptic loosening was 80% versus an outcome of 89% in the cases with a smaller defect. However, especially the patients who had a medial wall mesh and a lateral rim mesh in their study were unsatisfying, with only a survival of just over 50% at 15 years. This was also stated in the paper of Gilbody et al. [22] that was already cited before, although the overall outcome in this large study with over 300 acetabular reconstructions was satisfying, the outcome of the Paprosky type 3 defects were less satisfying. The same experience was reported before by van Haaren et al. [25], Iwase et al. [26] and Kostensalo et al. [27] who all reported a survival in the larger IIIA en IIIB defects of around 73% at 7 years follow-up. It is important to compare these less satisfying outcome with other techniques, who also have problems in these more extensive defects. Recently, a group from the Unites States started using this technique especially in these larger defects, as this is the only option to have a biological reconstruction and they showed satisfying results, although these are short term data [28].

Certainly, it has been suggested that Paprosky grade 3 defects may be better managed with other techniques. A solution could be to combine in these defects the technique of bone impaction grafting with tantalum or titanium metal augments [29, 30]. Short term results are promising, but the effect after long term has to be studied. Also stronger or better fitting meshes could be a solution to improve the outcome in these demanding cases as was shown by Stigbrand et al. [31].

Although the technique was started in combination with cemented cups, there are now data that this technique will also work with noncemented cup implants. This is important as in revisions with noncemented cups, and especially in the younger patients, bone reconstruction is also essential. Although one of the concerns was that not using cement would lead to higher migrations and more instability a recent RSA study proved that this assumption is not correct [32]. However, a caveat can be that in this study they used smaller sized bone chips. As stated before, cup stability is better when lager chips are used from 8 to 12 mm. Palm et al. [33] already reported about the use of bone impaction grafting with a noncemented cup. The extent of the graft was not extensive in all, but even in the case with a more extensive reconstruction the outcome at 7–11 years was satisfying. There are some other reports, but more information about the combination of impaction bone grafting is needed and this can also be a potent future reconstruction option leading to reconstruction of bone.

## Conclusions and Recommendations

Bone impaction grafting is one of the few biological methods to really reconstruct the bone loss as is often seen in revision surgery. This is important, and especially in the younger patients facing a future revision. Unfortunately, we will be confronted with more revisions in younger patients [34]. The process of incorporation of impacted bone grafts has been studied both in animal experiments and in human biopsies, with nearly complete incorporation of these grafts demonstrated. Satisfactorily outcomes of acetabular bone impaction grafting for the management of cavitary and simple segmental defects in revision procedures have been reported in many studies. However, in the Paprosky type IIIA and IIIB defects there certainly is a need for improvement of the outcomes. There are some guidelines to improve the outcome. First, one should start to get familiar with bone impaction grafting in the smaller and less demanding defects before starting to reconstruct extensive defects. It is important, especially in the larger defects to use larger chips from 8 to 12 mm. There is a need to improve the quality of the meshes, certainly in the situation larger superolateral defects. The limitations of the technique are unclear about how extensive the reconstruction can be. A thickness to a maximum of 3 cm seems to be safe. However, even in the case of a failed bone impaction grafting, even in a large defect, often the next revision is more easy as there will be more bone then at the first revision.

## References

1. Slooff TJ, Huiskes R, van Horn J, Lemmens AJ. Bone grafting in total hip replacement for acetabular protrusion. Acta Orthop Scand. 1984;55(6):593–6.
2. Hastings DE, Parker SM. Protrusio acetabuli in rheumatoid arthritis. Clin Orthop Relat Res. 1975;108:76–83.
3. McCollum DE, Nunley JA, Harrelson JM. Bone-grafting in total hip replacement for acetabular protrusion. J Bone Joint Surg Am. 1980;62(7):1065–73.
4. Jones LC, Hungerford DS. Cement disease. Clin Orthop Relat Res. 1987;225:192–206.
5. Bolder SB, Schreurs BW, Verdonschot N, van Unen JM, Gardeniers JW, Slooff TJ. Particle size of bone graft and method of impaction affect initial stability of cemented cups: human cadaveric and synthetic pelvic specimen studies. Acta Orthop Scand. 2003;74(6):652–7. https://doi.org/10.1080/00016470310018144.

6. Dunlop DG, Brewster NT, Madabhushi SP, Usmani AS, Pankaj P, Howie CR. Techniques to improve the shear strength of impacted bone graft: the effect of particle size and washing of the graft. J Bone Joint Surg Am. 2003;85-A(4):639–46.
7. Arts JJ, Verdonschot N, Buma P, Schreurs BW. Larger bone graft size and washing of bone grafts prior to impaction enhances the initial stability of cemented cups: experiments using a synthetic acetabular model. Acta Orthop. 2006;77(2):227–33. https://doi.org/10.1080/17453670610045957.
8. van der Donk S, Weernink T, Buma P, Aspenberg P, Slooff TJ, Schreurs BW. Rinsing morselized allografts improves bone and tissue ingrowth. Clin Orthop Relat Res. 2003;408:302–10.
9. Schimmel JW, Buma P, Versleyen D, Huiskes R, Slooff TJ. Acetabular reconstruction with impacted morselized cancellous allografts in cemented hip arthroplasty: a histological and biomechanical study on the goat. J Arthroplast. 1998;13(4):438–48.
10. van der Donk S, Buma P, Slooff TJ, Gardeniers JW, Schreurs BW. Incorporation of morselized bone grafts: a study of 24 acetabular biopsy specimens. Clin Orthop Relat Res. 2002;396:131–41.
11. Heekin RD, Engh CA, Vinh T. Morselized allograft in acetabular reconstruction. A postmortem retrieval analysis. Clin Orthop Relat Res. 1995;319:184–90.
12. Ibrahim MS, Raja S, Haddad FS. Acetabular impaction bone grafting in total hip replacement. Bone Joint J. 2013;95-B(11 Suppl A):98–102. https://doi.org/10.1302/0301-620X.95B11.32834.
13. Schreurs BW, Slooff TJ, Buma P, Gardeniers JW, Huiskes R. Acetabular reconstruction with impacted morsellised cancellous bone graft and cement. A 10- to 15-year follow-up of 60 revision arthroplasties. J Bone Joint Surg (Br). 1998;80(3):391–5.
14. Te Stroet MA, Keurentjes JC, Rijnen WH, Gardeniers JW, Verdonschot N, Slooff TJ, Schreurs BW. Acetabular revision with impaction bone grafting and a cemented polyethylene acetabular component: comparison of the Kaplan-Meier analysis to the competing risk analysis in 62 revisions with 25 to 30 years follow-up. Bone Joint J. 2015;97-B(10):1338–44. https://doi.org/10.1302/0301-620X.97B10.34984.
15. Schreurs BW, Luttjeboer J, Thien TM, de Waal Malefijt MC, Buma P, Veth RP, Slooff TJ. Acetabular revision with impacted morselized cancellous bone graft and a cemented cup in patients with rheumatoid arthritis. A concise follow-up, at eight to nineteen years, of a previous report. J Bone Joint Surg Am. 2009;91(3):646–51. https://doi.org/10.2106/JBJS.G.01701.
16. Mont MA, Domb B, Rajadhyaksha AD, Padden DA, Jones LC, Hungerford DS. The fate of revised uncemented acetabular components in patients with rheumatoid arthritis. Clin Orthop Relat Res. 2002;400:140–8.
17. Te Stroet MA, Rijnen WH, Gardeniers JW, van Kampen A, Schreurs BW. Satisfying outcomes scores and survivorship achieved with impaction grafting for revision THA in young patients. Clin Orthop Relat Res. 2015;473(12):3867–75. https://doi.org/10.1007/s11999-015-4293-y.
18. Lee PT, Lakstein DL, Lozano B, Safir O, Backstein J, Gross AE. Mid-to long-term results of revision total hip replacement in patients aged 50 years or younger. Bone Joint J. 2014;96-B(8):1047–51. https://doi.org/10.1302/0301-620X.96B8.31587.
19. Comba F, Buttaro M, Pusso R, Piccaluga F. Acetabular reconstruction with impacted bone allografts and cemented acetabular components: a 2- to 13-year follow-up study of 142 aseptic revisions. J Bone Joint Surg (Br). 2006;88(7):865–9. https://doi.org/10.1302/0301-620X.88B7.17227.
20. Cimbrelo G, et al. The survival and fate of acetabular reconstruction with impaction grafting for large defect. CORR. 2010;468:3304-3–13.
21. Fadulelmola A, Drampalos E, Hodgkinson J, Hemmady M. Survivorship analysis of eighty revised hip arthroplasties with the impaction grafting technique using whole femoral head allografts with the articular cartilage. J Arthroplast. 2017;32(6):1970–5. https://doi.org/10.1016/j.arth.2017.01.021.
22. Gilbody J, Taylor C, Bartlett GE, Whitehouse SL, Hubble MJ, Timperley AJ, Howell JR, Wilson MJ. Clinical and radiographic outcomes of acetabular impaction grafting without cage reinforcement for revision hip replacement: a minimum ten-year follow-up study. Bone Joint J. 2014;96-B(2):188–94. https://doi.org/10.1302/0301-620X.96B2.32121.

23. Buttaro MA, Comba F, Pusso R, Piccaluga F. Acetabular revision with metal mesh, impaction bone grafting, and a cemented cup. Clin Orthop Relat Res. 2008;466(10):2482–90. https://doi.org/10.1007/s11999-008-0442-x.
24. Garcia-Rey E, Madero R, Garcia-Cimbrelo E. THA revisions using impaction allografting with mesh is durable for medial but not lateral acetabular defects. Clin Orthop Relat Res. 2015;473(12):3882–91. https://doi.org/10.1007/s11999-015-4483-7.
25. van Haaren EH, Heyligers IC, Alexander FG, Wuisman PI. High rate of failure of impaction grafting in large acetabular defects. J Bone Joint Surg (Br). 2007;89(3):296–300. https://doi.org/10.1302/0301-620X.89B3.18080.
26. Iwase T, Ito T, Morita D. Massive bone defect compromises postoperative cup survivorship of acetabular revision hip arthroplasty with impaction bone grafting. J Arthroplast. 2014;29(12):2424–9. https://doi.org/10.1016/j.arth.2014.04.001.
27. Kostensalo I, Seppanen M, Virolainen P, Mokka J, Koivisto M, Makela KT. Acetabular reconstruction with impaction bone grafting and cemented polyethylene socket in total hip revision arthroplasty. Scand J Surg. 2015;104(4):267–72. https://doi.org/10.1177/1457496914568408.
28. Waddell BS, Boettner F, Gonzalez Della Valle A. Favorable early results of impaction bone grafting with reinforcement mesh for the treatment of paprosky 3B acetabular defects. J Arthroplast. 2017;32(3):919–23. https://doi.org/10.1016/j.arth.2016.09.037.
29. Borland WS, Bhattacharya R, Holland JP, Brewster NT. Use of porous trabecular metal augments with impaction bone grafting in management of acetabular bone loss. Acta Orthop. 2012;83(4):347–52. https://doi.org/10.3109/17453674.2012.718518.
30. Gill K, Wilson MJ, Whitehouse SL, Timperley AJ. Results using Trabecular Metal augments in combination with acetabular impaction bone grafting in deficient acetabula. Hip Int. 2013;23(6):522–8. https://doi.org/10.5301/hipint.5000053.
31. Stigbrand H, Gustafsson O, Ullmark G. A 2- to 16-year clinical follow-up of revision total hip arthroplasty using a new acetabular implant combined with impacted bone allografts and a cemented cup. J Arthroplast. 2018;33(3):815–22. https://doi.org/10.1016/j.arth.2017.10.006.
32. Mohaddes M, Herberts P, Malchau H, Johanson PE, Karrholm J. High proximal migration in cemented acetabular revisions operated with bone impaction grafting; 47 revision cups followed with RSA for 17 years. Hip Int. 2017;27(3):251–8. https://doi.org/10.5301/hipint.5000452.
33. Palm L, Jacobsson SA, Kvist J, Lindholm A, Ojersjo A, Ivarsson I. Acetabular revision with extensive allograft impaction and uncemented hydroxyapatite-coated implants. Results after 9 (7-11) years follow-up. J Arthroplast. 2007;22(8):1083–91. https://doi.org/10.1016/j.arth.2006.11.021.
34. Schreurs BW, Hannink G. Total joint arthroplasty in younger patients: heading for trouble? Lancet. 2017;389(10077):1374–5. https://doi.org/10.1016/S0140-6736(17)30190-3.

# Chapter 6
# Biological Repair of Acetabular Bone Defects and Cup Migration After Impaction Bone Grafting in Total Hip Arthroplasty

**Eduardo García-Rey and Eduardo García-Cimbrelo**

## Introduction

Cup loosening produces cup migration and acetabular bone defects. To be able to support a cup, there must be sufficient medial bone stock and supportive rims in the acetabulum. Reconstruction also require appropriate reconstruction of the anatomic center of rotation of the hip.

Different techniques and prostheses can be used to overcome the defects present at revision total hip arthroplasty surgery. Nowadays, many surgeons tend to replace the bone defects with large acetabular cups and metal augment if necessary with varying results [1]. Uncemented jumbo cups are used in large defects, so as to maximise prosthesis contact with host bone by using the larger cup size. Van Roth et al. report that the survival with end point re-revision for any reason at 20 years was 83%, and using aseptic loosening as end point 88% at the same period [2]. When a defect is not restored in a biological manner, one could assume that the absence of sufficient bone stock could jeopardize further revisions. If a defect is just filled with a larger cup, without restoring the acetabular bone stock, especially in young patients, it cause serious problems when there is no bone left for proper reconstruction of the acetabulum [1].

## Impaction Bone Grafting Outcome

We must choose between using more metal to reconstruct these acetabular defects or biological reconstruction techniques that should create a stable situation with good long-term results [1] (Fig. 6.1). Different studies have evaluated the use of

E. García-Rey (✉) · E. García-Cimbrelo
Orthopaedic Surgery Department, Hospital Universitario La Paz-IdiPaz,
Madrid, Spain



E. García-Rey, E. García-Cimbrelo (eds.), *Acetabular Revision Surgery in Major Bone Defects*, https://doi.org/10.1007/978-3-319-98596-1_6

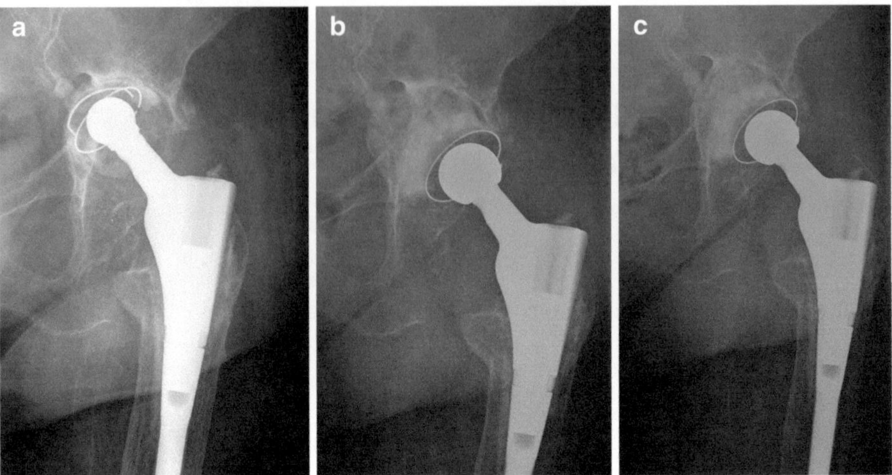


**Fig. 6.1** (**a**) Anteroposterior radiograph of hip shows a cemented loosened cup. (**b**) Postoperative radiograph 3 months after impacting allograft bone grafting with a cemented cup used in revision surgery. (**c**) Radiograph three years after operattion. We can follow remodelling of the allograft

impacting bone grafting (IBG) combined with an uncemented total hip arthroplasty (THA). Lie et al. reported inferior results in uncemented revision THA with IBG when compared with other revision techniques at a relatively short follow-up [3]. In contrast, over the past few years, advances have been made in the porous coating, and the results of uncemented cups combined with IBG have improved subsequently [4–6]. The Nijmegen group has repeatedly reported favorable long-term results using IBG with cemented cup technique [7, 8].

Different studies have shown that many of the mechanical failures in acetabular revisions occur within the first years postoperatively [9–11]. Early migration of the cup might be a risk of applying IBG, as it takes time for the bone, cement and graft to interlock and form a stable construction (Fig. 6.2). Schreurs et al. report that partial post-operative weight-bearing postoperatively after large reconstructions with IBG is important [9]. However, Ornstein et al. found no significant differences in migration of the cup between immediate full weight-bearing and partial weight-bearing [12], however in their group, only one patient had an extensive acetabular defect and all the other acetabular defects were less extensive. Overall, it is not known what the most optimal postoperative protocol should be, although histological studies show that during the first weeks and months postoperatively, the bone-graft-cement interface is remodeling and subject to many changes [13]. Especially in the large reconstructions with meshes, one can imagine that immediate full weight-bearing might increase the chances of early failure [1]. In contrast to cemented THA without IBG, patients are not allowed immediate full weight-bearing and are instructed to use some weight-bearing support [1]. During the first three post-operative months, as it takes some time for the bone graft to become stable, probably by fibrous armoring and later on incorporation [14].

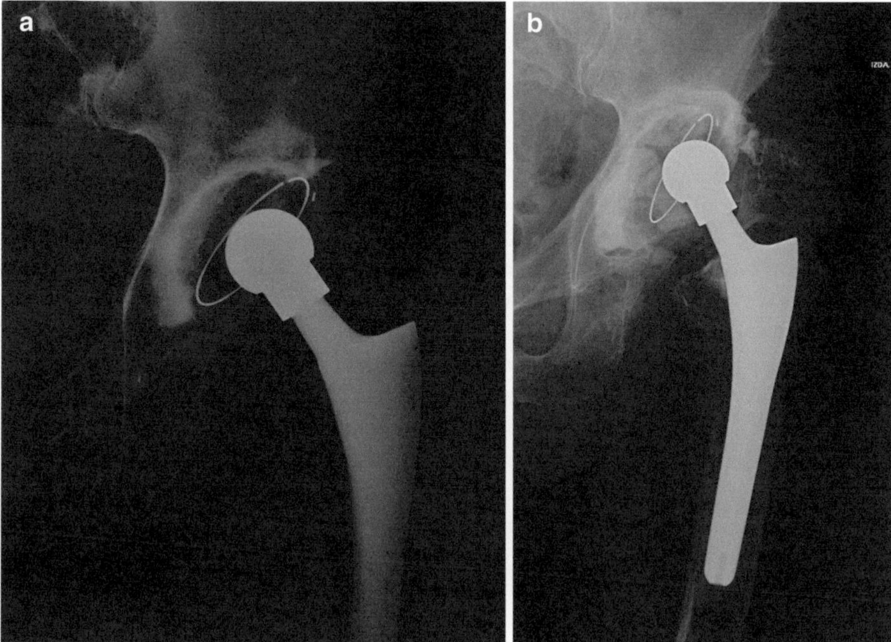

**Fig. 6.2** (**a**) Postoperative radiograph after impacting allograft bone grafting with a cemented cup used in revision surgery. (**b**) Postoperative radiographs at 10 years after operation. A cup tilt is observed but the clinical outcome is very good

Waddell et al. report their American experience after an average 47-month follow-up in 21 patients with Paprosky 3B acetabular defect who underwent revision THA using IBG [15]. One patient has had radiographic loosening and no symptoms at 120 months postoperatively and no patients have been revised for any reason related to the arthroplasty. However, radiographic assessment revealed cephalad cup migration of 2.29 mm and medial migration of 1.57 mm. The authors concluded that impacting bone grafting is a reliable technique for the treatment of Paprosky 3B acetabular defects. It restores bone stock like no other available for addressing these defects.

Although it is difficult to interpret radiographic findings after the use of the impacted bone allograft with cement in an acetabular revision, the cup and graft remodeling are clearly stable [16]. Although bone graft resorption has been described in areas of substantial weight bearing, most hips present uniform radiodensity of the graft and host bone. Histologic studies of cup loosening in humans report bone substitution, but at a slower rate than in animal models [13, 17]. The open structure of the cancellous bone graft, associated with cement, permits good vascularization, with apposition preceding resorption in the new bone, and bone substitution takes place without mechanical loosening [18]. Although the importance of the presence of radiolucent lines adjacent to acetabular components has already been established in cemented prostheses. Radiolucent lines are quite infrequent in most series [7, 16, 19]. When a cup is in close contact with well-vascularized bone, the stability of the cup is comparable to fixation in primary surgery [13].

Many factors may be responsible for acetabular cup loosening. A finite-element analysis of a protruded acetabulum has shown that stress on a deficient medial wall varies directly with medial placement of the cup [20]. Different authors suggest it is important for good long-term results that deficient acetabulum be corrected to the anatomic position [16, 18, 19]. Theoretically, the location of the center of rotation of the hip affects the load with a higher and more medial position resulting in greater loads than a lower placement. In these series, the anatomic rotation center of the hip was improved in all assessed parameters in both Paprosky bone defect grades. However, the change in the distance from the approximate rotation center of the hip to the center of the prosthetic femoral head is greater in hips with Paprosky 3B bone defects [21], which also had a greater preoperative distance [16] (Fig. 6.3). Waddell et al. show that cup migration and bone graft resorption are some of the limitations after acetabular impaction bone grafting in revision surgery when used for large segmental defects [15]. Loosening and bone resorption are more frequent in cases with a large segmental defect of the acetabular roof in which a large metal mesh cannot avoid the cranial migration of the femoral head [22].

We have analysed 330 consecutive hips that had received acetabular IBG and a cemented cup in revision surgery with large bone defects (Paprosky types 3A and 3B) in our institution. Fresh-frozen femoral head allograft was morselized manually. The mean follow-up after re-revision was 15 years (5–26). The radiological analysis showed cup migration in 40 hips. The mean time of appearance was 4.3 years (range, 1–25). Migration was progressive and painful in 27 hips (67.5%) requiring cup revision. Lateral mesh was more frequently used in migrated cups. Cup tilt adn cranial migration were found in all migrated cups and survival with further cup revision for aseptic loosening was78.3% (95%confidence interval: 68.7–87.9). In all surviving re-revisions trabecular incorporation was observed without radiolucent lines. In this study bone graft resorption and cup migration were not frequent and, in one-third part of the cases, they were not progressive. Cup migration was more frequent in cases with segmental roof defect in which a lateral mesh was used.

The magnitude of this migration probably depends on the grafting technique used, including factors such as the quality of donor bone, size of the bone chips and the surgical technique employed to achieve impaction. First, different types of bone mills have been used. The importance of bone chip size is not addressed in most published papers. The true size and location of the bony defect, the quality of the graft, the amount of graft used and the final amount of living bone facing the implant or the cement are probably all factors with a more or less pronounced influence on cup fixation. Ornstein et al. [12], using RSA studies, confirmed similar good clinical results using this surgical technique at mid-term follow-up, although the high migration rates as measured with RSA might be a cause for concern regarding the longevity of this type of cup revision. Mohaddes et al., also using RSA, studied that cemented fixation with bone grafting in acetabular revision surgery results in higher proximal migration [6]. Better results for cemented

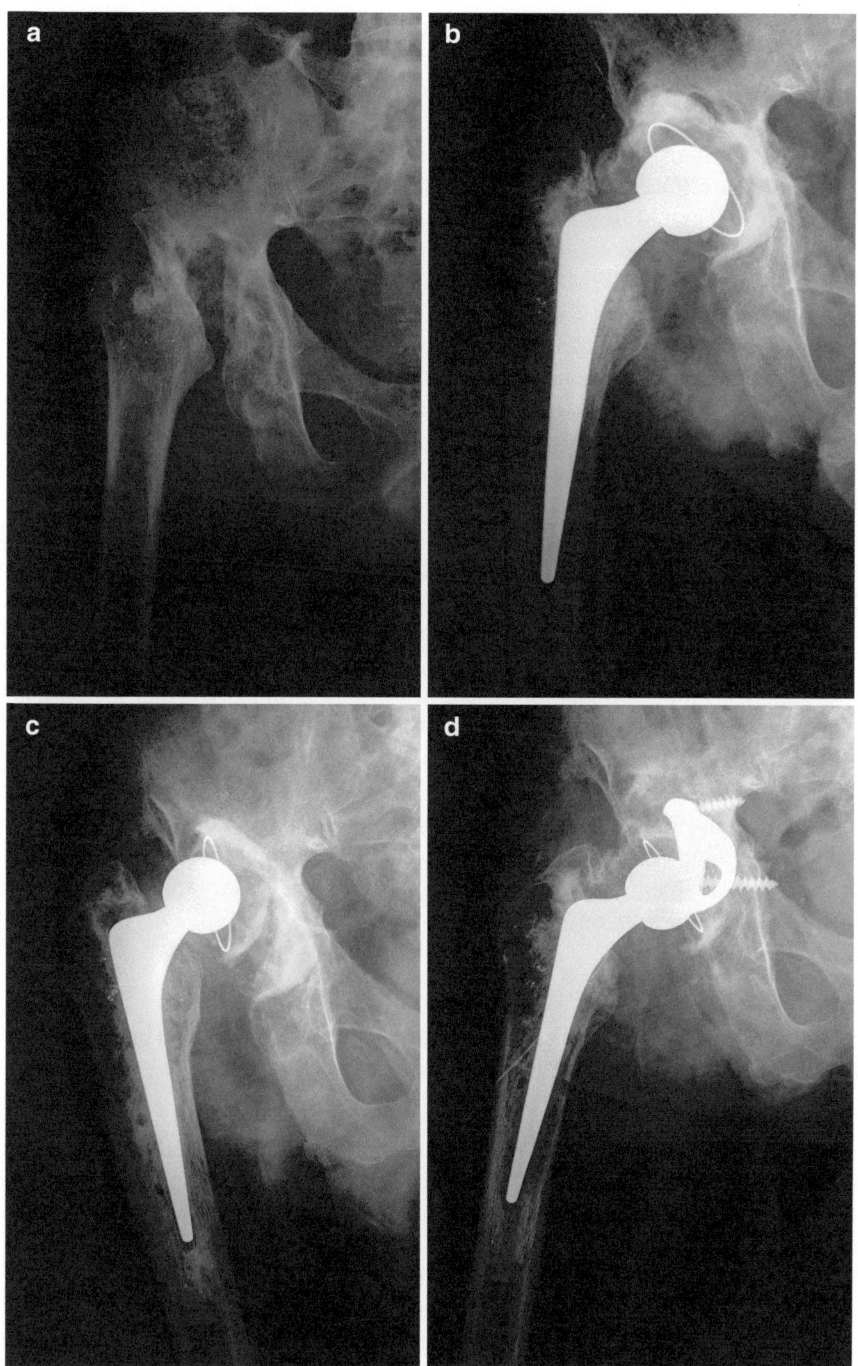


**Fig. 6.3** (**a**) preoperative radiograph shows a resection-arthroplasty after an infected total hip arthroplasty. (**b**) Impacting bone grafting was used in both components in revision surgery. (**c**) Postoperative radiograph. (**c**) Postoperative radiograph at 10 years shows symptomatic cup migration. (**d**) Impacting bone grafting associted with a tantalum augment was used in re-revision surgery

fixation could probably be obtained if bigger graft particles and a more consistent impaction technique had been used. It could also be argued that the increased proximal migration of the cemented acetabular components is due to a different pattern of bone remodelling when cemented fixation is used in conjunction with bone impaction grafting. These hypotheses should most certainly be addressed in future studies [6]. García-Rey et al. establish differences in long-term results according to the type of defect and use of lateral mesh [22]. Survivorship analysis at 15 years was 89.1 ± 14% when no mesh was required, 84.9 ± 12% when only medial mesh was required, 79.6 ± 12% whith lateral mesh, and 53.9 ± 22% in cases when both meshes were required (log Rank-Mantel Cox P = 0.008). But some aspects are still not clearly defined, and future studies should focus on them. The influence of sex, including sex-related differences in bone quality and/or activity, the relationship of prior surgery (both type and number) on the results of the procedure, and the size of allograft fragments must all be examined. Future studies should likewise be large enough to stratify results according to the type and severity of the bone defects being treated.

We need to pay particular attention to those situations in which IBG fails. In these cases, porous trabecular metal augments could be used associated with IBG [23–25]. The combination of biological fixation offered by tantalum and impaction grafting could generate adequate cranial support for the cemented cup (Fig. 6.4). Comparisons between impacting bone grafting and these implants may represent a good topic for future investigations. We need to ascertain is whether metallic augments can improve long-term results in 3B/lateral/segmental defects, which are difficult to treat. We also might consider evaluating the combination of porous metal augments with impacting bone grafting. Finally, we must perform more prospective comparative, and ideally, randomized studies examining impacting bone grafting versus metal augments, as well as the results of impacting bone grafting with and without these augments. Longer follow-ups are also necessary to assess the potential deterioration of fixation.

## Impacting Bone Grafting Facilitates Future Acetabular Re-revisions

Long-term follow-up studies have shown that impaction bone grafting can be used to perform actual biological repair of acetabular bone defects and hence facilitate future revisions [8]. Schmitz et al. report no osteolysis after 30 years, showing that the fact the use of this technique in revision reconstruction can make these reconstructions last for over 30 years [8]. Another advantage of this technique is that in case of reconstruction failure, a cemented cup and impaction bone grafting can again be used to perform a re-revision (Fig. 6.3). Technically, this can be done since the remaining bone stock can still be used to perform a new reconstruction. If the cement fixation into the graft deteriorates with time, the new bone is likely to facilitate re-revision surgery (Fig. 6.5).

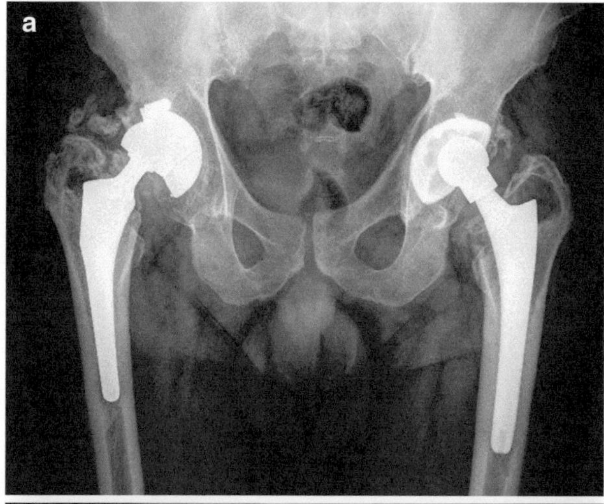


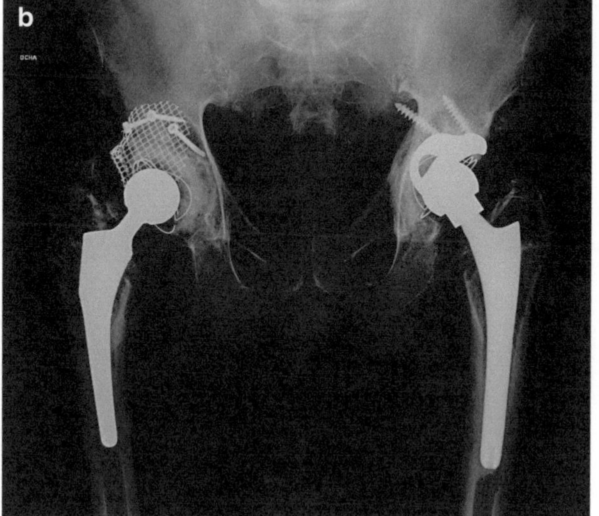


**Fig. 6.4** (**a**) Preoperative radiograph shows bilateral cementless loosened cups. (**b**) The rigth cup was revised using impacting bone grafting with cemented cup, and the left hip was revised using a impacting bone grafting associated with a tantalum augment

Few studies analyse the clinical and radiographic outcome of acetabular re-revisions using IBG and a cemented polyethylene cup after a follow-up of 5–15 years [26]. Consequently, we decided to study the outcome of the re-revisions again using IBG and a cemented cupin 34 hips in our institution. Radiological failure was defined as migration of more than 5 mm in any direction or progressive radiolucent lines in all three zones. We assessed progressive radiolucent lines around the cup and changes in different radiographic parameters, such as abcetabular abduction angle, anteversion angles, horizontal distance, vertical distance and distance from the prosthetic femoral head center to the anatomic rotation center of the hip according Ranawat et al. [27]. In these 34 hips we found migration in 11 hips, of these migration appeared before the first year postoperation in five, between the

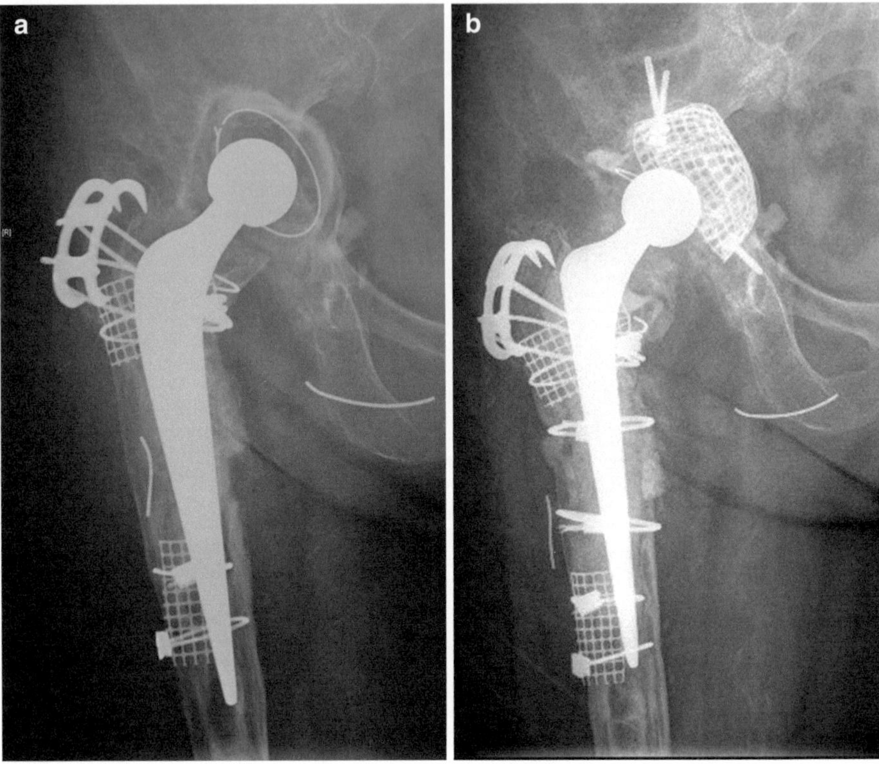


**Fig. 6.5** (**a**) Preoperative radiograph of teh hip shows a failed impacting bone grafting used in cup revision surgery. (**b**) The hip was re-revised using a new impacting bone grafting with metallic mesh with a good clinical result

1st and 5th years in five and, only one case, at 6 years postoperation. Intraoperative bone defect was improved after the first failed revision. At the first revision there were 14 hips with Paprosky bone defect type 3 A and 20 with Paprosky type 3B. At the re-revision there were five hips with Paproky 2B, 21 with Paprosky type 3A and eight with type 3B. The mean time for the appearance of migration was 25 months (range, 3–72). In three cups, migration was progressive and painful requiring re-revision. Cup tilt was found in all migrated hips. There were one dislocation requiring a cemented dual mobility cup associated with IBG and one infection solved with resection-arthroplasty. Survival with further cup revision for aseptic loosening was 80.7% (95% CI 57.4–100). In all surviving re-revisions trabecular incorporation was observed without radiolucent lines.

This outcome seems to confirm that IBG and cement can restore bone stock loss and normal biomechanics thus allowing future revisions. In all patients the technique could be repeated again, so no special implants were needed and hence a relatively inexpensive standard cup implant was used [26]. A main limitation of our study is that the number of patients is small, but we believe our findings are significant and we concur with other studies that using IBG [26], facilitates future re-revisions. A weakness of the outcome studies of acetabular bone impacting in revision surgery is the large number of patients lost to follow-up [28]; the reason is that the average ageis relatively high in these patients so by review many had died of different causes.

According to Schreurs et al. the key in revision surgery is restoration of the bone stock defects [26], using biological reconstructive techniques and we agree. Some studies have reported a high rate of failure with the use of structural allografts [29, 30], and IBG would be the appropriate biological reconstrucive technique to reconstruct bone defects. As in other reconstructive techniques the outcome of IBG is less optimal in larger defects: Buttaro et al. [10] have shown that metal mesh, IBG and a cemented acetabular component result in a favorable outcome in uncontained acetabular defects of medium severity, but the outcome in more extensive combined deficiencies is less successful. The postoperative treatment protocol is especially importantin these demanding cases. We used a very conservative postoperative treatment protocol including a three weeks bedrest period when there had been with extensive acetabular bone defects, in this group with very large reconstructions at 10 years after surgery, an excellent survival has been reported with IBG, but these large reconstructions are technically very demanding [31]. Also it is very important in acetabular reconstruction that large sized bone chips of 8–12 mm be used [32]. Experience shows that even successive acetabular reconstructions using IBG and a cemented polyethylene cup are possible with satisfying 6-years survivorship. Impaction bone grafting seems to be especially effective in younger patients, as they have a long life expectancy and will possibly will outlive even their revision implants [26]. IBG is our standard approach for acetabular reconstructions with bone stock loss.

## References

1. Colo E, Rijnen WH-C, Schreurs BW. The biological approach in acetabular revision surgery: impaction bone grafting and a cemented cup. Hip Int. 2015;25(4):361–7.
2. von Roth P, Abdel MP, Harmsen WS, Berry DJ. Uncemented jumbo cups for revision total hip arthroplasty: a concise followup, at a mean of twenty years, of a previous report. J Bone Joint Surg Am. 2015;97(4):284–7.
3. Lie SA, Havelin LI, Furnes ON, Engesaeter LB, Vollset SE. Failure rates for 4762 revision total hip arthroplasties in the Norwegian arthroplasty register. J Bone Joint Surg Br. 2004;86(4):504–9.
4. Lee JM, Nam HT. Acetabular revision total hip arthroplasty using an impacted morselized allograft and a cementless cup: minimum 10-year follow-up. J Arthroplasty. 2011;26(7):1057–60.
5. Palm L, Jacobsson SA, Kvist J, Lindholm A, Ojersjö A, Ivarsson I. Acetabular revision with extensive allograft impaction and uncemented hydroxyapatite-coated implants. Results after 9 (7–11) years follow-up. J Arthroplasty. 2007;22(8):1083–91.
6. Mohaddes M, Herberts P, Malchau, Johanson P-E, Kärrholm J. High proximal migration in cemented acetabular revisions operated with bone impaction grafting; 47 revision cups followed with RSA for 17 years. Hip Int. 2017;27(3):251–8.

7. Schreurs BW, Keurentjes JC, Gardeniers JW, Verdonschot N, Slooff TJ, Veth RP. Acetabular revision with impacted morsellised cancellous bone grafting and a cemented acetabular component: a 20- to 25-year follow-up. J Bone Joint Surg Br. 2009;91(9):1148–53.
8. Schmitz MWJL, Hannink G, Gardeniers JWM, Verdonschot N, Slooff TJJH, Schreurs BW. Acetabular reconstruction with impaction bone-greafting and a cemented cup in patients younger than 50 years of age. A concise follo-up, at 27 to 35 years, of a previous report. J Bone Joint Surg Am. 2017;99(19):1440–6.
9. Schreurs BW, Luttjeboer J, Thien TM, de Waal Malefijt MC, Buma P, Veth RPH, Slooff TJJH. Acetabular revision with impacted morselized cancellous bone graft and a cemented cup in patients with rheumatoid arthritis. A concise followup, at eight to nineteen years, of a previous report. J Bone Joint Surg Am. 2009;91(3):646–51.
10. Buttaro MA, Comba F, Pusso R, Piccaluga F. Acetabular revision with metal mesh, impaction bone grafting, and a cemented cup. Clin Orthop Relat Res. 2008;466(10):2482–90.
11. Van Haaren EH, Heyligers IC, Alexander FGM, Wuisman PIJM. High rate of failure of impaction grafting in large acetabular defects. J Bone Joint Surg Br. 2007;89:296–300.
12. Ornstein E, Franzén H, Johnsson R, Stefánsdóttir A, Sundberg M, Tägil M. Five-year follow-up of socket movements and loosening after revision with impacted morselized allograft bone and cement. A radiostereometric and radiographic analysis. J Arthroplasty. 2006;21:975–84.
13. Buma P, Lamerigts N, Schreurs BW, Gardeniers J, Verslayen D, Slooff TJJH. Impacted graft incorporation after cemented acetabular revision. Histological evaluation in 8 patients. Acta Orthop Scand. 1996;67:536–40.
14. Tägil M, Aspenberg P. Fibrous tissue armoring increases the mechanical strength of an impacted bone graft. Acta Orthop Scand. 2001;72(1):78–82.
15. Waddell BS, Boettner F, Gonzalez Della Valle A. Favorable early results of impaction bone grafting with reinforcement mesh for the treatment of Paprosky 3B acetabular defects. J Arthroplasty. 2017;32:919–23.
16. Garcia-Cimbrelo E, Cruz-Pardos A, Garcia-Rey E, Ortega-Chamarro J. The survival and fate of acetabular reconstruction with impaction grafting for large defects. Clin Orthop Relat Res. 2010;468:3304–13.
17. Schimmel JW, Buma P, Versleyen D, Huiskes R, Slooff TJJH. Acetabular reconstruction with impacted morcellized cancellous allografts in cemented hip arthroplasty: A histologic and biomechanical study on the goat. J Arthroplasty. 1998;13:438–48.
18. Slooff TJ, Schimmel JW, Buma P. Cemented fixation with bone grafts. Orthop Clin North Am. 1993;24:667–77.
19. Comba F, Buttaro M, Pusso R, Piccaluga F. Acetabular reconstruction with impacted bone allografts and cemented acetabular components: a 2- to 13-year followup study of 142 aseptic revisions. J Bone Joint Surg Br. 2006;88:865–9.
20. Crowninshield RD, Brand RA, Pedersen DR. A stress analysis of acetabular reconstruction in protrusion acetabuli. J Bone Joint Surg Am. 1983;65:495–9.
21. Paprosky WG, Perona PG, Lawrence JM. Acetabular defect classification and surgical reconstruction in revision arthroplasty: a 6-year follow-up evaluation. J Arthroplasty. 1994;9:33–44.
22. García-Rey E, Madero R, García-Cimbrelo E. THA revisions using impaction allografting with mesh is durfor medial but not lateral acetabular defects. Clin Orthop Relat Res. 2015;473:3882–91.
23. Borland WS, Bhattacharya R, Holland JP, Brewster NT. Use of porous trabecular metal augments with impaction bone grafting in management of acetabular bone loss. Early to mediumtrem results. Acta Orthop. 2012;83(4):347–52.
24. Gehrke T, Bangert Y, Schwantes B, Gebauer M, Kendoff D. Acetabular revision in THA using tantalum augments combined with impaction bone grafting. Hip Int. 2013;23:359–65.
25. Gill K, Wilson MJ, Whitehouse SL, Timperley AJ. Results using trabecular metal augments in combination with acetabular impaction bone grafting in deficient acetabula. Hip Int. 2013;23(6):522–8.

26. Schreurs BW, te Stroet MAJ, Rijnen WHC, Gardeniers JWM. Acetabular re-revision with impaction bone grafting and a cemented polyethylene cup; a biological option for successive reconstructions. Hip Int. 2015;25(1):44–9.
27. Ranawat CS, Dorr LD, Inglis AE. Total hip arthroplasty in protrusio acetabuli of rheumatoid arthritis. J Bone Joint Surg Am. 1980;62:1059–65.
28. Schreurs BW, Slooff THHJ, Gardeniers JWM, Buma P. Acetabular reconsruction with bone impaction grafting and a cemented cup. 20 years' of experience. Clin Orthop Relat Res. 2001;393:202–15.
29. Hooten JP Jr, Engh CA Jr, Engh CA. Failure of structural acetabular allografts in cementless revision hip arthroplasty. J Bone Joint Surg Br. 1994;76(3):419–22.
30. Shinar AA, Harris WH. Bulk structural autogenous grafts and allografts for reconstruction of the acetabulum in total hip arthroplasty. Sixteen-year-average follow-up. J Bone Joint Surg Am. 1997;79(2):159–68.
31. van Egmond N, De Kam DC, Gardeniers JW, Schreurs BW. Revisions of extensive acetabular defects with impaction grafting and a cement cup. Clin Orthop Relat Res. 2011;469(2):562–73.
32. Bolder SB, Schreurs BW, Verdonschot N, van Unen JM, Gardeniers JW, Slooff TJ. Particle size of bone graft and method of impaction affect initial stability of cemented cups: human cadaveric and synthetic pelvic specimen studies. Acta Orthop Scand. 2003;74(6):652–7.

# Chapter 7
# Revision Surgery After Fractures of Ceramic Components

**Luigi Zagra and Enrico Gallazzi**

## Introduction

Ceramic on Ceramic (CoC) bearings for Total Hip Arthroplasty (THA) were introduced with the aim of reducing wear associated with polyethylene (PE) components, thus limiting osteolysis and increasing the longevity of the implant especially in young and active patients. The first attempts of utilizing a ceramic cup with a ceramic head were made in the 1970 by Pierre Boutin in France with cemented liners and in 1974 by Heinz Mittelmeier in Germany with cementless all ceramic threaded cups and skirted heads. Both systems were burdened by high failure rates related to poor mechanical properties of the first generation of alumina (low strength resistance due to the grain size), and to materials and design faults (direct contact of the ceramic to the bone, as alumina has no osseointegration capability, and skirted heads creating impingement). Since then, several new compounds with new generations of alumina (with smaller and more uniform grains) were introduced with good to excellent results [1–3]. Nowadays the most commonly used ceramics is the alumina matrix composite (AMC) (Biolox Delta™; CeramTech AG, Plochingen, Germany).

A brief explanation of the characteristics of the ceramics used in medical devices could be helpful to better understand the issues related to its utilization. Ceramics is defined, in material science, as a non-metallic, solid material comprising an inorganic compound of metal, non-metal and metalloid atoms primarily held in ionic and covalent bonds. Since the beginning, the ceramics used for medical purposes is composed of Alumina (Al), an oxide of Aluminum, the same material that composes the crystalline structure of Ruby and Sapphire. Al was chosen for its chemical inertness and biocompatibility: given its high oxidative state, the material does not tend to oxidize further in the body, and therefore its particles do not generate oxidative

L. Zagra (✉) · E. Gallazzi
Hip Department, IRCCS Istituto Ortopedico Galeazzi, Milano, Italy
e-mail: luigi.zagra@fastwebnet.it



E. García-Rey, E. García-Cimbrelo (eds.), *Acetabular Revision Surgery in Major Bone Defects*, https://doi.org/10.1007/978-3-319-98596-1_7

stress and inflammatory reaction. Moreover, thanks to its crystalline structure, Al ceramics has a very "smooth" surface, that provides a very low friction coefficient and an extremely low wear rate. Concerning its mechanical proprieties, as a covalently linked, crystalline structure, Al has the characteristics of a "hard" material: a high compressive strength (>4500 MPa) and a high Young's (elastic) modulus (400GPa); on the other hand, it has a low flexural strength (around 600 MPa) and low deformation capacities [4]. Thus, in this material fractures tend to occur before any plastic deformation can take place. The intrinsic porosity of the material has a role in fracture generation: the pores act as a stress concentrator, thus reducing tensile stress and facilitating the crack propagation. Since mechanical fragility was clearly a weak point of this bearing, industry tried to overcome it with different technical solutions. To further increase the hardness and strength of the material, Zirconium oxide (ZrO), Strontium oxide (SrO) and Chromium oxide (CrO) were added to the Al matrix during the sintering process (Alumina Composite Matrix, AMC). In particular, ZrO particles play an important role in reducing the fracture propagation. These particles are less dense and are evenly distributed in the Al matrix; when a fracture appears, it propagates towards these less dense ZrO areas, that react to the fracture by changing their spatial phase (from tetragonal to monocyclic); this change is associated with an increase in density of the area, that in turn creates compressive forces that ultimately limit the fracture propagation. As a result, AMC ceramics almost doubles flexural strength (and hardness) compared to the Al ceramics, while maintaining the same elastic modulus and compressive strength [5].

While these technological advancements improved the mechanical properties of CoC bearings, dramatically reducing the fracture rates, nevertheless ceramic fracture remains a cause of concern as revision for ceramic fracture can lead to catastrophic failures and severe complications due to third body wear, caused by ceramic fragments [6, 7].

## Epidemiology, Risk factors and Causes of Ceramic Fractures

According to the Australian Registry data, 99.8% of ceramics used in THA is CeramTech Biolox products [8]. However, this data may not reflect all the markets in different countries (such as in France or in Spain). Anyway, Manufacturer's data on recorded events can help to understand the frequency of occurrence of ceramic fractures. Concerning Delta Ceramics, the reported fracture rate for the head is 1 in 100.000 (0.001%), while for the liner is 22 in 100.000 (0.022%). The fracture rate is higher for the old Forte™ Ceramics, being 21 in 100.000 (0.021%) for the head and 46 in 100.000 (0.046%) for the liner (CeramTech, Unpublished Data, 2017); while Forte Ceramics is no longer used for new THAs, it is important to know the risk of fracture of this material since it was widely used until few years ago. In a recent analysis of the National Joint Registry for England, Wales, Northern Ireland and Isle of Man (NJR), the percentage of ceramic fractures were found to be slightly higher than reported by the Company: 7 of 79,442 (0.009%) Biolox Delta heads, 38 of 31,982 (0.119%) Biolox Forte heads, 101 of 80,170 (0.126%) Biolox Delta liners and 35 of 31,258 (0.112%) Biolox Forte liners. Interestingly, regression analysis revealed that the two most important risk factors for fracture were smaller heads (in particular the 28 mm Forte head) and high BMI of the patient [9]. Most of the other published data reports similar fracture rates [10], the only outliers being single center studies [11, 12] that reported a prevalence of liner fracture of 0.9–1.1% with Delta Ceramics; however, since in both studies the same cup was used, it is possible that the higher fracture rates reported depends more on technical issues related to component design of the metal back rather than on the ceramic material itself [6].

Head fractures are nowadays less frequent than liner ones. Direct impact is a very rare cause of head fracture, while a more common mechanism is fatigue break due to taper mismatch, scratches on the taper and third bodies between the head and the taper. The only identified risk factor for head breakage in large clinical series is the 28 mm diameter head with short neck, as previously mentioned by NJR data and confirmed by a systematic review [13].

Liner fractures are almost never related to trauma as well, but rather depend on two main reasons: the former is the edge loading and the impingement due to the cup positioning, while the latter is the misalignment of the liner during insertion in the metal back or a metal back damage [14]. Edge loading occurs when the hip contact force vector moves over the edge of the liner or when the stress concentrates on a limited area; when this occurs, the increased stress both on the liner and on the head surfaces increases the risk of damage. A steep cup could reduce the contact area between components, therefore increasing the force transmitted at the edge. Another mechanism that provokes edge loading is neck impingement that causes a diametrically opposed sub-luxation of the head over the liner edge (Fig. 7.1). Poor orientation or bad rim design can create such a neck impingement and sub-

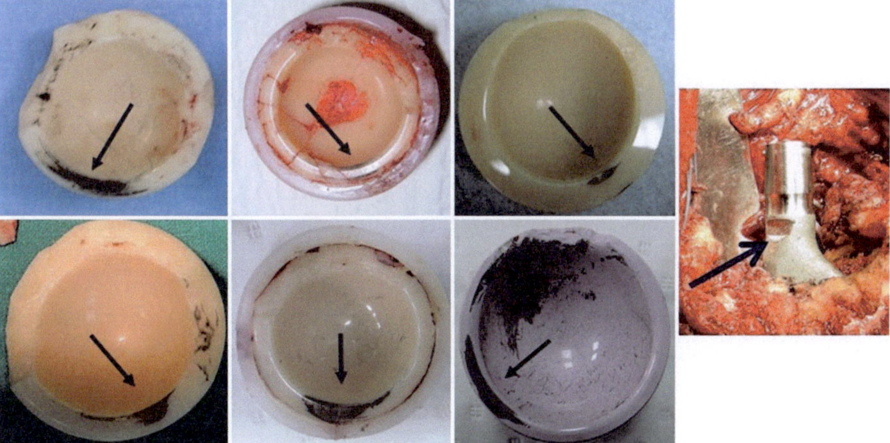

**Fig. 7.1** Retrieval samples of fractured ceramic liners. Black arrows indicates the area of impingement against the neck of the stem, on the opposite side of the broken rim of the liner. In the last panel to the right, the blue arrow point to the damaged neck that impinged on the liner

dislocation on the opposite side of the liner with very small contact of the head on the rim as a consequence, leading to grain detachment, third body wear and crack propagation [14]. This model of fracture was confirmed by the clinical observation of Traina et al. that found a higher risk of fracture in cups with anteversion over the range [15], thus confirming previous studies [16] and finite element analysis [17]. Therefore clean positioning of the components is fundamental [18]. A particular situation of edge loading occurs when the acetabular liner is not correctly seated in the metal back. This could be due to a metal back rim damage or even a deformation during the insertion: titanium shell can deform by 0.6 mm during impaction, consequently generating a two-point support of the liner [19]. Another reason for that can be simply an incorrect handling of the ceramic liner during insertion jammed in a wrong position by the surgeon. Thus, a careful preparation of the acetabulum and assessment with trial insert is required when using a ceramic liner. Again, each implant must be checked intra-operatively for correct engaging of the liner into the metal back and of the head on the stem taper prior to the final reduction of the prosthesis [20]. Finally, screws protruding in the metal back have been described as a risk factor of the same phenomenon of incorrect seating of the ceramic liner, thus leading to the risk of later liner breakage [21].

Finally, a fracture of the liner can lead to a secondary breakage of the head. In any case the head is usually deeply damaged by the break of the liner.

## Clinical Features and Diagnosis

The clinical picture of a fracture of ceramic head is straightforward. The breakage is usually sudden, complete and noisy. The patient immediately realizes that something has happened. X-Rays is mandatory, and the fragmented head is usually clearly visible and easy to be recognized.

The clinical picture of a ceramic liner fracture, differently, can be subtle and underestimated, thus a high level of consideration in suspicious events by the clinician is required to make the correct diagnosis. A careful history should be collected, with particular attention to pain, discomfort and noises. In patients with risk factors for ceramic fracture, such as cup malpositioning, a strict (i.e. yearly) follow up with X-Rays is suggested, and in case of new increasing noises a ceramic fracture should be suspected [22]. Onset of symptoms is not clear every time, so they could be underestimated both by the patient and by the physician. X-Rays are the first level of investigation, even if their diagnostic accuracy can be quite low. Fragments of the fractured liner could be visible on X-Rays as radiopaque areas that can be confused with heterotopic ossifications. Once the diagnosis of ceramic fracture is suspected, confirmative exam should be performed. CT-scan is helpful in this context: the fragments are usually visible in the soft tissues, and the liner can show cracks or chipping at the rim. Some studies suggested that the microanalysis by SEM (Scanning Electronic Microscope) of synovial fluid with the evaluation of ceramic particles can be useful in diagnosing ceramic fractures [23, 24]. However this exam is not readily available in most centers.

## Revision Surgery

### *Timing*

Once the diagnosis of ceramic fracture is made, the surgeon should be aware that the treatment cannot be postponed. Early revision is indicated for two main reasons: first, with time the ceramic fragments spread around into the soft tissues, and thus their complete removal becomes more and more difficult; retaining of fragments in the tissues could compromise the outcome of the revised prosthesis, because of third body wear. Secondly, the metal components, especially the titanium taper of the stem in case of head breakage, could be rapidly damaged with metallosis, leading to the need to revise a well-fixed stem (or even the cup), making the revision surgery much more complex and heavy for the patient (Fig. 7.2).

### *Planning*

Despite the "relative urgent" condition of a ceramic fracture, the revision surgery should be carefully planned. Information about the prosthesis manufacturer, type and size, should be obtained. The timing of the fracture is also important, since more distant is the time of the fracture, more fragments could be found in the soft tissues. Preoperative X-Rays should be used to evaluate components orientation, in particular of the cup: if cup malpositioning is shown that can be the cause of failure, cup revision should be planned before surgery; if areas of osteolysis or cup/stem

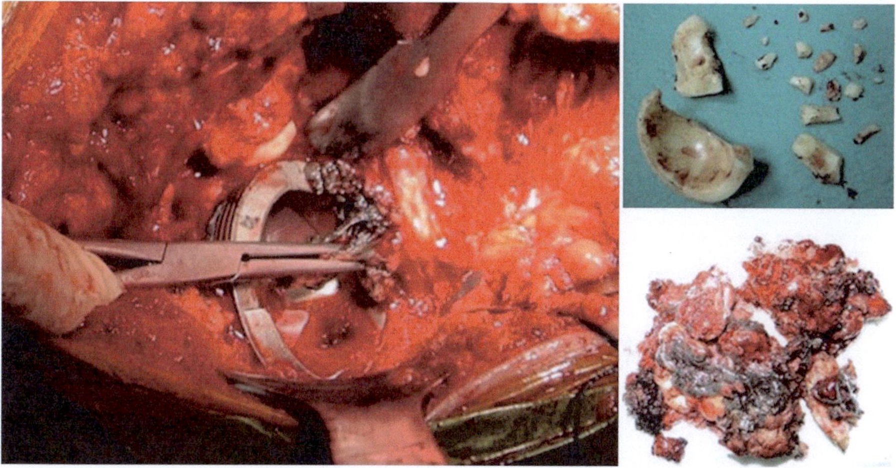

**Fig. 7.2** Ceramic on ceramic fragments in soft tissues following a fracture of the liner. Left Panel: Removal of soft tissues with small ceramics fragments and metallosis due to Ti damage caused by AI. Top Right Panel: retrieved fragments of the liner; Bottom Right Panel: Removed soft tissues with metallosis

instability are suspected before surgery, a revision of the unstable component should be planned. The surgeon should be familiar with hip revision and with the approach that is intended to be used [25].

## *Surgical Technique*

Surgical technique is of course of major importance. The goal of revision surgery is the positioning of a stable prosthesis that can have a long term survival without any early or late bearing problem. Therefore, the first step of the surgery is an aggressive soft tissue debridement and synoviectomy, with the ultimate goal of removing all the ceramic fragments or at least as much as possible (Fig. 7.2). For this purposes some Authors proposed in the past a double approach to the hip [26].

The second step is the removal of the broken head and/or liner, followed by the evaluation of stability, orientation and damage of the metal back and of the stem. If the metal back is in a satisfactory position and it is intra-operatively stable and not damaged, a new PE liner can be inserted (or cemented) if available for the cup in situ. Placement of a new ceramic liner in a previous metal back (even if well fixed, correctly oriented and apparently not damaged) is not acceptable as ceramic is too much sensitive to even small metal back damages, as outlined before. In case of isolated liner fracture, the change of the head is suggested in any case because, as mentioned before, a damage of the head surface is always relevant. If the taper is not damaged, according to manufacturer's recommendations, which is sometimes not so easy to be evaluated, a new head should be used without revising the stem. The decision between a major revision with removal of well-fixed components slightly damaged and retaining of those, should be anyway balanced on the age, general conditions, life expectancy and activity of the single patient. In case the stem is retained, the surgeon should be aware that nowadays when using a ceramic head it is mandatory to implant the one specifically developed for revision surgery (Biolox Option™, CeramTech, Plochingen, Germany). This type of head (Delta ceramic with a titanium sleeve) offers the possibility to select different head diameter and neck length, and can fit on different taper angles as provided by different prosthesis manufacturers. Anyway if the taper or the metal back damages have major damages, revision of those components is necessary to ensure long term survival of the implant.

## *Which Bearing Couple?*

Few studies evaluated the outcomes of the various bearing surfaces in revision surgery after ceramic fracture [7, 26–30]. Several case reports highlighted massive wear of the metal head used after ceramic fracture including severe Co and Cr poisoning of the patients [7, 26, 29–33]. The hypothesis that metal is more susceptible to wear in presence of ceramic particles was confirmed in laboratory wear as well. Ceramic particles up to 5 mm of diameter were placed between the head and liner with three different couplings: Ceramic/Polyethilene, Ceramic/Cross-Linked Polyethilene (C/XLPE) and Metal/Cross-Linked Polyethilene (M/XLPE); while the two combination of ceramics showed a wear of 0.56 and 0.31 mg/million cycles, the wear of Met-XLPE coupling was 316 mg/million cycles, several magnitudes higher [34]. The use of Cer/Cer coupling after ceramic fracture was evaluated in a series of 30 cases by Traina et al., that reported a survival of 93.3% at a 3.3 years follow up [28]. While the use of a Cer/Cer bearing is a valid option after ceramic fracture, probably the most used for the scratch resistance to third body wear, Cer/PE is the Author's preferred option. Retrieval analysis showed how ceramics fragments can impact in PE liners (Fig. 7.3), rather than remaining free bodies between the two hard ceramic surfaces, thus probably causing less wear. Moreover, for the patient the proposal of a bearing that already failed could be not the most favorable option. In a series of 12 patients revised for ceramic fracture with Cer/XPE coupling, at a mean follow up of 6 years only one patient was revised again for PE wear, with an overall survival of 93.7% (Fig. 7.4). Interestingly, in this series the rate of early dislocation was very high (33.3%), probably because of the aggressive soft tissue release. Therefore we suggest to be very careful during surgery: to use a bigger diameter head possibly with longer neck, and in case of major instability, a dual mobility can be suggested with a ceramic liner instead of a metal one (construct composed by modular ceramic liner-mobile PE-ceramic head) that could reduce the risk of dislocation [27]. A judicious postoperative course is strongly recommended.

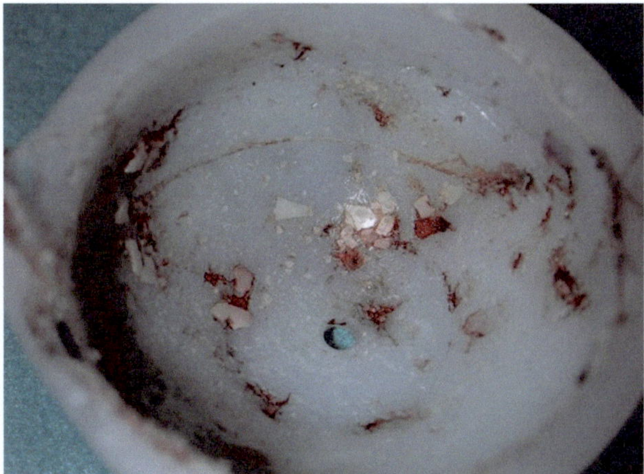

**Fig. 7.3** Fragments of broken ceramics impacted in a PE par of a sandwich liner

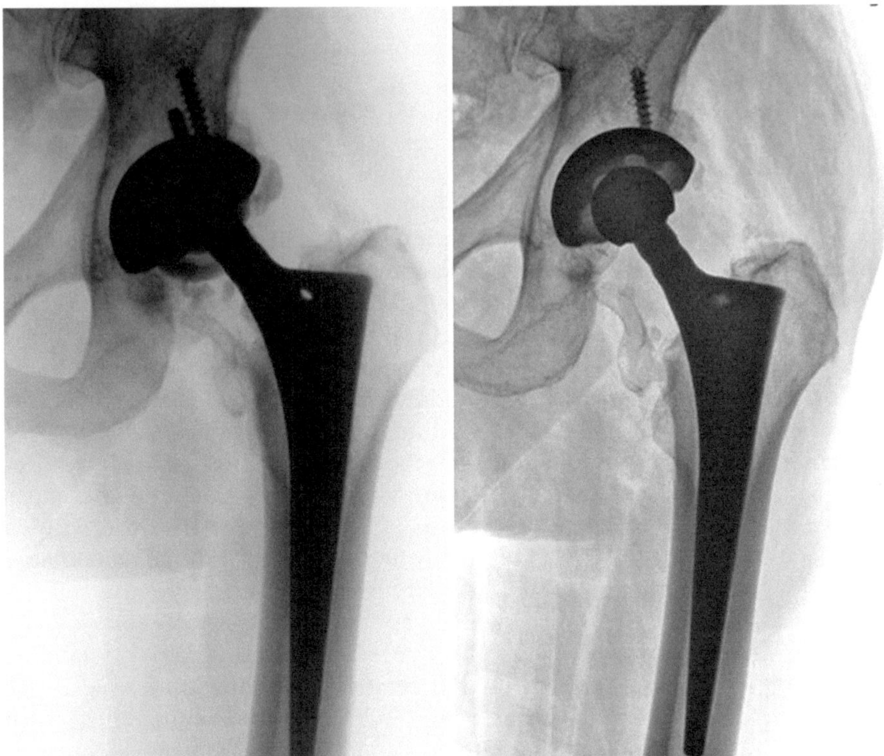

**Fig. 7.4** Panel A: male, 74 years, fracture of PE sandwich ceramic liner. Panel B: same patient, with a Cer-PE bearing, at 10-year follow up. No signs of wear or osteolysis can be found

## Conclusions

Ceramic on Ceramic bearing is a good option in young and active patients due to the excellent wear resistance and the high biocompatibility of the material. Compared to soft bearings, Cer/Cer coupling is more sensitive to handling of the components and implant positioning. While rare, ceramic fracture is a catastrophic event, with high rate of complications. In case of ceramic breakage, accurate fragments removal and synoviectomy, replacement of damaged components and correction of malpositioning and impingement are the key points. At the moment there is no clear evidence on which is the bearing of choice in case of revision for ceramic breakage, but metal must be absolutely avoided. Revision using ceramic heads, with Ti sleeves in case of retained stem, on PE liners or on ceramic liners, can yield favorable results.

## References

1. Kang BJ, Ha YC, Ham DW, Hwang SC, Lee YK, Koo KH. Third-generation alumina-on-alumina total hip arthroplasty: 14 to 16-year follow-up study. J Arthroplast. 2015;30(3):411–5.

2. Petsatodis GE, Papadopoulos PP, Papavasiliou KA, Hatzokos IG, Agathangelidis FG, Christodoulou AG. Primary cementless total hip arthroplasty with an alumina ceramic-on-ceramic bearing: results after a minimum of twenty years of follow-up. J Bone Joint Surg Am. 2010;92(3):639–44.
3. Sedel L, Walter WL, Pitto RP. Clinical faceoff: ceramic-on-ceramic THA: do the advantages outweigh the limitations? Clin Orthop Relat Res. 2014;472(10):2927–31.
4. Macdonald N, Bankes M. Ceramic on ceramic hip prostheses: a review of past and modern materials. Arch Orthop Trauma Surg. 2014;134(9):1325–33.
5. Hannouche D, Zingg M, Miozzari H, Nizard R, Lubbeke A. Third-generation pure alumina and alumina matrix composites in total hip arthroplasty: what is the evidence? EFORT Open Rev. 2018;3(1):7–14.
6. Zagra L. CORR insights((R)): do the reasons for ceramic-on-ceramic revisions differ from other bearings in total hip arthroplasty? Clin Orthop Relat Res. 2016;474(10):2200–1.
7. Koo KH, Ha YC, Kim SY, Yoon KS, Min BW, Kim SR. Revision of ceramic head fracture after third generation ceramic-on-ceramic total hip arthroplasty. J Arthroplast. 2014;29(1):214–8.
8. Association AO. Australian arthroplasty register 2016. Available from: https://aoanjrr.sahmri.com/annual-reports-2016.
9. Howard DP, Wall PDH, Fernandez MA, Parsons H, Howard PW. Ceramic-on-ceramic bearing fractures in total hip arthroplasty: an analysis of data from the National Joint Registry. Bone Joint J. 2017;99-b(8):1012–9.
10. D'Antonio JA, Sutton K. Ceramic materials as bearing surfaces for total hip arthroplasty. J Am Acad Orthop Surg. 2009;17(2):63–8.
11. Hamilton WG, McAuley JP, Dennis DA, Murphy JA, Blumenfeld TJ, Politi J. THA with delta ceramic on ceramic: results of a multicenter investigational device exemption trial. Clin Orthop Relat Res. 2010;468(2):358–66.
12. Hamilton WG, McAuley JP, Blumenfeld TJ, Lesko JP, Himden SE, Dennis DA. Midterm results of delta ceramic-on-ceramic total hip arthroplasty. J Arthroplast. 2015;30(9 Suppl):110–5.
13. Traina F, De Fine M, Di Martino A, Faldini C. Fracture of ceramic bearing surfaces following total hip replacement: a systematic review. Biomed Res Int. 2013;2013:157247.
14. Dalla Pria P, Zagra L, Esopi P, Masoni D. Breakage and noises in ceramic on ceramic couplings. Eur Orthop Traumatol. 2010;1(2):53–9.
15. Traina F, De Fine M, Bordini B, Toni A. Risk factors for ceramic liner fracture after total hip arthroplasty. Hip Int. 2012;22(6):607–14.
16. Johansson HR, Johnson AJ, Zywiel MG, Naughton M, Mont MA, Bonutti PM. Does acetabular inclination angle affect survivorship of alumina-ceramic articulations? Clin Orthop Relat Res. 2011;469(6):1560–6.
17. Elkins JM, Pedersen DR, Callaghan JJ, Brown TD. Fracture propagation propensity of ceramic liners during impingement-subluxation: a finite element exploration. J Arthroplast. 2012;27(4):520–6.
18. Jeffers JR, Walter WL. Ceramic-on-ceramic bearings in hip arthroplasty: state of the art and the future. J Bone Joint Surg Br. 2012;94(6):735–45.
19. Squire M, Griffin WL, Mason JB, Peindl RD, Odum S. Acetabular component deformation with press-fit fixation. J Arthroplast. 2006;21(6 Suppl 2):72–7.
20. Zagra L, Gallazzi E. Bearing surfaces in primary total hip arthroplasty. EFORT Open Rev. 2018;3(5):217–24.
21. Lee SC, Jung KA, Nam CH, Kim TH, Ahn NK, Hwang SH. Acetabular screw head-induced ceramic acetabular liner fracture in cementless ceramic-on-ceramic total hip arthroplasty. Orthopedics. 2010;33(5)
22. Parvizi J, Adeli B, Wong JC, Restrepo C, Rothman RH. A squeaky reputation: the problem may be design-dependent. Clin Orthop Relat Res. 2011;469(6):1598–605.
23. Toni A, Traina F, Stea S, Sudanese A, Visentin M, Bordini B, et al. Early diagnosis of ceramic liner fracture. Guidelines based on a twelve-year clinical experience. J Bone Joint Surg Am. 2006;88(Suppl 4):55–63.
24. Stea S, Traina F, Beraudi A, Montesi M, Bordini B, Squarzoni S, et al. Synovial fluid microanalysis allows early diagnosis of ceramic hip prosthesis damage. J Orthop Res. 2012;30(8):1312–20.

25. Zagra L, Maccario C, Mondini A, Bianchi L. Treatment of failures related to articulation material in THA. A comprehensive algorithm of surgical options and open questions. Hip Int. 2014;24(Suppl 10):S48–57.
26. Sharma V, Ranawat AS, Rasquinha VJ, Weiskopf J, Howard H, Ranawat CS. Revision total hip arthroplasty for ceramic head fracture: a long-term follow-up. J Arthroplast. 2010;25(3):342–7.
27. Zagra L, Bianchi L, Giacometti Ceroni R. Revision of ceramic fracture with ceramic-on-polyethylene in total hip arthroplasty: medium-term results. Injury. 2016;47(Suppl 4):S116–s20.
28. Traina F, Tassinari E, De Fine M, Bordini B, Toni A. Revision of ceramic hip replacements for fracture of a ceramic component: AAOS exhibit selection. J Bone Joint Surg Am. 2011;93(24):e147.
29. Gozzini PA, Schmid C, Dalla PP. Massive wear in a CoCrMo head following the fracture of an alumina head. Hip Int. 2002;12(1):37–42.
30. Allain J, Roudot-Thoraval F, Delecrin J, Anract P, Migaud H, Goutallier D. Revision total hip arthroplasty performed after fracture of a ceramic femoral head. A multicenter survivorship study. J Bone Joint Surg Am. 2003;85-a(5):825–30.
31. Sharma OP, Lochab J, Berkovich Y, Safir OA, Gross AE. Severe metallosis leading to femoral head perforation. Orthopedics. 2013;36(2):e241–3.
32. Ikeda T, Takahashi K, Kabata T, Sakagoshi D, Tomita K, Yamada M. Polyneuropathy caused by cobalt-chromium metallosis after total hip replacement. Muscle Nerve. 2010;42(1):140–3.
33. Zywiel MG, Brandt JM, Overgaard CB, Cheung AC, Turgeon TR, Syed KA. Fatal cardiomyopathy after revision total hip replacement for fracture of a ceramic liner. Bone Joint J. 2013;95-b(1):31–7.
34. Hintner M, Kaddick C, Usbeck S, Scheuber L, Streicher RM. What an orthopedic surgeon should know: selection of a bearing couple in case of revision after a fractured ceramic component. Semin Arthroplast. 2012;23(4):241–7.

# Chapter 8
# Antiprotrusio Cages for Acetabular Revision

**Antonio Coscujuela, Jose Luis Agullo, and Daniel Rodriguez-Perez**

## Introduction

The bone defect determines the surgical technique in acetabular revision surgery. Different studies report the necessity of restoring acetabular anatomy and the anatomical center of rotation of the hip to enable stable prosthetic component fixation, especially in revision surgery for cases with deficient bone stock [1]. Loss of acetabular bone also makes it difficult to place a new component in an optimal position on bone of sufficient strength and quality as to provide secure fixation [2]. Uncemented sockets have some limitations in acetabular revision, especially when the loss of bone stock is more extensive, comprising more than 50% of the weight-bearing surface; in this situation, primary stability cannot be achieved without the use of structural allografts. Several techniques have been proposed to compensate for acetabular deficiency, including bone grafting in conjuction with cemented [3, 4] or uncemented cups [5], Müller reinforcement metal rings [6] and tantalum augments [7–11]. Antiprotrusio cages are considered when the extent and geometry of the bone loss do not favour an uncemented porous socket. Various antiprotrusio cages are available. The Burch-Schneider antiprotrusio cage (BSAC) has been the most used and the one with the most published clinical data (Fig. 8.1). Other acetabular reinforcement designs include the Ganz cup, the Link cage, the Contour cage and the Gap cup.

An antiprotrusio cage that was larger than the Müller acetabular reinforcement ring was developed by Burch and Schneider [12]. The Swiss orthopedic surgeon Dr. Hans-Beat Burch created the cage after becoming involved in the treatment of a

A. Coscujuela (✉) · J. L. Agullo · D. Rodriguez-Perez
Department of Orthopaedic Surgery and Trauma, Hospital Universitari de Bellvitge, L'Hospitalet de Llobregat (Barcelona), Barcelona, Spain
e-mail: 20798acm@comb.cat



E. García-Rey, E. García-Cimbrelo (eds.), *Acetabular Revision Surgery in Major Bone Defects*, https://doi.org/10.1007/978-3-319-98596-1_8

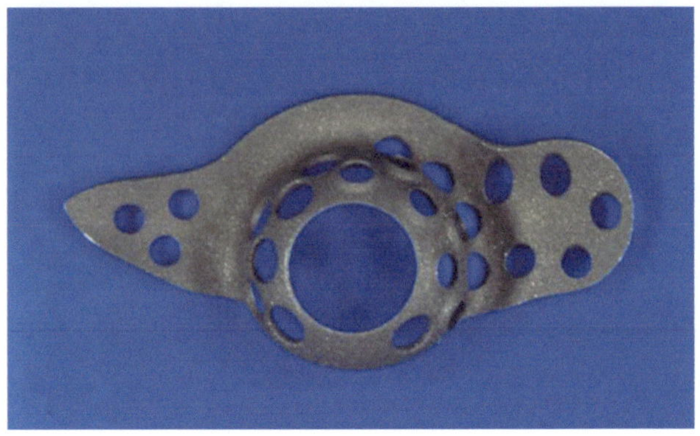

**Fig. 8.1** The Burch-Schneider antiprotusio cage (BSAC)

patient with an older, unhealed acetabular fracture. The prototype was developed especially for the treatment of this patient and implanted by Dr. Burch in 1974 in the Cantonal Hospital of Fribourg, Switzerland. Dr. Robert Schneider from Biel, Switzerland, took up the idea of bridging acetabular defects and developed it further, emphasizing the necessity of proximal screw fixation of the implant to the iliosacral joint, and suggested impacting the distal plate in the ischial bone. Steel was initially used as the implant material. Since 1987, titanium has become available for this type of acetabular component. Primary stability of the implant is achieved by fixation of the proximal flange to the ilium with screws while, distally, the flange is inserted into the ischium. In order to restore the centre of rotation to an ideal level, the implant should generally be placed in the acetabular floor (which is preserved in most cases). If necessary, defects in the acetabular roof are compensated by bone grafts (structural or morcellised), which should then be secured by screws that are directed through the anchorage holes of the flange in a horizontal or slightly descending direction. Finally, the polyethylene inlay is cemented in place at an optimal inclination of 40° with a 10–15° antetorsion, independently of the cage position.

Since the introduction of antiprotrusio cages for acetabular revision surgery of different bone defects at the beginning of the eighties, their use has been more or less widespread [13]. In North America the cages were considered a cemented reconstruction and their use was restricted after the disappointing results of cemented revisions at mid-term follow up become known [14].

Meanwhile, reasonable midterm results with antiprotrusio cages were reported from Europe when used in the presence of marked bone loss [15, 16]. That conceptual facet made the reinforcement device an extraordinary tool. The advantages of antoprotrusio cages are that the reinforcement device seems to protect grafts from overstress, distribute load, help to restore the appropriate centre of rotation of the hip and support the cemented polyethylene cup [17, 18]. With experience, more has been learned about the limitations of antiprotrusio devices. They are more difficult to implant than hemispheric cups. A wide approach is needed and it is not exempt from serious neurovascular complications [19]. Most designs have no potential for biologic bone ingrowth and, with time, particularly in younger patients, they may fail.

## Technical Data

Between 1996 and 2004, the BSAC was implanted in 96 patients (53 women and 38 men), undergoing acetabular revision in our institution. Cause of the revision was aseptical loosening (62 patients), sepsis (14 patients), severe osteolysis (10 patients), acetabular malposition (6 patients) and others (4 patients). The mean age at surgery was 67.3 years (range, 35–85 years). Including criteria were to use a BSAC in revision acetabular surgery whenever there is deficient acetabular stock (Fig. 8.2). Eleven patients passed away from causes unrelated to the operation and 17 patients have been lost to follow-up. Of the remaining 68 hips, three cages had to be removed: two due to deep infection and one due to aseptic loosening. Thus, the complete cohort consists of 65 hips (61 patients) that were available for clinical and radiological review at an average follow-up of 8.1 years (range 5–13 years). The right hip was operated in 42 cases and the left hip in 54 cases. The revised acetabular component was cemented in 36% of cases and uncemented in 54%. The femoral component was revised in 48% of cases. Preoperative bone defects were assessed according to Paprosky classification [20]: type 2A (nine hips); type 2B (31 hips); type 2C (20 hips); type3A (25 hips): and type 3B (11 hips).

A standard operative technique was employed in all cases. Most patients were operated on by the senior author (A.C.-M.), and, in most cases (86%), the anterolateral approach was used. A posterolateral approach with extended femoral osteotomy was carried out (14%) when the femoral component had to be revised, as well. The acetabular cavity was always meticulously prepared. Bone grafting was performed in 38 cases (39.5%; 29 allograft, 7 autologous, and 2 combined auto-allograft). The BSAC was adapted to the acetabular defect and surrounding bone after the bone graft was placed to fill the defect. In all cases, the cage was placed by driving its inferior flange into the inferior acetabulum so that it lodged in the ischium. This trick is not easy. In our series inferior flange was finally, lodged outside the ischium in more than 35% of cases. The superior flange was fixed to the

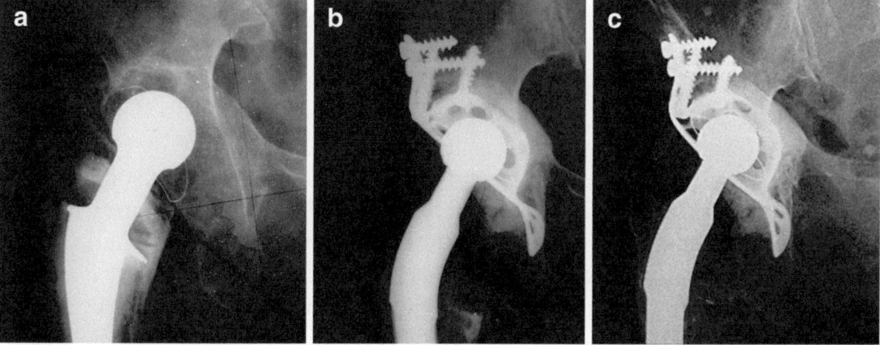


**Fig. 8.2** (**a**) Radiograph showing aseptic loosening both components in a 69 year-old woman with rheumatoid arthritis. (**b**) Post-operative radiograph with a BSAC without graft and Wagner stem. (**c**) X-ray control at 12 years. Good clinical situation

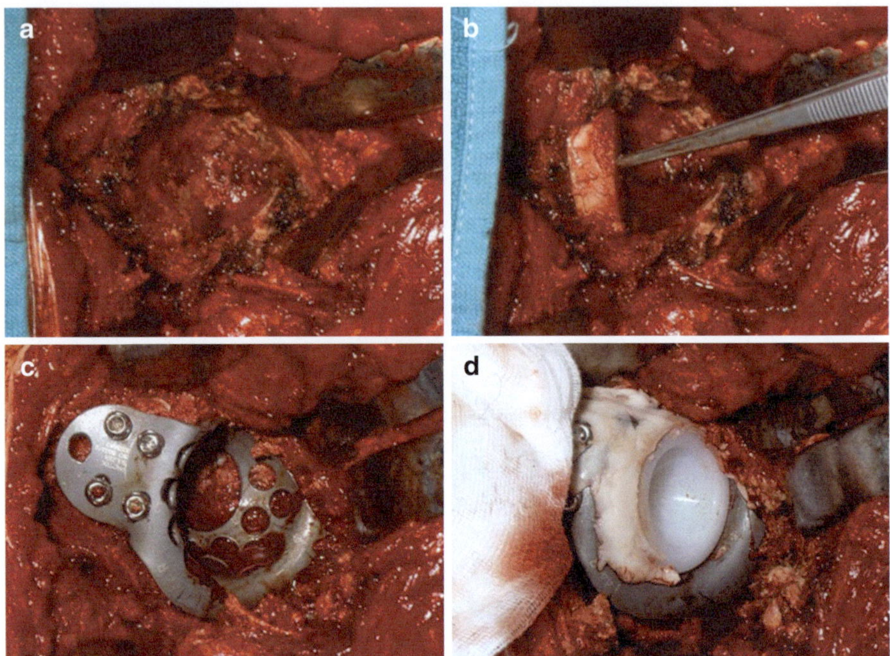


**Fig. 8.3** (**a**) The failed acetabular component is removed and the acetabular bed was thoroughly debrided until achieving healthy and bleeding bone beds. (**b**) Bone grafting. The specific type of graft used is determined by the shape and size of the defect. (**c**) Cage placement. (**d**) Cementing all-poly into the cage. The socket can be oriented slightly independant of the cage position

outside of the ilium with 3–6 cortical screws. A size 44 antiprotrusio cage was implanted in 38 hips, a size 50 in 51 hips, a size 56 in 3, and the largest, a size 62, in 4 hips. An all-polyethylene cup (28- and 32-mm diameter low profile UHMW polyethylene cups; Sulzer Orthopaedics, Baar, Switzerland) was cemented into the cage (Fig. 8.3). The patients were mobilised after 3–7 days depending on their bone quality, and remained on crutches for not less than 3 months. Antibiotic prophylaxis (1 g cefazolin every 6 h) was administered for 48 h. Routine preventive measures for thromboembolism were employed under the strict protocol of our hospital Haematology Department.

Clinical results were evaluated using the Merle d'Aubigné-Postel score [21]. Patients were asked to express their subjective opinion on the outcome of the operation as in Johnston et al. [22]. Clinical failure was defined as re-revision or removal of the cup, pain (grade 4 or worse), or both. Thigh pain was not considered evidence of clinical acetabular failure, whereas groin and buttock pain were recorded as signs of clinical failure resulting from acetabular loosening [23]. Any radiolucent line around the cup was assessed according to the three DeLee-Charnley zones [24].

Of 68 cages, three had to be removed: two for deep infection and the other for aseptic loosening after 7 years and it was revised with another BSAC. The mean preoperative Merle D'Aubigné score of 8.8 points had increased to 15.1 points at final follow-up. Differences between the preoperative and postoperative scores as evaluated with the Wilcoxon test for paired samples were highly significant ($P < 0.001$) for both for the overall Merle D'Aubigné score as well as for pain, hip motion, and walking ability. The results were excellent and good in 69% of the hips, regular in 22% and fair in 9%. In addition, 46 patients stated that they were very satisfied, 13 were satisfied, and 6 were dissatisfied. Overall, about 71% of patients reported satisfactory results. Radiographic analysis showed that the mean inclination of the antiprotrusio cage was 47.3° (range, 27–72°) after implantation and that the mean inclination at follow-up was 46.9°. The mean proximal and medial migrations of the antiprotrusio cage were 0.8 mm and 0.9 mm respectively. Using the Nunn technique [25] the hip rotation centre was descended an average of 4.3 mm and lateralised an average of 1.3 mm in the post revision study. In the most severe cases (Paprosky 2C, 3A and 3B) the respective corrections were 7.8 mm and 0.8 mm. Broken screws were seen in two cases and an inferior flange fracture in one case. Although both are criteria of definite loosening, there was no cage migration nor had pain been reported. Three cages were considered loose according to Gill criteria [26], indicating a mechanical failure index of 6.1% for the whole series at the end of follow-up. Although graft remodelling is difficult to evaluate with the antiprotrusio cage, according to Gerbert criteria [27], 76.3% of the grafts appeared to have incorporated, 21.6% seemed not to have changed and 2.1% showed resorption. The Kaplan-Meier survivorship analysis [28], using estimated radiological loosening and revision for mechanical failure of the antiprotrusio cage as the survivorship endpoint, showed a survival rate of 92.4% (95% confidence interval, 85.1–99.8%) after 13 years for the antiprotrusio cage.

There have been six acute infections (6.2%), which were treated with debridement and antibiotics without further problems in four cases while two cases required two- stage revision. There were 11 dislocations (11.4%), 6 during the first 3 months and 5 late dislocations. Nine were treated by closed reduction and two needed open reduction. One patient developed recurrent dislocation, which was treated by replacing the socket with a constrained cemented component. There was another revision for aseptic loosening of the polyethylene socket after 1 year that was revised with another cemented socket. There were six sciatic nerve palsies, three temporary and three definitive.

## Discussion

Bone defects determine the surgical technique in acetabular revision surgery. Cementless cups have been widely used in revision surgery for these patients, and several series have reported good results [29–32]. However, other series have reported poor results for revisions associated with massive bone defects greater than 50% (Paprosky grade 3B) [33, 34–36]. Various techniques have been described for managing large acetabular defects, including placement of an large uncemented acetabular component [37], placement a cup at a high hip centre [38], oblong or bilobed cups [39–41] and impacted bone graft and cement [3, 4]. Antiprotusio cages, one of the systems used for handling these situations, have been used for a long time, especially in Europe, and the long-term experience to provide sufficient data to explore the results and define their current indications even though comparison of cage results is difficult because patient populations are mixed, are treated with different devices and present varying degrees of bone loss.

Berry and Müller [2] report a 24% failure rate 5 years after implantation, but, bone grafts were not used in the early series. Gill et al. [26, 42] published on the use of acetabular reinforcement devices. Their most recent study included 37 hips in 35 patients. Bulk structural allograft was used in association with 30 BSAC and seven Müller reinforcement rings. The mean follow-up period was 7.1 years. Excellent or good patient satisfaction was reported by 91.9%. No survivorship data were given. The BSAC can be used with morcellised or bulk graft, protecting the graft from forces which may contribute to its failure. All series report the best results using metal rings in association with grafting [2, 16, 42–44]. Healing and probable graft incorporation, without significant resorption, have usually been seen [17, 45]. A recent study by van der Linde [46] reported the outcome of using ring or cage devices. The series included 42 hips in 40 patients. Using a criterion similar to ours, the authors used some type of reinforcement device for all acetabular revisions whenever there was deficient acetabular stock, including type I and II (AAOS) defects. They reported four failures: three due to infection, and one due to aseptic loosening. Their survival was 90.5% at a mean follow-up of 10 years. After an average follow-up period of 7.3 years, Winter et al. [47] observed no cage loosening or migration and incorporation of the cancellous allograft into host bone in 38 cases. They concluded that a close fit between the graft and the acetabulum in addition to mechanical stability was crucial to their successful results. Recently, Regis et al. [48] have published excellent results in one of the series with greater follow-up in patients with severe Paprosky 3A and 3B defects. The cumulative survival rates at 18.9 years with removal for any reason or X-ray migration of the cage and aseptic or radiographic loosening as the end points were 80.0% and 84.6% respectively.

Postoperative implant instability is more frequent after prosthesis revision, reaching 23%. Dual mobility technology has proven its efficacy in preventing dislocations. Schneider et al. [49] suggest an original technique for surgical acetabular revision associating acetabular reconstruction antiprotrusio cages and cemented dual mobility cups. In their series had a dislocation rate of 10.4%. A constrained cemented cup was suggested in selected cases [29, 50].

Using the Nunn technique [25], the hip rotation centre was descended an average of 4.3 mm and lateralised an average of 1.3 mm in our series. Overall, and only considering the most severe cases (Paprosky 2C, 3A and 3B defects) the respective corrections were 7.8 mm and 0.8 mm. Although no attempt was made to implant the component at the level of the anatomical centre of rotation, there was an improvement in the vertical hip centre. In their series, Schneider et al. [49] obtain better corrections although using different reconstruction devices. A mean lowering

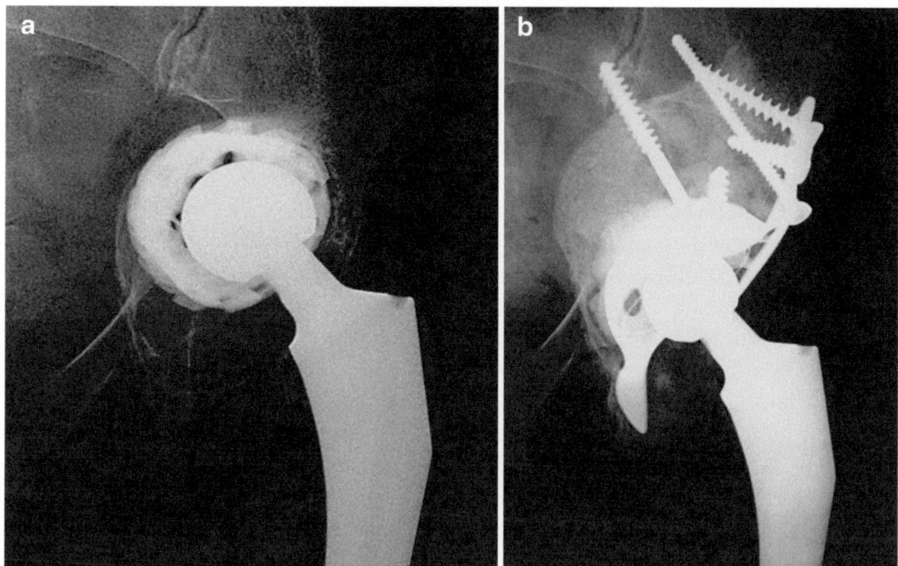


**Fig. 8.4** (**a**) Anteroposterior radiograph showing a failed THA with pelvic discontinuity in a 72 year–old man, 12 years after surgery. (**b**) 5 years after revision with BSAC and morcellised bone allograft

of 15.6 mm and a 9.4 mm lateralization compared to the preoperative position. Our findings have also been supported by other series and have lead some authors to use BSAC in situations of pelvic discontinuity [2, 17]. Pelvic discontinuity is always difficult to solve. In the current series four patients had pelvic discontinuity; acetabular defect size was estimated to choose an appropriate anti-protrusion cage to span the defect from ilium to ischium and the defect filled with morcellised allograft (Fig. 8.4). Bulk allografts and the Burch-Schneider cage were effective in the management of 18 pelvic discontinuities and associated periprosthetic bone deficiency, with a cumulative 72.2% survival rate at 16.6 years [51]. All patients show a good result at the end of the study period.

There are few references to models other than the Burch-Schneider antiprotusio cage. Recently, Vigdorchik et al. [52] reports a series of 42 Contour cages with a follow-up of 42.5 months. The clinical outcomes are similar to those with the BSAC, with comparable rates in regard to complications, loosening, and failure [53]. The biomechanical analysis of retrieved antiprotrusio cages (APC) gives interesting with radiographic and clinical data to determine which factors influence or predict APC failure. Hosny et al. [54] reports 100% revision free surviving hip at mean follow-up of a 49 months using a GAP II cage and impaction bone grafting.

The most important problem with cages is that they are not made of a material that allows osseo-integration and, consequently, there is a high incidence of hardware failure due to screw breakage or ischial flange migration [50, 55]. New materials, like tantalum, could provide greater long-term success than the traditional antiprotusio cages because they would permit bony ingrowth and so achieve stability [8–11]. Early and mid-term results with this material are encouraging; however, there are no long-term results as yet [56, 57].

Today, it is difficult to propose the current indications for these new implants but we would suggest that antiprotrusio cages are a resourceful option for cases in which there can be no confidence in initial or secondary stability of a reconstruction with porous-coated uncemented devices, and there is pelvic discontinuity, a need to protect allografts, an irradiated host bone or the patient is elderly subjects with little functional strain.

Based on our long-term results, we can conclude that use of a BSAC in acetabular revision surgery provides a viable treatment option for the reconstruction of different bone defects, including pelvic discontinuity, it has proven clinical efficacy and good mid to long term survival. Antiprotrusio cages are a valuable tool providing successful stability at mid and long-term reconstruction of severe acetabular bone deficiencies in revision hip replacement, but always providing that three basic principles are maintained in their use: initial mechanical stability, restoration of the hip centre of rotation and the use bone grafting in the acetabular bone deficiencies.

**Funding Support** No benefits in any form have been received or will be received from a commercial party related directly to the subject of this article. No funds were received in support of this study.

## References

1. Pagnano MW, Hanssen AD, Lewallen DG, Shaughnessy WJ. The effect of superior placement of the acetabular component on the rate of loosening after total hip arthroplasty: long-term results in patients who have Crowe type-II congenital dysplasia of the hip. J Bone Joint Surg Am. 1996;78A:1004–14.
2. Berry DJ, Müller ME. Revision arthroplasty using an atiprotusio cage for masive acetabular bone deficiency. J Bone Joint Surg Br. 1992;74B:711–5.
3. Slooff TJJH, Huiskes R, Van Horn J, Lemmens AJ. Bone grafting in total hip replacement for acetabular protrusion. Acta Orthop Scand. 1984;55:593–66.
4. Slooff TJJH, Schimmel JW, Buma P. Cemented fixation with bone grafts. Orthop Clin North Am. 1993;24:667–77.
5. Hungerford DS, Jones LC. The rationale of cementless revision of cemented arthroplasty failures. Clin Orthop Relat Res. 1988;235:12–24.
6. Müller ME. Acetabular revision. In: The hip. Proc 9th meeting of the hip society. St Louis: CV Mosby; 1981. p. 45–56.
7. Hanssen AD, Lewallen DG. Modular acetabular augments: composite void fillers. Orthopedics. 2005;28:971–2.
8. Nehme A, Lewallen DG, Hanssen AD. Modular porous metal augments for treatment of severe acetabular bone loss during revision hip arthroplasty. Clin Orthop Relat Res. 2004;429:201–8.
9. Weeden SH, Schmidt RH. The use of tantalum porous implants for Paprosky 3A and 3B defects. J Arthroplast. 2007;22:151–5.

10. Flecher A, Sporer S, Paprosky W. Management of severe bone loss in acetabular revision using a trabecular metal shell. J Arthroplast. 2008;23:949–55.
11. Lakstein D, Backstein D, Safir O, Kosashvili Y, Gross AE. Trabecular metal™ cups for acetabular defects with 50% or loss host bone cement. Clin Orthop Relat Res. 2009;467:2318–24.
12. Schneider R. Total prosthetic replacement of the hip: a biomechanical concept and its consequences. Toronto: Hans Huber; 1989.
13. Berry DJ. Antiprotusio cages for acetabular revision. Clin Orthop Relat Res. 2004;420:106–12.
14. Possai KW, Dorr LD, McPherson EJ. Metal ring supports for deficient acetabular bone in total hip replacement. In: Pritchard DJ, editor. Instr course lect, vol. 45. Rosemont: AAOS; 1996. p. 161–9.
15. Peters CL, Curtain M, Samuelson KM. Acetabular revision with the Burch-Schneider antiprotusio cage and cancellous allograft bone. J Arthroplast. 1995;10:307–12.
16. Rosson J, Schatzker J. The use of reinforcement rings to reconstruct deficient acetabula. J Bone Joint Surg Br. 1992;74B:270–5.
17. Berry DJ. Acetabular anti-protusio rings in revision total hip arthroplasty. Sem Arthroplasty. 1995;6:68–75.
18. Gross AE, Wong P, Saleh KJ. Don't throw away the ring: Indications and use. J Arthroplast. 2002;17(4 Suppl 1):162–6.
19. Lavernia CJ, Cook CC, Hernandez RA, Sierra RJ, Rossi MD. Neurovascular injuries in acetabular reconstruction cage surgery: an anatomical study. J Arthroplast. 2007 Jan;22(1):124–32.
20. Paprosky WG, Perona PG, Lawrence JM. Acetabular defect classification and surgical reconstruction in revision arthroplasty. A 6-year follow-up evaluation. J Arthroplast. 1994;9:33–44.
21. Merle d'Aubigné R, Postel M. Functional results of hip arthroplasty with acrylic prosthesis. J Bone Joint Surg Am. 1954;36A:451–75.
22. Johnston RC, Fitzgerald RH Jr, Harris WH, Poss R, Muller ME, Sledge CB. Clinical and radiographic evaluation of total hip replacement: a standard system of terminology for reporting results. J Bone Joint Surg Am. 1990;72A:161–8.
23. Pupparo F, Engh CA. Comparison of porous-threaded and smooth-threaded acetabular components of identical design. Two-to four-year results. Clin Orthop Relat Res. 1991;271:201–6.
24. DeLee JG, Charnley J. Radiological demarcation of cemented sockets in total hip replacement. Clin Orthop Relat Res. 1976;121:20–32.
25. Nunn D, Freeman MAR, Hill PF, Evans SJW. The measurement of migration of the acetabular component of hip prosthesis. J Bone Joint Surg Br. 1989;71B:629–31.
26. Gill TJ, Sledge JB, Muller ME. The Burch-Schneider anti-protrusio cage in revision total hip arthroplasty: indications, principles and long-term results. J Bone Joint Surg Br. 1998;80B:946–53.
27. Gerber SD, Harris WH. Femoral head autografting to augment acetabular deficiency in patients requiring total hip replacement: a minimum five-year and an average seven-year follow-up study. J Bone Joint Surg. 1986;68A:1241–8.
28. Kaplan EL, Meier P. Nonparametric estimation from incomplete observation. J Am Stat Assoc. 1958;53:457–81.
29. Udomkiat P, Dorr LD, Won YY, Longjohn D, Wan Z. Technical factors for success with metal ring acetabular reconstruction. J Arthroplast. 2001;16:961–9.
30. Padgett DE, Kull L, Rosenberg A, Sumner DR, Galante JO. Revision of the acetabular component without cement after total hiparthroplasty. Three to six-year follow-up. J Bone Joint Surg Am. 1993;75A:663–73.
31. Tanzer M, Drucker D, Jasty M, McDonald M, Harris WH. Revision of the acetabular component with an uncemented Harris-Galante porous-coated prosthesis. J Bone Joint Surg Am. 1992;74A:987–94.
32. Paprosky WG, Magnus RE. Principles of bone grafting in revision total hip arthroplasty: acetabular technique. Clin Orthop Relat Res. 1994;298:147–55.
33. Kwong LM, Jasty M, Harris WH. High failure rate of bulk femoral head allografts in total hip acetabular reconstructions at 10 years. J Arthroplast. 1993;8:341–6.

34. Hooten JP Jr, Engh CA Jr, Engh CA. Failure of structural acetabular allografts in cementless revision hip arthroplasty. J Bone Joint Surg Br. 1994;76B:419–22.
35. Garbuz D, Morsi E, Gross A. Revision of the acetabular component of a total hip arthroplasty with a massive structural allograft. Study with a minimum five-year follow-up. J Bone Joint Surg Am. 1996;78A:693–7.
36. Garcia-Cimbrelo E. Porous-coated cementless acetabular cups in revision surgery. A 6- to 11-year follow-up study. J Arthroplast. 1999;14:397–406.
37. Brooks PJ. The jumbo cup: the 95% solution. Orthopedics. 2008;31:971–2.
38. Hendricks KJ, Harris WH. High placement of noncemented acetabular components in revision total hip arthroplasty. A concise follow-up, at a minimum of fifteen years, of a previous report. J Bone Joint Surg Am. 2006;88A:2231–6.
39. Berry DJ, Sutherland CJ, Trousdale RT, Colwell CW Jr, Chandler HP, Ayres D, et al. Bilobed oblong porous coated acetabular components in revision total hip arthroplasty. Clin Orthop Relat Res. 2000;371:154–60.
40. Chen WM, Engh CA Jr, Hooper RH Jr, McAuley JP, Engh CA. Acetabular revision with use of a bilobed component inserted without cement in patients who have acetabular bone-stock deficiency. J Bone Joint Surg Am. 2000;82A:197–206.
41. Moskal JT, Shen FH. The use of bilobed porous-coated acetabular components without structural bone graft for type III acetabular defects in revision total hip arthroplasty. J Arthroplast. 2004;19:867–73.
42. Gill TJ, Sledge JB, Muller ME. The management of sever acetabular bone loos using structural allograft and acetabular reinforcement devices. J Arthroplast. 2000;15:1–7.
43. Zehntner MK, Ganz R. Midterm results (5.5–10 years) of acetabular allograft reconstruction with the acetabular reinforcement ring during total hip revision. J Arthroplast. 1994;9:469–79.
44. Watchtl SW, Jung M, Jakob RP, et al. The Burch-Schneider anti-protusio cage in acetabular revisión surgery; a mean follow-up of 12 years. J Arthroplast. 2000;15:959–63.
45. Pieringer H, Auersperg V, Böhler N. Reconstruction of severe acetabular bone-deficiency: the Burch-Schneider antiprotrusio cage in primary and revision total hip arthroplasty. J Arthroplast. 2006;21(4):489–96.
46. van der Linde M, Tonino A. Acetabular revisión with impacted grafting and a reinforcement ring: 42 patients followed for a mean of 10 years. Acta Orthop Scand. 2001;72:221–7.
47. Winter E, Piert M, Volkmann R, Maurer F, Eingartner C, Weise K, et al. Allogeneic cancellous bone graft and a Burch-Schneider ring for acetabular reconstruction in revision hip arthroplasty. J Bone Joint Surg Am. 2001;83-A:862–7.
48. Regis D, Sandri A, Ingrid Bonetti I. Acetabular reconstruction with the Burch-Schneider antiprotrusio cage and bulk allografts: minimum 10-year follow-up results. Biomed Res Int. 2014;2014:194076., 9 p.
49. Schneider L, Philippot R, Boyer B, Farizon F. Revision total hip arthroplasty using a reconstruction cage device and a cemented dual mobility cup. Orthop Traumatol Surg Res. 2011;97:807–13.
50. Goodman S, Saastamoinen H, Shasha N, Gross A. Complicationsof ilioischial reconstruction rings in revision total hiparthroplasty. J Arthroplast. 2004;19:436–46.
51. Regis D, Sandri A, Bonetti I, Bortolami O, Bartolozzi P. A minimum of 10-year follow-up of the Burch-Schneider cage and bulk allografts for the revision of pelvic discontinuity. J Arthroplast. 2012;27(6):1057–63.
52. Vigdorchik JM, Yoon RS, Gilbert SL, Lipman JD, Bostrom MP. Retrieval and radiographic analysis of the Contour antiprotusio cage. Hip Int. 2017;27(4):378–81.
53. Bostrom MP, Lehman AP, Buly RL, Lyman S, Nestor BJ. Acetabular revision with the Contour antiprotrusio cage: 2- to 5-year follow up. Clin Orthop Relat Res. 2006;453:188–94.
54. Hosny HAH, El-Bakoury A, Fekry H, Keenan J. Mid-term results of graft augmentation prosthesis II cage and impacted allograft bone in revision hip arthroplasty. J Arthroplasty. 2017. pii: S0883–5403(17)31065–3.

55. Gross AE, Goodman S. The current role of structural grafts and cages in revision arthroplasty of the hip. Clin Orthop Relat Res. 2004;429:193–200.
56. Beckmann NA, Weiss S, Klotz MC, Gondan M, Jaeger S, Bitsch RG. Loosening after acetabular revision: comparison of trabecular metal and reinforcement rings. Asystematic review. J Arthroplasty. 2014;29(1):229–35.
57. Mäkinen T, Kuzyk P, Safir O, Backstein D, Gross AE. Role of cages in revision arthroplasty of the acetabulum. J Bone Joint Surg Am. 2016;98:233–42.

# Chapter 9
# Revision Arthroplasty of the Acetabulum Using Structural Allograft and a Cage: State-of-the-Art

**E. Gibon, L. Kerboull, and M. Hamadouche**

## Introduction

The demand for total lower limb joint replacement is increasing at a staggering rate. Data from past studies [1, 2] and projection studies [3, 4] shows that the number of revision total hip arthroplasty (THA) will increase 137% over the next 25 years in the US. Similar trends have been observed in the UK and Australia [5, 6]. Among revision THA, Bozic et al. [7] have shown that acetabular component revision was the third most common procedure (12.7%) after femoral component revision (13.2%) and all-component revision (41.1%). Major breakthroughs have been made in manufacturing new bearing surfaces. Among these, ceramics and first- and second-generation highly crossed-linked polyethylene (HXLPE) are now available for primary THAs dramatically decreasing wear and osteolysis [8–11]. However, although markedly mitigated, osteolysis is still responsible for up to 11% of the revision THAs [7, 12]. DeLee and Charnely created a way to locate osteolysis on the acetabular side by dividing it in three different zones [13]. This classification is still in use today. Two lines, one vertical and one horizontal, cross at the center of the prosthetic femoral head. Zone I is superolateral, zone III is inferomedial and zone II is in between. Chiang et al. [14] have shown that the pattern of osteolysis differs between cemented and cementless acetabular component. For cemented components, osteolysis predominantly occurs in DeLee zones III and I whereas it is mostly observed in DeLee zones II and III for cementless components.

The severity of the osteolysis can be categorized through different classifications. The Engh classification focuses on the integrity of the rim and the bed [15]. The Gustilo and Pasternak classification is based on the integrity of the acetabular

E. Gibon (✉) · L. Kerboull · M. Hamadouche
Clinical Orthopaedic Research Center, Centre Hospitalo-Universitaire Cochin-Port Royal, Paris, France
e-mail: moussah@club-intrnet.fr



E. García-Rey, E. García-Cimbrelo (eds.), *Acetabular Revision Surgery in Major Bone Defects*, https://doi.org/10.1007/978-3-319-98596-1_9

walls [16]. D'Antonio et al. described a classification based on acetabular segmental and cavitary deficiencies with special types for pelvic discontinuity and arthrodesis as well [17]. This classification is now known as the AAOS classification [18]. Gross et al. [19] described a classification with contained/uncontained bone loss including the percentage of bone defect of the acetabulum. The Saleh classification [20] describes bone defects after removal of the acetabulum implant. Finally, the Paprosky classification [21] relies on the presence or absence of key supporting structures of the acetabulum. Those classifications are further detailed in Chap. 2.

Reconstruction techniques of the damaged acetabulum are guided by the extension of the bone loss. Studies have shown that when a contact between a viable bleeding host bone greater than 50% of a porous-coated acetabular implant and initial mechanical stability can be obtained, then a reliable osseointegration is expected [22–26]. On the other hand, when 50% of contact cannot be achieved between host bone and the acetabular implant, studies showed that an acetabular reinforcement ring is indicated [27–29].

In this chapter, we will be reviewing different techniques of reconstruction of the severely damaged acetabulum (Paprosky III) following primary THA. First, we will discuss the use of a structural allograft only. Second, we will present techniques using a structural allograft and an acetabular reinforcement ring with proximal fixation. And in the last section, we will review the use of a structural allograft and an acetabular reinforcement ring with proximal and distal fixation.

## Structural Allografts Only

The use of a structural allograft alone for acetabular reconstruction in revision THAs has been studied since the 1990s. Different results have been reported depending on the severity of the initial bone loss. The major concern is the fate of the allograft with subsequent risk of failure due to resorption and collapse leading to implant loosening. When used for minor acetabular bone defects (involving less than 50% of the acetabulum), results are controversial. Morsi et al. [30] reported a successful rate of 86% at mean of 7.1 years, Woodgate et al. [31] showed a cup survival of 80.6% at almost 10 years and Lee et al. [32] had survival of 61% and 55% at 15- and 20 years, respectively.

For major acetabular deficiencies (more than 50% of the acetabulum) a structural allograft needs to be use. This allograft is provided by a bone bank and can be either a femoral head, as described by Harris [33, 34] or part of the distal femur [35]. Early on, Harris and colleagues warned of catastrophic failures. Jasty and Harris [36] reported a failure rate of 32% at 6 years with a mean time to failure of 5.4 years. Failure was attributed to marked resorption of the graft in all but one of the failure cases. Interestingly, they also showed that the extent of the acetabular cover provided by the allograft had a positive correlation with acetabular implant loosening. Moreover, the more severe the resorption was, the more frequent the loosening was. Similarly, in a minimum 2 year follow-up study, Pollock et al. [37] showed 28.6% of migration and 30% of gross loosening. Further studies [38, 39] confirmed early catastrophic failures. Paprosky et al. [40] emphasized those outcomes showing as high as 70% failures at a mean of 5.1 years in revision THAs with Paprosky IIIB acetabular defects. Garbuz et al. [41] in a series of 38 hips showed successful results at a mean of 7.5 years when an acetabular reinforcement device supported the structural allograft whereas most of the reconstructions without such a device failed. Therefore they advocated the use of an acetabular reinforcement ring in association with a structural allograft. Latest reports showed a survival of 74% and 72% at a mean 10- and 21 years, respectively, for Paprosky type IIIA acetabular defects revised with a structural allograft only [42, 43].

## Cup Cage

This technique was first developed by Hanssen and Lewallen and reported in 2005 [44]. It consists in a trabecular metal (TM) acetabular shell and an ilioischial anti-protusio cage placed over the cup (full cup-cage reconstruction) (Fig. 9.1). The technique has been later modified and can be used in its half cup-cage version. It is somehow the reverse technique of a cage placed first in the acetabulum and then a cup is cemented into it. The rational of this construct was based on the fact that no bone ingrowth could be achieved into the cage whereas a TM acetabular shell allows and promotes bone ingrowth when placed first. Kosashvili et al. [45] reported on a series of 26 cases of acetabular revision including 24 patients with pelvic discontinuity (PD) and severe acetabular bone loss (a mean of 15.8% contact with bleeding host bone). After filling the defects with morsellised bone graft, the cup-cage construct was put in place and a polyethylene liner cemented into the cage. At a mean of 3.7-year follow-up, the authors reported three (11.5%) migrations. Later on, the same group presented an extended follow-up study of the initial series and compared it with a group of PD cases reconstructed with a conventional cage [46]. At a mean follow-up of 6.8 years and 5.75 years for the cup-cage and conventional cage

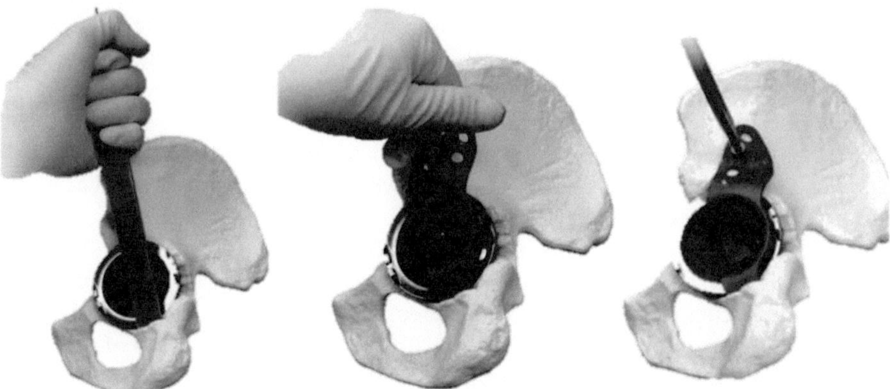

**Fig. 9.1** The cup-cage construct. (Courtesy of Zimmer-Biomet)

groups respectively, the survivorship was significantly different. The cup-cage group had a survivorship of 87.2% whereas the conventional cage group had a survivorship of 49.9%. Four migrations occurred in the cup-cage group and three of them were revised. Similar results were reported by Amenabar et al. [47] who treated Gross type IV (uncontained loss of bone stock involving >50% of the acetabulum and affecting both columns) and Gross type V (PD) acetabular deficiencies. The authors showed a 10-year survival rate of 85%. As stated earlier, the full cup-cage construct can be modified to a half cup-cage construct by removing the inferior flange of the cage. This evolution was reported by Sculco et al. [48]. The reasons for such an evolution, as mentioned by the authors, are numerous: (1) slotting the ischial flange of the cage into the ischium may lead to a PD, (2) the ischium might be obliterated and (3) the risk of damaging the sciatic nerve while dissecting the ischium. To investigate the outcomes of the half cup-cage construct, the authors compared 27 revision THAs performed with this technique to 30 revision THAs with the full cup-cage construct. Acetabular defects were graded as Paprosky IIB through IIIB including 60% of PD. No significant differences were found between the two groups. Two sciatic nerve injuries occurred in the full cup-cage group whereas none were reported in the half cup-cage group. At a mean follow-up of 4.6 years the survivorship was 83% and 96% for full and half cup-cage groups, respectively. Although a relatively new technique, the cup-cage construct appears to be a viable and reliable method for revision THAs with major acetabular defects.

## Proximal Fixation

### *The Müller Ring*

The Müller ring became available in the 1980s and is still in use by some teams across the world. The Müller ring can be used either in primary or revision THA. The design of the ring is cup-shaped with a flange around the posterior two-thirds of the cup edge. The ring accepts screw fixation on its superior lip. Three to five 6.5 fully threaded cancellous screws are generally necessary. To ensure a strong fixation, the ring must have support from the posterior pillar, the medial wall and the superior acetabular lip [49]. Therefore, bone grafting is most of the time mandatory to achieve these requirements. The literature is very scarce regarding the use of the Müller ring in revision THA with severe bone loss. Early studies [49, 50] showed good and promising results but the follow-up was limited to 3–4 years and accurate description of the extension of bone loss in revision cases was absent. Therefore it is uncertain to draw any conclusions from those studies. Later, Zehntner and Ganz [51] investigated the outcomes of the Müller ring in AAOS type III (combined cavitary and segmental defects) acetabular defect associated with structural allograft from a fresh frozen femoral head. Their results showed that at a mean of 7.2 years of follow-up, 45% of the component failed and migrated. The authors concluded that additional internal fixation should be used in case of AAOS type III defects.

Thereafter, Korovesis et al. [52] showed no failure at a mean of 9-year of follow-up after revision THA using the Müller ring and bone allograft. However, their series was very small with only eight hips having AAOS type III defects. Similar results were found by van de Linde and Tonino [53] but again, their series was limited to 13 cases of AAOS type III acetabular defects and they randomly used either the Müller ring or the Burch Shneider cage. Schlegel et al. [54] followed a series of 164 revision THAs reconstructed with fresh frozen femoral head allograft and the Müller ring. Among them, 56% had AAOS type III acetabular defects and 5% had AAOS type IV acetabular defects (pelvic discontinuity). The survival rate was 98% at 5 years but no difference was made between regarding the severity of the acetabular defects. Massin et al. [55] used the Müller ring in combination with structural allograft to treat segmental or important cavitary roof defects. Using aseptic loosening as the end point, the authors showed a survival rate of 55% at 11 years. They reported that mechanical failures were related to the resorption of structural bone grafts.

The Müller ring has not been extensively investigated to treat large acetabular defects. From the small data available in the literature, the Müller ring appears to be insufficient for revision THAs with severe acetabular defects.

## Proximal and Distal Fixation

### *The Ganz Ring*

The design of the Ganz ring is similar to the Müller ring. The additional feature of the Ganz ring is an inferior hook meant to be placed under the inferior margin of the acetabulum providing a reliable way to restore the anatomic center of the hip (Fig. 9.2). The Ganz ring was initially used for primary THAs in developmental dysplasia of the hip [56]. The first study of its use for revision THAs was performed by Siebenrock et al. [57] in Germany, a group including Dr. Ganz, the designer of the ring. The authors revised 57 hips, among them, 36 hips had enough data to be incorporated in the study and most of them (n = 19) had a combined segmental and cavitary defect and three cases had a pelvic discontinuity. At a mean follow-up of 11.4 years, 8% of the hips undergone re-revision, two for aseptic loosening and one for septic loosening. Later on, Gerber et al. [58] used the Ganz ring for AAOS Type II, III and IV acetabular defects. Fifty hips were analyzed and defects were filled with morselized allograft bone. Their results showed seven failures due to aseptic loosening and the survivorship at 10 years was 81%. Further analysis showed that inadequate fixation of the ring at the revision was the only significant predictor of failure and the authors also concluded that the ring might not be appropriate for AAOS Type IV defects or segmental defects affecting the medial wall. Likewise, a Japanese team [59] evaluated the outcomes of the Ganz ring associated with bone allograft in 30 revision THAs. They used their own acetabular defect classification, which makes it difficult to compare to other studies. Moreover, they introduced a

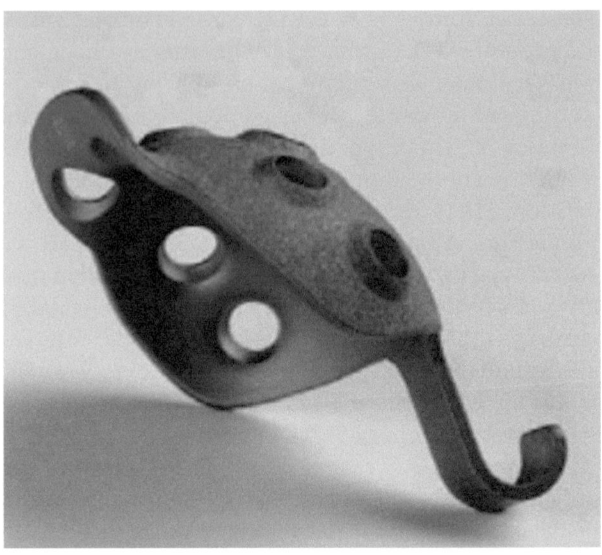

**Fig. 9.2** The Ganz® ring. (Courtesy of Zimmer-Biomet)

special technique for massive bone defect, which consisted in screwing two or three cancellous screws ("strut screws") in the allograft prior to installation of the ring. The authors reported five aspetic loosenings but none of them required re-revision and the survival rate using loosening, as the end point was 80.2% at 10 years. As previously shown by Gerber et al. the Japanese team also highlighted the critical importance of a reliable primary stability of the ring as 75% of the hips with mal-positioning of the ring (hook out of position) failed. Lately, Hourscht et al. [60] investigated the outcomes of the Ganz ring with structural allograft in revision THAs with AAOS Type III and IV acetabular defects. Additionally, the Types IV were reinforced with a plate. The authors showed that the AAOS type of acetabular defect was the only independent risk factor of failure according to a multivariate Cox regression; the Type IV being at a significant higher risk for failure. The 5-year survival rate using revision for any reason was 86% and 57% in Type III and IV, respectively. Therefore, the authors concluded the Ganz ring should not be used when there is a pelvic discontinuity.

Taken together, these data show that the Ganz ring is reliable for minor acetabular defects but should not be used for AAOS Type IV acetabular defects or segmental defects affecting the medial wall.

## *The Kerboull Acetabular Reinforcement Device and Its Evolution*

In the early 1970s, at the authors' institution, pelvic discontinuities associated with acetabular bone loss were present in some cases of metal on metal total hip arthroplasty. To fix the fracture and implant a new socket in one stage, in 1974 Marcel

**Table 9.1** Comparative data regarding the Kerboull device used in major acetabular defects

| Studies (authors) | Year | AAOS defect type (number of hip) | Mean follow-up (years) | Device used in the study | Survival/end point[a] |
|---|---|---|---|---|---|
| Kim et al. [62] | 2015 | n = 40<br>III (37); II (3) | 12.8 | KT + bulk allograft + HA | 94.9%/revision for loosening (type III) |
| Hori et al. [63] | 2011 | n = 32<br>IV (3); III (29) | 7.5 | KT + bulk or morselised allograft | 92.3%/revision for loosening or rx loosening |
| Akiyama et al. [64] | 2011 | n = 40<br>III (23); II (17) | 6.7 | KT + bulk or morselised allograft | 87%/revision for loosening or rx loosening |
| Okano et al. [65] | 2010 | n = 31<br>III (29); II (2) | 6.3 | KT + bulk or morselised allograft | NA |
| Kawanabe et al. [66] | 2007 | n = 42<br>IV (1); III (28)<br>II (13) | 8.7 | KT + bulk or morselised allograft | 53%/failure of acetabular implant (morsellised allograft)<br>82%/failure of acetabular implant (bulk allograft) |
| Tanaka et al. [61] | 2003 | n = 21<br>III (16); II (5) | 5.3 | KT + HA ± morselised allograft | NA |
| Kerboull et al. [67] | 2000 | n = 60<br>IV (12); III (48) | 8 | Kerboull cage (original) + bulk allograft | 92.1%/loosening of the acetabular implant |

[a]Survival at the mean follow-up of the series
*NA* non available, *KT* Kerboull-Type device, *HA* hydroxyapatite, *rx* radiographic

Kerboull conceived a special acetabular armature, hemispheric cross shaped, with four arms, an inferior hook, and a superior plate. First intended for this indication, this device was used later as a guide and reinforcement with bulky frozen femoral head allografts in almost all acetabular reconstructions. This device can also be employed in primary THAs when dealing with fragile bone or altered anatomy such as is frequently the case following an acetabular fracture or a pelvic osteotomy. Series of reconstruction using the original device have been mainly reported from France, whereas a modification to its design has been made by Chiaki Tanaka [61] to adapt to Japan with favorable results. It should be emphasized that most of the early failures are related to inadequate surgical technique. Comparative data regarding the Kerboull device used in major acetabular defects are seen in Table 9.1.

## Mechanical Principles

The Kerboull acetabular reinforcement device (KARD) is a semi-rigid and open component allowing prevention from graft overloading during the initial osseo-integration process that starts with osteoclastic resorption. Also, because of its

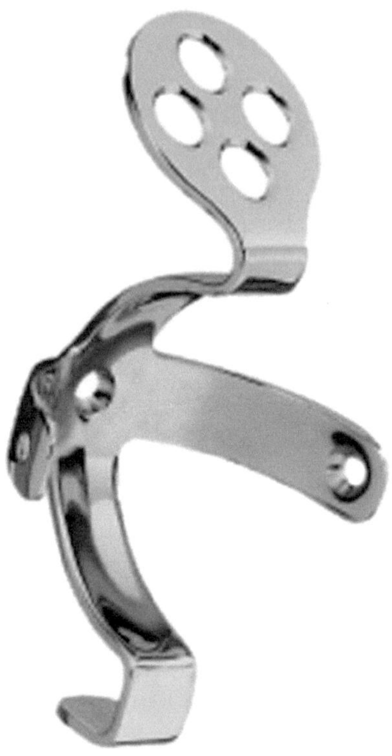

**Fig. 9.3** The original Kerboull device. (Courtesy of Zimmer-Biomet)

specific design, when correctly positioned, one can expect to accurately reconstruct the acetabular defect and orient the acetabular component. To achieve this goal, it is of major importance to choose the adequate size of the KARD, and to not modify its shape, that would alter its mechanical properties.

## The KARD Evolution

The original KARD (Fig. 9.3) consists of a four-branched hemispheric cross, made of 316 L stainless steel. Its shape results from the orthogonal crossing of two hemispheric plates. The vertical plate ends distally with a hook which must be inserted under the teardrop, and proximally with a rounded plate perforated by four holes for iliac screw fixation above the acetabulum. The horizontal plate is asymmetric: its anterior branch being shorter than the posterior determines a 10° anteversion of the opening plane of the device. A left and a right series of the device are available in six sizes in which sockets with an outer diameter of 37–54 mm can be cemented (Fig. 9.4). Three holes, one at the crossing of the plates and one at each extremity of the horizontal plate, allow direct fixation of the allograft fragments to the device with 3.5-mm screws.

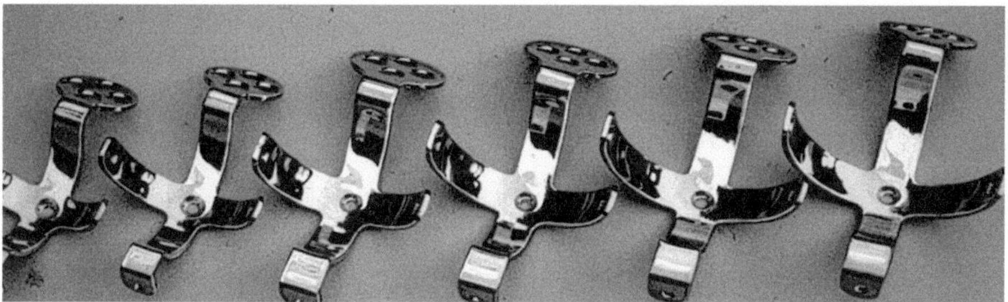

**Fig. 9.4** The original KARD displayed in a series of six sizes

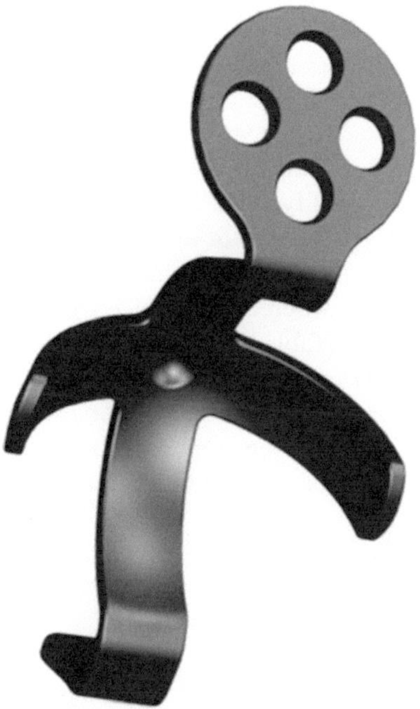

**Fig. 9.5** The modified Kerboull device. (Courtesy of Medacta)

In some Paprosky III acetabular defects involving the tear drop requiring its reconstruction to place the socket in an anatomic situation, we have observed a high risk of proximal and medial migration of the KARD. Indeed, primary stability of the KARD including its the hook is of paramount importance for long-term survival. For this reason, we have recently modified the KARD (Kerboull Cage, Medacta International SA, Castel San Pietro, Switzerland). The general design and the number of sizes have not been modified, as can be seen in Fig. 9.5. However, based upon the results from Tanaka et al. [61] this new device is made of Grade 4 Titanium (ASTM F67) in order to increase the resistance to fatigue, whilst keeping the same rigidity by slightly increasing its thickness from 2 to 2.5 mm and remove the holes that were present on the branches and at their crossing. The finite element

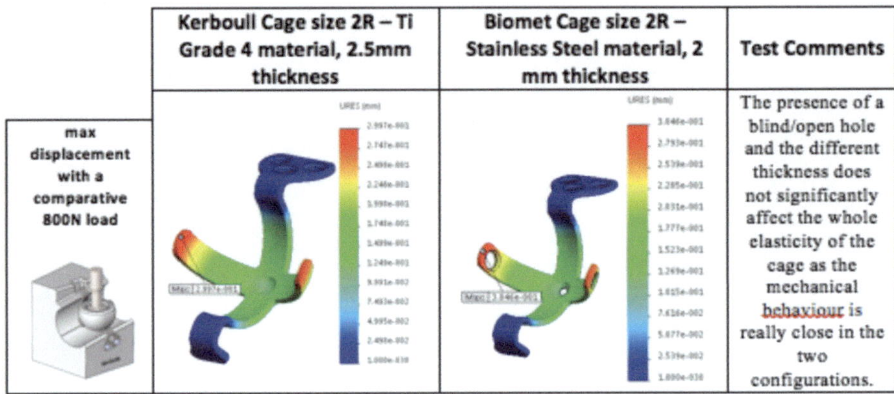


**Fig. 9.6** Comparative fatigue resistance test between the new KARD (left) and the original KARD (right)

analysis indicated that taken together, these modifications did not modify the general rigidity of the device. We have also demonstrated in vitro that the fatigue resistance (Fig. 9.6) of the new design was greater than that of the original one. Indeed, the original version showed breakage at a maximal load of 800 N over 0.57 million cycles, whereas the new design did not exhibit failure at 1500 N up to eight million cycles (Table 9.2).

Also, the outer convex surface of the device has a sand-blasted finish in order to promote fixation to host bone where direct contact occurs.

Finally, the hook has been made larger in order to accommodate situations where the inferior margin is partially destroyed in order to increase its primary stability.

## Surgical Technique

This section will not discuss the optimal approach to achieve the prerequisite goals but a wide exposure of the acetabular cavity is necessary to completely remove the loosened socket and the cement fragments when present. Of major importance is the complete excision of the fibrous membrane adherent to the socket and the granulation tissue filling in the defects. Also, remnant osteophytes and fibrous tissue present around the inferior margin should be completely excised in order to clearly visualize this region. The acetabular cavity is thereafter washed with pulsatile lavage. No reaming of the cavity is performed because of the fragility of the acetabular walls related to the bone stock loss.

The size of the device to choose should be anticipated on preoperative radiograph when the opposite hip is un-operated. Otherwise, intraoperatively it should

**Table 9.2** Outcomes of fatigue resistance tests for the original KARD (Biomet) and the new KARD (Medacta)

| Medacta Kerboull cage | | | | Biomet CMK reinforcement cage | | | |
|---|---|---|---|---|---|---|---|
| Sample | Load(N) | TOT cycles | Result | Sample | Load(N) | TOT cycles | Result |
| 1.1 | 3400 | 5140 | Fracture | 1.1 (step 1) | 3400 | 574 | Deformation |
| 1.2 (step 1) | 3400 | 3478 | Fracture | 1.2 (step 3) | 800 | 1.58 milion | Fracture |
| 1.3 (step 2) | 2300 | 21,406 | Fracture | 1.3 (step 3) | 800 | 0.52 milion | Fracture |
| 1.4 (step 3) + locati | 800 | 5 milion | No failure | 1.4 (step 3) | 800 | 0.57 milion | Fracture |
| | 900 | 5.5 milion | | | | | |
| | 1000 | 6 milion | | | | | |
| | 1100 | 6.5 milion | | | | | |
| | 1200 | 7 milion | | | | | |
| | 1300 | 7.5 milion | | | | | |
| | 1400 | 8 milion | | | | | |
| | 1500 | 8 milion | Fracture | | | | |
| 1.5 (step 3) + locati | 800 | 5 milion | No failure | 1.5 (step 3) | 800 | 0.63 milion | Fracture |
| | 900 | 5.5 milion | | | | | |
| | 1000 | 6 milion | | | | | |
| | 1100 | 6.5 milion | | | | | |
| | 1200 | 7 milion | | | | | |
| | 1300 | 7.5 milion | | | | | |
| | 1400 | 8 milion | | | | | |
| | 1500 | 8 milion | Fracture | | | | |
| 1.6 (step 3) + locati | 800 | 5 milion | No failure | | | | |
| | 900 | 5.5 milion | | | | | |
| | 1000 | 6 milion | | | | | |
| | 1100 | 6.5 milion | | | | | |
| | 1200 | 7 milion | | | | | |
| | 1300 | 7.3 milion | Fracture | | | | |

Courtesy of Medacta

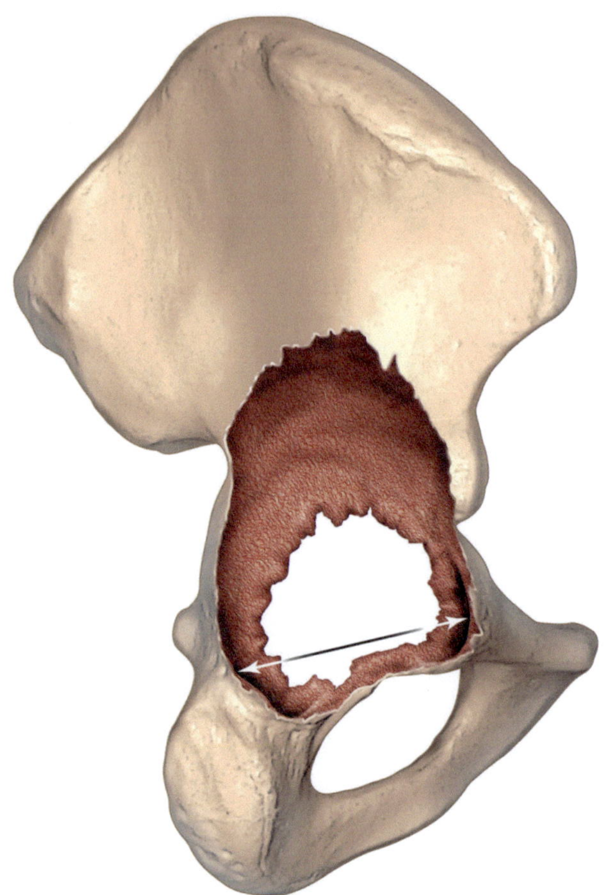

**Fig. 9.7** Assessing the anatomic osseous size of the acetabulum

be based upon the anatomic osseous size of the acetabulum in the inferior part (Fig. 9.7).

The hook of the acetabular device must be placed under the teardrop in its posterior portion, near the ischium (Fig. 9.8). The acetabular device is then tilted 40–45° of abduction (Fig. 9.9). Once placed in its correction position, the device allows to assess the extent and location of bone defects and the required shape of bone graft. The plate must never be opened or bent to adapt to the bone loss. Bone loss reconstruction usually starts with acetabular roof restoration. This superior bone defect is reconstructed whenever possible, by one allograft block shaped from a fresh frozen femoral head allograft (Fig. 9.10). Then, the recon-

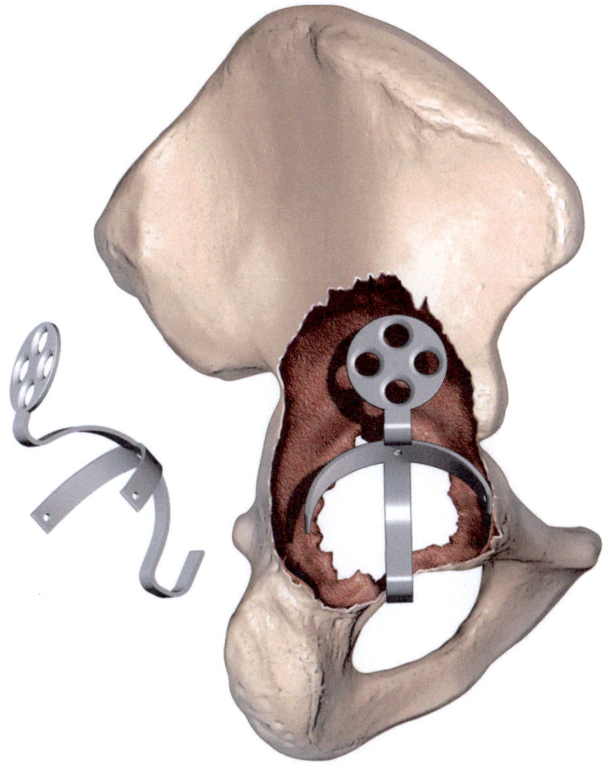

**Fig. 9.8** The hook of the acetabular device must be placed under the teardrop in its posterior portion, near the ischium

struction of the medial wall is performed with an adequate slice cut from a femoral head. The plate then was fixed to the iliac host bone with 5-mm screws (Fig. 9.11). At least two screws are used to obtain sufficient stability, always starting with the inferior screw. The latter must be tightened again, once all screws are placed. Reconstruction of the anterior and posterior walls is performed using allograft fragments wedged in between the residual walls and the horizontal branches of the acetabular device (Fig. 9.12). Finally, the reconstruction is completed by morselized cancellous bone packed in the cavitary defects of the pubis and the ischium and in the gaps between the different allograft fragments to avoid any cement leak.

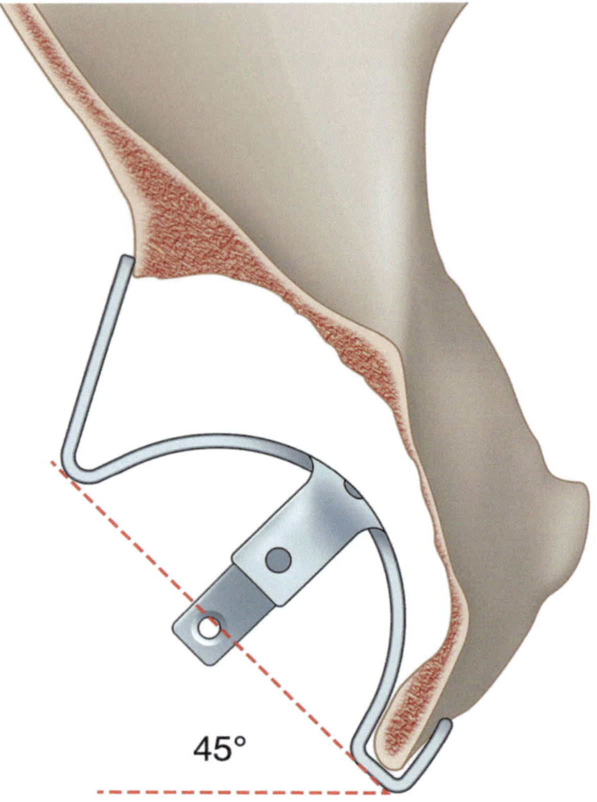


**Fig. 9.9** The acetabular device is tilted 40–45° of abduction

## *The Gap Ring*

Published data on the outcomes of the GAP ring (Graft Augmentation Prosthesis) are scarce. The design of this device is special as it combines an inferior hook to be placed under the teardrop and two superior plates for screw fixation to the pelvis (Fig. 9.13). The outside surface is made of grit blasted titanium with HA (hydroxyapatite) coating. Duffy et al. [68] investigated the GAP ring in revision THA. Within their series of 17 patients, they had 11 cases of severe acetabular bone loss graded AAOS type III. Six patients received bulk femoral heads. The average follow-up was 6.5 years, and at the latest follow-up, 7 of the 12 still alive patients were revised. Five cases were revised for fatigue failure of the GAP ring including four cases of breakage at the bone-plate junction. The authors concluded that "this device should not be used unless it is adequately supported by the host bone." In a similar study,

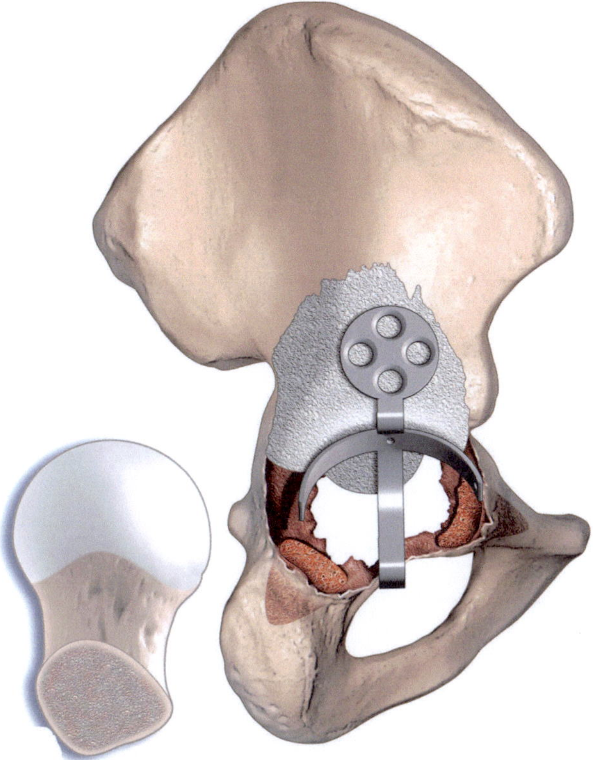

**Fig. 9.10** This superior bone defect is reconstructed whenever possible, by one allograft block shaped from a fresh frozen femoral head allograft

Buttaro et al. [69] also found catastrophic early failure. In their work, they reviewed 24 cases of AAOS type III and IV acetabular defects treated with the GAP ring and bone allograft. At 34 months, the survival rate was 67%. Nine failures occurred at the last follow-up and they reported five fractures of the ring at the plate-cup junction. Eventually, the authors abandoned its use for the treatment of severe acetabular defects, especially AAOS type IV.

## *The Burch Schneider Cage and Its Evolution*

The Burch Schneider cage is discussed in Chap. 9.

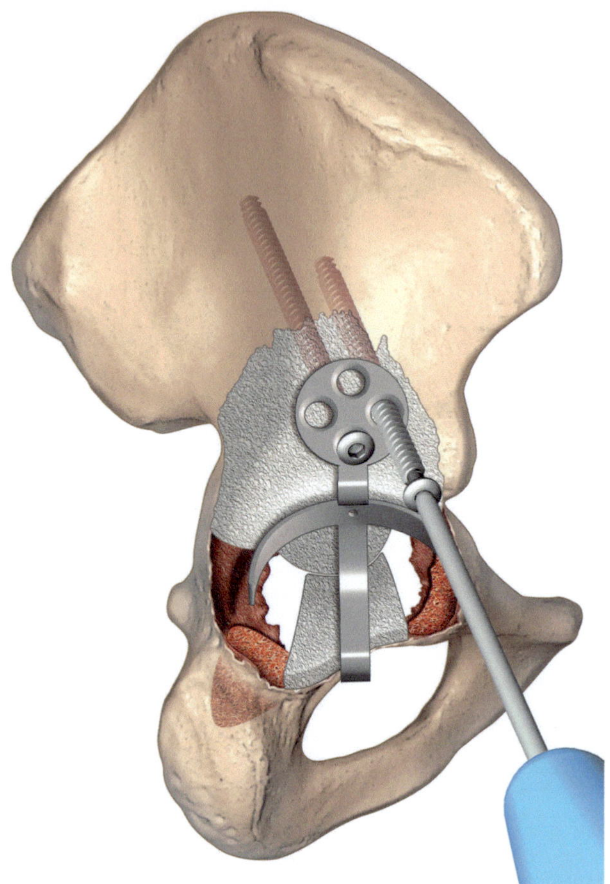

**Fig. 9.11** The plate is fixed to the iliac host bone with 5-mm screws. At least two screws are used to obtain sufficient stability, always starting with the inferior screw

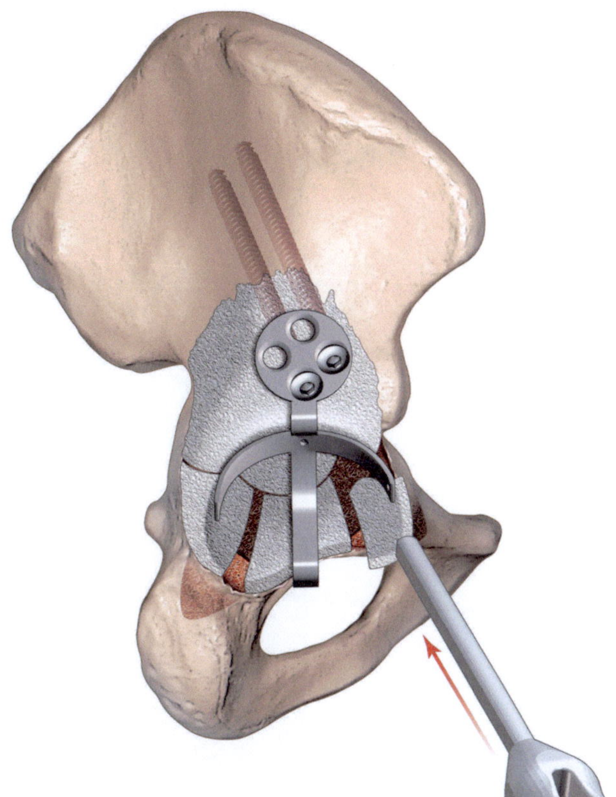

**Fig. 9.12** Reconstruction of the anterior and posterior walls is performed using allograft fragments wedged in between the residual walls and the horizontal branches of the acetabular device

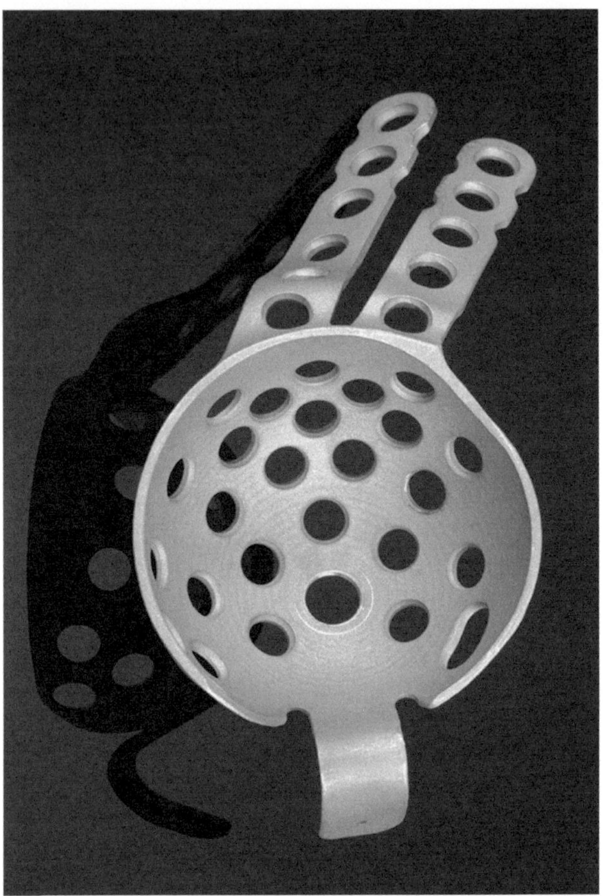

**Fig. 9.13** The Gap II® ring. (Courtesy of Stryker)

## Conclusion

Reconstruction of major acetabular defects is a surgical challenge. Nowadays, there are numerous acetabular reinforcement devices available on the market as well as various reconstruction techniques, with or without bone graft. The top priorities are to restore the anatomic center of rotation of the hip and ensure a long-term success of the reconstruction. Several solutions based upon the literature review and depending on the surgeon's own experience can be proposed to deal with these complex cases.

## References

1. Kurtz SM, Ong KL, Schmier J, Zhao K, Mowat F, Lau E. Primary and revision arthroplasty surgery caseloads in the United States from 1990 to 2004. J Arthroplast. 2009;24(2):195–203.
2. Kurtz S, Mowat F, Ong K, Chan N, Lau E, Halpern M. Prevalence of primary and revision total hip and knee arthroplasty in the United States from 1990 through 2002. J Bone Joint Surg Am. 2005;87(7):1487–97.

3. Kurtz SM, Ong KL, Lau E, Bozic KJ. Impact of the economic downturn on total joint replacement demand in the United States: updated projections to 2021. J Bone Joint Surg Am. 2014;96(8):624–30.
4. Kurtz S, Ong K, Lau E, Mowat F, Halpern M. Projections of primary and revision hip and knee arthroplasty in the United States from 2005 to 2030. J Bone Joint Surg Am. 2007;89(4):780–5.
5. Inacio MCS, Graves SE, Pratt NL, Roughead EE, Nemes S. Increase in total joint arthroplasty projected from 2014 to 2046 in Australia: a conservative local model with international implications. Clin Orthop Relat Res. 2017;475(8):2130–7.
6. Patel A, Pavlou G, Mújica-Mota RE, Toms AD. The epidemiology of revision total knee and hip arthroplasty in England and Wales: a comparative analysis with projections for the United States. A study using the National Joint Registry dataset. Bone Joint J. 2015;97-B(8):1076–81.
7. Bozic KJ, Kurtz SM, Lau E, Ong K, Vail TP, Berry DJ. The epidemiology of revision total hip arthroplasty in the United States. J Bone Joint Surg Am. 2009;91(1):128–33.
8. Hanna SA, Somerville L, McCalden RW, Naudie DD, MacDonald SJ. Highly cross-linked polyethylene decreases the rate of revision of total hip arthroplasty compared with conventional polyethylene at 13 years' follow-up. Bone Joint J. 2016;98-B(1):28–32.
9. Shen C, Tang ZH, Hu JZ, Zou GY, Xiao RC, Yan DX. Does cross-linked polyethylene decrease the revision rate of total hip arthroplasty compared with conventional polyethylene? A meta-analysis. Orthop Traumatol Surg Res. 2014;100(7):745–50.
10. Bitsch RG, Loidolt T, Heisel C, Ball S, Schmalzried TP. Reduction of osteolysis with use of Marathon cross-linked polyethylene. A concise follow-up, at a minimum of five years, of a previous report. J Bone Joint Surg Am. 2008;90(7):1487–91.
11. Epinette J-A, Jolles-Haeberli BM. Comparative results from a National Joint Registry hip data set of a new cross-linked annealed polyethylene vs both conventional polyethylene and ceramic bearings. J Arthroplast. 2016;31(7):1483–91.
12. Delaunay C, Hamadouche M, Girard J, Duhamel A, So FG. What are the causes for failures of primary hip arthroplasties in France? Clin Orthop Relat Res. 2013;471(12):3863–9.
13. DeLee JG, Charnley J. Radiological demarcation of cemented sockets in total hip replacement. Clin Orthop Relat Res. 1976;121:20–32.
14. Chiang PP, Burke DW, Freiberg AA, Rubash HE. Osteolysis of the pelvis: evaluation and treatment. Clin Orthop Relat Res. 2003;417:164–74.
15. Engh CA, Glassman AH, Griffin WL, Mayer JG. Results of cementless revision for failed cemented total hip arthroplasty. Clin Orthop Relat Res. 1988;235:91–110.
16. Gustilo RB, Pasternak HS. Revision total hip arthroplasty with titanium ingrowth prosthesis and bone grafting for failed cemented femoral component loosening. Clin Orthop Relat Res. 1988;235:111–9.
17. D'Antonio JA, Capello WN, Borden LS, Bargar WL, Bierbaum BF, Boettcher WG, et al. Classification and management of acetabular abnormalities in total hip arthroplasty. Clin Orthop Relat Res. 1989;243:126–37.
18. Sheth NP, Nelson CL, Springer BD, Fehring TK, Paprosky WG. Acetabular bone loss in revision total hip arthroplasty: evaluation and management. J Am Acad Orthop Surg. 2013;21(3):128–39.
19. Gross AE, Allan DG, Catre M, Garbuz DS, Stockley I. Bone grafts in hip replacement surgery. The pelvic side. Orthop Clin North Am. 1993;24(4):679–95.
20. Saleh KJ, Holtzman J, Gafni Asaleh L, Jaroszynski G, Wong P, Woodgate I, et al. Development, test reliability and validation of a classification for revision hip arthroplasty. J Orthop Res. 2001;19(1):50–6.
21. Paprosky WG, Perona PG, Lawrence JM. Acetabular defect classification and surgical reconstruction in revision arthroplasty. A 6-year follow-up evaluation. J Arthroplast. 1994;9(1):33–44.
22. Della Valle CJ, Berger RA, Rosenberg AG, Galante JO. Cementless acetabular reconstruction in revision total hip arthroplasty. Clin Orthop Relat Res. 2004;420:96–100.
23. Hallstrom BR, Golladay GJ, Vittetoe DA, Harris WH. Cementless acetabular revision with the Harris-Galante porous prosthesis. Results after a minimum of ten years of follow-up. J Bone Joint Surg Am. 2004;86-A(5):1007–11.

24. Park DK, Della Valle CJ, Quigley L, Moric M, Rosenberg AG, Galante JO. Revision of the acetabular component without cement. A concise follow-up, at twenty to twenty-four years, of a previous report. J Bone Joint Surg Am. 2009;91(2):350–5.
25. Templeton JE, Callaghan JJ, Goetz DD, Sullivan PM, Johnston RC. Revision of a cemented acetabular component to a cementless acetabular component. A ten to fourteen-year follow-up study. J Bone Joint Surg Am. 2001 2001/11//;83-A(11):1706–11.
26. Trumm BN, Callaghan JJ, Liu SS, Goetz DD, Johnston RC. Revision with cementless acetabular components: a concise follow-up, at a minimum of twenty years, of previous reports. J Bone Joint Surg Am. 2012;94(21):2001–4.
27. Boscainos PJ, Kellett CF, Maury AC, Backstein D, Gross AE. Management of periacetabular bone loss in revision hip arthroplasty. Clin Orthop Relat Res. 2007;465:159–65.
28. Garcia-Cimbrelo E. Porous-coated cementless acetabular cups in revision surgery: a 6- to 11-year follow-up study. J Arthroplast. 1999;14(4):397–406.
29. Goodman S, Saastamoinen H, Shasha N, Gross A. Complications of ilioischial reconstruction rings in revision total hip arthroplasty. J Arthroplast. 2004;19(4):436–46.
30. Morsi E, Garbuz D, Gross AE. Revision total hip arthroplasty with shelf bulk allografts. A long-term follow-up study. J Arthroplast. 1996;11(1):86–90.
31. Woodgate IG, Saleh KJ, Jaroszynski G, Agnidis Z, Woodgate MM, Gross AE. Minor column structural acetabular allografts in revision hip arthroplasty. Clin Orthop Relat Res. 2000;371:75–85.
32. Lee PTH, Raz G, Safir OA, Backstein DJ, Gross AE. Long-term results for minor column allografts in revision hip arthroplasty. Clin Orthop Relat Res. 2010;468(12):3295–303.
33. Harris WH. Allografting in total hip arthroplasty: in adults with severe acetabular deficiency including a surgical technique for bolting the graft to the ilium. Clin Orthop Relat Res. 1982;162:150–64.
34. Harris WH, Crothers O, Oh I. Total hip replacement and femoral-head bone-grafting for severe acetabular deficiency in adults. J Bone Joint Surg Am. 1977;59(6):752–9.
35. Sporer SM, O'Rourke M, Chong P, Paprosky WG. The use of structural distal femoral allografts for acetabular reconstruction. Surgical technique. J Bone Joint Surg Am. 2006;88(Suppl 1 Pt 1):92–9.
36. Jasty M, Harris WH. Salvage total hip reconstruction in patients with major acetabular bone deficiency using structural femoral head allografts. J Bone Joint Surg Br. 1990;72(1):63–7.
37. Pollock FH, Whiteside LA. The fate of massive allografts in total hip acetabular revision surgery. J Arthroplast. 1992;7(3):271–6.
38. Hooten JP, Engh CA, Engh CA. Failure of structural acetabular allografts in cementless revision hip arthroplasty. J Bone Joint Surg Br. 1994;76(3):419–22.
39. Kwong LM, Jasty M, Harris WH. High failure rate of bulk femoral head allografts in total hip acetabular reconstructions at 10 years. J Arthroplast. 1993;8(4):341–6.
40. Paprosky WG, Magnus RE. Principles of bone grafting in revision total hip arthroplasty. Acetabular technique. Clin Orthop Relat Res. 1994;298:147–55.
41. Garbuz D, Morsi E, Gross AE. Revision of the acetabular component of a total hip arthroplasty with a massive structural allograft. Study with a minimum five-year follow-up. J Bone Joint Surg Am. 1996;78(5):693–7.
42. Brown NM, Morrison J, Sporer SM, Paprosky WG. The use of structural distal femoral allograft for acetabular reconstruction of paprosky type IIIA defects at a mean 21 years of follow-up. J Arthroplast. 2016;31(3):680–3.
43. Sporer SM, O'Rourke M, Chong P, Paprosky WG. The use of structural distal femoral allografts for acetabular reconstruction. Average ten-year follow-up. J Bone Joint Surg Am. 2005;87(4):760–5.
44. Hanssen AD, Lewallen DG. Modular acetabular augments: composite void fillers. Orthopedics. 2005;28(9):971–2.

45. Kosashvili Y, Backstein D, Safir O, Lakstein D, Gross AE. Acetabular revision using an anti-protrusion (ilio-ischial) cage and trabecular metal acetabular component for severe acetabular bone loss associated with pelvic discontinuity. J Bone Joint Surg Br. 2009;91(7):870–6.
46. Abolghasemian M, Tangsaraporn S, Drexler M, Barbuto R, Backstein D, Safir O, et al. The challenge of pelvic discontinuity: cup-cage reconstruction does better than conventional cages in mid-term. Bone Joint J. 2014;96-B(2):195–200.
47. Amenabar T, Rahman WA, Hetaimish BM, Kuzyk PR, Safir OA, Gross AE. Promising mid-term results with a cup-cage construct for large acetabular defects and pelvic discontinuity. Clin Orthop Relat Res. 2016;474(2):408–14.
48. Sculco PK, Ledford CK, Hanssen AD, Abdel MP, Lewallen DG. The evolution of the cup-cage technique for major acetabular defects: full and half cup-cage reconstruction. J Bone Joint Surg Am. 2017;99(13):1104–10.
49. Haentjens P, Handelberg F, Casteleyn PP, Opdecam P. The Müller acetabular support ring. A preliminary review of indications and clinical results. Int Orthop. 1986;10(4):223–30.
50. Schatzker J, Glynn MK, Ritter D. A preliminary review of the Müller acetabular and Burch-Schneider antiprotrusio support rings. Arch Orthop Trauma Surg Arch Orthopadische Unfall-Chir. 1984;103(1):5–12.
51. Zehntner MK, Ganz R. Midterm results (5.5–10 years) of acetabular allograft reconstruction with the acetabular reinforcement ring during total hip revision. J Arthroplasty. 1994;9(5):469–79.
52. Korovessis P, Stamatakis M, Baikousis A, Katonis P, Petsinis G. Mueller roof reinforcement rings. Medium-term results. Clin Orthop Relat Res. 1999;362:125–37.
53. van der Linde M, Tonino A. Acetabular revision with impacted grafting and a reinforcement ring: 42 patients followed for a mean of 10 years. Acta Orthop Scand. 2001;72(3):221–7.
54. Schlegel UJ, Bitsch RG, Pritsch M, Clauss M, Mau H, Breusch SJ. Mueller reinforcement rings in acetabular revision: outcome in 164 hips followed for 2–17 years. Acta Orthop. 2006;77(2):234–41.
55. Massin P, Tanaka C, Huten D, Duparc J. Treatment of aseptic acetabular loosening by reconstruction combining bone graft and Müller ring. Actuarial analysis over 11 years. Rev Chir Orthop Reparatrice Appar Mot. 1998;84(1):51–60.
56. Gill TJ, Siebenrock K, Oberholzer R, Ganz R. Acetabular reconstruction in developmental dysplasia of the hip: results of the acetabular reinforcement ring with hook. J Arthroplast. 1999;14(2):131–7.
57. Siebenrock KA, Trochsler M, Sadri H, Ganz R. Hooked roof cup in revision of difficult loose hip prosthesis cups. Results after a minimum of 10 years. Orthopade. 2001;30(5):273–9.
58. Gerber A, Pisan M, Zurakowski D, Isler B. Ganz reinforcement ring for reconstruction of acetabular defects in revision total hip arthroplasty. J Bone Joint Surg Am. 2003;85-A(12):2358–64.
59. Uchiyama K, Takahira N, Fukushima K, Yamamoto T, Moriya M, Itoman M. Radiological evaluation of allograft reconstruction in acetabulum with Ganz reinforcement ring in revision total hip replacement. J Orthop Sci. 2010;15(6):764–71. https://doi.org/10.1007/s00776-010-1549-y.
60. Hourscht C, Abdelnasser MK, Ahmad SS, Kraler L, Keel MJ, Siebenrock KA, et al. Reconstruction of AAOS type III and IV acetabular defects with the Ganz reinforcement ring: high failure in pelvic discontinuity. Arch Orthop Trauma Surg. 2017;137(8):1139–48.
61. Tanaka C, Shikata J, Ikenaga M, Takahashi M. Acetabular reconstruction using a Kerboull-type acetabular reinforcement device and hydroxyapatite granules: a 3- to 8-year follow-up study. J Arthroplast. 2003;18(6):719–25.
62. Kim Y, Tanaka C, Kanoe H. Long-term outcome of acetabular reconstruction using a Kerboull-type acetabular reinforcement device with hydroxyapetite granule and structural autograft for AAOS type II and III acetabular defects. J Arthroplasty. 2015;30(10):1810–4. https://doi.org/10.1016/j.arth.2015.04.034.

63. Hori J, Yasunaga Y, Yamasaki T, Yoshida T, Oshima S, Yamasaki K, Matsuo T, Ochi M. Mid-term results of acetabular reconstruction using a Kerboull-type acetabular reinforcement device. Int Orthop. 2012;36(1):23–6. https://doi.org/10.1007/s00264-011-1248-0.
64. Akiyama H, Yamamoto K, Tsukanaka M, Kawanabe K, Otsuka H, So K, Goto K, Nakamura T. Revision total hip arthroplasty using a Kerboull-type acetabular reinforcement device with bone allograft: minimum 4.5-year follow-up results and mechanical analysis. J Bone Joint Surg Br. 2011;93(9):1194–200. https://doi.org/10.1302/0301-620x.93b9.26598.
65. Okano K, Miyata N, Enomoto H, Osaki M, Shindo H. Revision with impacted bone allografts and the Kerboull cross plate for massive bone defect of the acetabulum. J Arthroplasty. 2010;25(4):594–9. https://doi.org/10.1016/j.arth.2009.04.003.
66. Kawanabe K, Akiyama H, Onishi E, Nakamura T. Revision total hip replacement using the Kerboull acetabular reinforcement device with morsellised or bulk graft: results at a mean follow-up of 8.7 years. J Bone Joint Surg Br. 2007;89(1):26–31. https://doi.org/10.1302/0301-620x.89b1.18037.
67. Kerboull M, Hamadouche M, Kerboull L. The Kerboull acetabular reinforcement device in major acetabular reconstructions. Clin Orthop Relat Res. 2000;378:155–68.
68. Duffy GP, O'Connor MI, Brodersen MP. Fatigue failure of the GAP ring. J Arthroplast. 2007;22(5):711–4.
69. Buttaro MA, de la Rosa DM, Comba F, Piccaluga F. High failure rate with the GAP II ring and impacted allograft bone in severe acetabular defects. Clin Orthop Relat Res. 2012;470(11):3148–55.

# Chapter 10
# Total Hip Replacement Revision Using a Dual Mobility Cup Cemented into a Metallic Ring

**Pascal Bizot**

## Introduction

The number of patients undergoing THA is constantly increasing. This trend is reported worldwide and results from multiple factors, including the progresses made in the field of hip surgery, the quality of the functional results, the increasing patient life span, the higher functional demand, and the enlargement of THA indications to younger patients and older patients as well. Consequently, the number of patients undergoing THA revision also increased significantly with time [4, 18, 19, 32]. For Kurtz et al. [18, 19], the total number of procedures in the United States from 2009 to 2010 increased by 6.0% for primary total hip arthroplasty, and 10.8% for revision total hip arthroplasty. The number of THA will increase from 174% in 2030, and the number of THA revision will double in 2026. In the same way, Bozic et al. [4], reported an increase of THA revision by 23% between 2005 and 2010 in the US.

However, THA revision remains a challenging procedure for the orthopedic surgeon. The survival rate after THA revision is lower than that after of primary THA, and the complications (mainly loosening, instability, infection, and fracture) are significantly more frequent. Instability is one of the main complications in THA revisions, and also one of the most common cause for re revision [1, 4, 10, 16, 27]. Dislocation generally occurs early, within 2–3 years post operatively. After primary THA, the rate of instability ranged from 0.2 to 7%, whereas after revision surgery, it can increase up to 35% [1, 10, 16, 25, 27].

P. Bizot
Department of Orthopaedic Surgery, Lariboisière Teaching Hospital, Paris, France

Laboratoire Bioingénierie et Bioimagerie ostéo-articulaire (B20A) CNRS UMR7052, University of Paris Diderot, Paris, France
e-mail: pascal.bizot@aphp.fr



E. García-Rey, E. García-Cimbrelo (eds.), *Acetabular Revision Surgery in Major Bone Defects*, https://doi.org/10.1007/978-3-319-98596-1_10

In a retrospective analysis conducted on 539 hips undergoing revision THA done for instability, Jo et al. [16] reported a cumulative risk of re-dislocation and re-revision for all cause of 34.5% and 45.9% at 15 years, respectively.

The mechanism is often multifactorial, and due to impingement and/or soft tissues insufficiencies, which depends on the patient characteristics (age, gender, initial diagnosis, associated diseases), the surgical technique (approach, implant positioning), the implant design (head, neck, cup), and the rehabilitation.

Treatment of instability does remain a challenging procedure. Several surgical options are available, including soft tissues procedures (abductor muscles reconstruction), increase hip length and offset, use of constraint acetabular implants and use of larger femoral heads (in order to increase the range of motion (ROM) before impingement, the head-neck ratio, and the jump distance). Constrained implants restrict the ROM and cause high stress transmission responsible of liner damage, locking mechanism failure, dislocation and loosening. Larger heads increase volumetric wear and reduce PE thickness, and may cause fractures of thin PE liners, tribo-corrosion generated by large torsional forces at the trunnion-head junction, and groin pain secondary to impingement against the iliopsoas muscle. Finally, none appears clearly superior over others, and the literature showed quite disappointing results with these options, especially in patients with high risk of instability [1, 10].

## Dual Mobility Cup

Dual Mobility (DM) is a concept first introduced by Gilles Bousquet in France during the 1970s. DM cup combines two bearings: a small joint between the prosthetic head and the mobile PE component, and a large one between the mobile PE component and the inner surface of the metal cup. It is a non-constraint device which provides a greater effective head size and head-to-neck ratio, and is expected to improve the ROM to impingement and joint stability. Mobility occurs at the two bearings, but preferentially at the inner bearing, the outer bearing engages only at the extremes of motion. The original cementless design has been significantly improved: the original cylindro-spherical design has been modified in order to improve the ROM free of impingement, and to avoid psoas tendon-to-cup impingement. The coating of the shell has been also modified by adding either a double coating (hydroxyapatite and titanium plasma spray) or a porous metal coating, to improve bone fixation (Fig. 10.1).

Contemporary DM THA outperforms large diameter heads and constrained liners in terms of wear, stability and survival. Clinical reports on the use of the first generation of implants have shown encouraging results, with survival rates of 81% at 15 years and 75% over 20 years [3, 12]. With improved designs, survivorship has been reported superior to 95% at 6–8 years, but, nowadays, survivorship over 10 years with modern implants are not yet available [7, 8, 12].

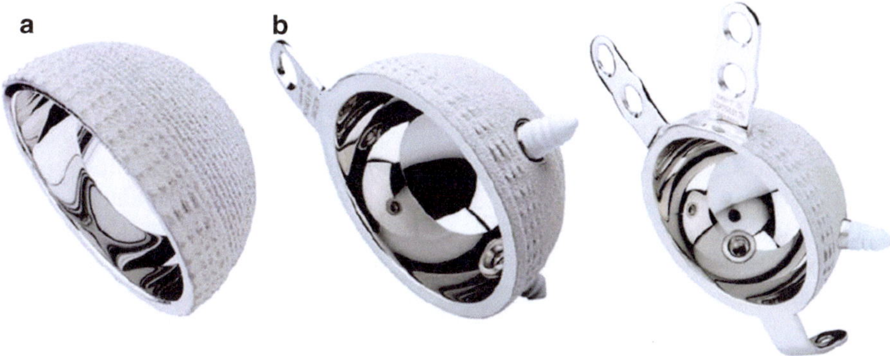

**Fig. 10.1** Uncemented dual mobility cups. (Novae®, Serf-Dedienne, France). (**a**) Primary case. (**b**) Revision case

Many series have shown the efficiency of DM in preventing postoperative dislocation both for primary and revision procedures. In primary THA using DM cups, the dislocation rate ranged from 0% to 4.6% even in patients at risk for dislocation, without increase with time [12, 14, 26, 30, 31]. In unstable THA, reports have demonstrated low rates of re-dislocation, ranging from 0% to 5.5% [15, 16, 20, 24]. DM has been also reported with low dislocation rates in revision THA, ranging from 0% to 5% [7, 8, 25, 26]. In a systematic review of the literature including a total of 17,908 DM THAs, De Martino et al. [8] reported a mean rate of dislocation and intra-prosthetic dislocation (IPD) (the prosthetic head dislodges from the mobile PE component) of 0.9% and 0.7% in primary THA, and 3.0% and 1.3% in revision THA. On the same way, Darrith et al. [7] reported for a total of 10,783 primary DM THAs, rates of aseptic loosening, IPD and dislocation of 1.3%, 1.1% and 0.46% respectively, with an overall survivorship of 98.0% at of 8.5 years. For 3008 revisions DM THAs, the rates of aseptic acetabular loosening, IPD and dislocation were 1.4%, 0.3% and 2.2% respectively and the survival was 96.6% at 5.4 years. Both concluded that the use of DM cups is effective in minimizing the risk of instability after both primary and revision THA.

Concerns about increased wear compared to conventional bearings and IPD have been nearly solved with modern designs. IPD is a specific failure which has been noted with the first generation of implants with an incidence of 2–4% [3, 12, 23, 30]. The main mechanism resulted from PE wear at the retentive rim of the component. With improvements of the head-neck geometry, PE damage in the retentive area decreased, and consequently the incidence of IPD decreased ranging from 0% at 6 years to 0.28% at 10 years with the newer generation of implants [7, 8, 31]. The linear penetration rate, used to estimate volumetric wear in conventional metal-on-PE bearings, is ineffective for estimating wear on DM cups because of the presence of two bearings. Wear measurements from retrieved first-generation DM implants have confirmed low wear rates [3, 12]. For Boyer et al. [3], the two articulations of the DM THA do not cause more wear. The median wear rate was 38 $mm^3$/year, similar to that of cemented PE liners and lower than equivalent cementless liners. On the same way, Gaudin et al. [11] showed that in vitro wear for conventional PE was comparable between a standard and a dual mobility cup, confirming the very good long-term clinical results observed with DM bearing.

Specific DM cups have been designed to secure the cementless fixation in cases of poor bone stock, poor bone quality and in revision cases, with additional pegs, supra-acetabular screws, hook and flanges, and recently with a modular cup for screw fixation and a metallic liner (Fig. 10.1). However, in cases of THA revisions with severe bone loss, uncemented fixation might be compromised, especially if the acetabular implant is placed close to its original position, as it has been recommended for long term maintenance of the hip function. Although other uncemented options have been proposed, sometimes with acceptance of a high hip center (bi lobed cup, tri flanged and jumbo cups, reconstructive cup with trabecular metal), the use of cement may become necessary.

In cemented revision THR, acetabular reconstruction using unsupported structural allografts has been associated with a high rate of failure. In contrast, when supported by an acetabular reinforcement device, a low rate of failure has been reported [2, 17, 33, 35]. Use of DM cemented directly into the bone without a reinforcement device has encountered controversies. Although Haen et al. [13] have recently reported a rate of loosening of only 1.5% and a 5-year survival rate of 98%, most of the series have reported a high rate of loosening [5, 15, 29]. Therefore, the use of cemented DM implants into a reinforcement may be an interesting option. Many metallic reinforcement devices are available (Müller ring, Bursch ring, Link reinforcement, Kerboull cross). The choice is mainly based on the surgeon habits and the severity of the acetabular lesions. The Kerboull Cross (KC) is an open device, flexible enough to conform with the elasticity of the acetabular bone, and resistant enough to assume a strong fixation. It is composed of two branches. The vertical branch ends distally with a hook that must be inserted under the inferior margin of the acetabulum, and proximally with a rounded plate for ilium screw fixation. The horizontal branch is asymmetrical, shorter forward, which generates a ten degrees ante version. It facilitates restoration of the hip's center of rotation and gave very satisfactory results at long term in THA revision with acetabular reconstruction [17].

## Surgical Technique

The revision procedure offers the possibility to restore hip anatomy and mechanic, which involves restoring the bone stock, implanting the components in a correct position with durable bone fixation, and achieving joint stability.

The operation is performed using posterolateral approach or lateral approach with trochanteric osteotomy. A large exposure is necessary in order to remove the initial acetabular components, the cement if present, the granuloma and fibrous membrane. Caution is necessary not to enlarge acetabular bone damage during this step. The degree of acetabular bone defects, assessed preoperatively on radiographs and/or CT scan, is reevaluated per operatively. The stem may be remove or retain, according to its position and fixation. However, if the stem is retained, make sure that the head is modular and can fit to the new DM PE insert.

The first step is to determine the good position and the appropriate size of the KC (Figs. 10.4 and 10.5). Its outer diameter should be not too large (if not the antero-posterior axis does not fit), and close to that of the undamaged acetabulum (possibly measured on the opposite side). One must pay attention that the KC must allow cementing of the DM shell, which means that its inner diameter should be 2 mm superior to that of DM cup. It is paramount to fix the KC in a correct position. The KC must be fixed inferiorly at the superior margin of the obturator foramen by the hook, and superiorly through the round plate with three to four screws to the ilium, at 45° of abduction angle and vertically, which means that the upper plate should not be bent and not shifted anteriorly nor posteriorly. The screws of the plate should be inserted at an angle >40° and posteriorly within 0–10°. In practice, templates are useful to determine the correct size and position of the KC, and also to determine the need for acetabular reconstruction. It is often necessary to reconstruct the roof with a structural allograft. Remaining acetabular defects are treated, either with impaction bone grafting using bone chips, or with structural allografts, possibly supplemented by cement.

Once the acetabular reconstruction is achieved and the final KC is fixed, the correct position of the device (especially the hook) must be verified on an intra operative radiograph before cementing the dual mobility cup. The dual mobility cup is cemented into the KC, with 10 to 15° of ante version and 45° of abduction. The metal shell has circumferential and longitudinal grooves to improve cementing (Figs. 10.2 and 10.3). Its size should be 2 mm inferior to the inner diameter of the KC, in order to preserve a minimal cement mantel of 2 mm. The technique of cementing is a determining factor for fixation quality and device stability with time. The use of cement added with gentamycin and standard viscosity is recommended.

Finally, the modular head (preferentially 28 mm diameter) is inserted into the mobile PE insert. The whole is impacted on the stem trunnion and the hip is finally reduced.

Postoperative treatment involves routinely prophylactic anticoagulation, careful mobilization of the hip and early full weight bearing with two crutches for 6 weeks (Figs. 10.4 and 10.5).

## Results

Between July 2007 and April 2011, we performed 40 THA revisions using a dual mobility cup cemented in a KC, in 38 consecutive patients (21 females, 17 males) (Figs. 10.6 and 10.7). The mean age of the patients at the procedure was 74 years (18–90). The number of previous THA per patient ranged from 1 to 6 with a mean of 1.8. The causes of THA revision were mainly aseptic loosening with or without

**Fig. 10.2** Cemented dual mobility cup into a Kerboull cross. (*Quattro*®, Lépine, France)

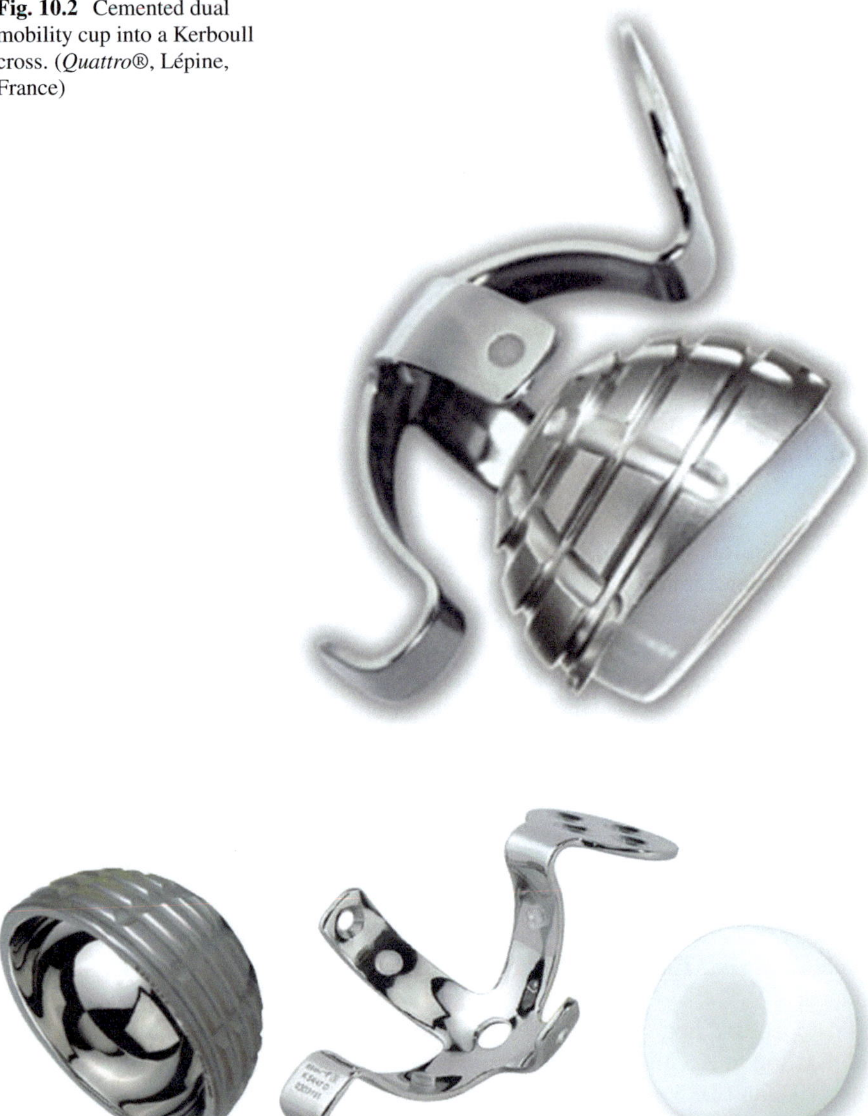

**Fig. 10.3** Cemented dual mobility cup with the corresponding Kerboull cross and mobile PE insert. (*Novae Stick*®, Serf-Dedienne, France)

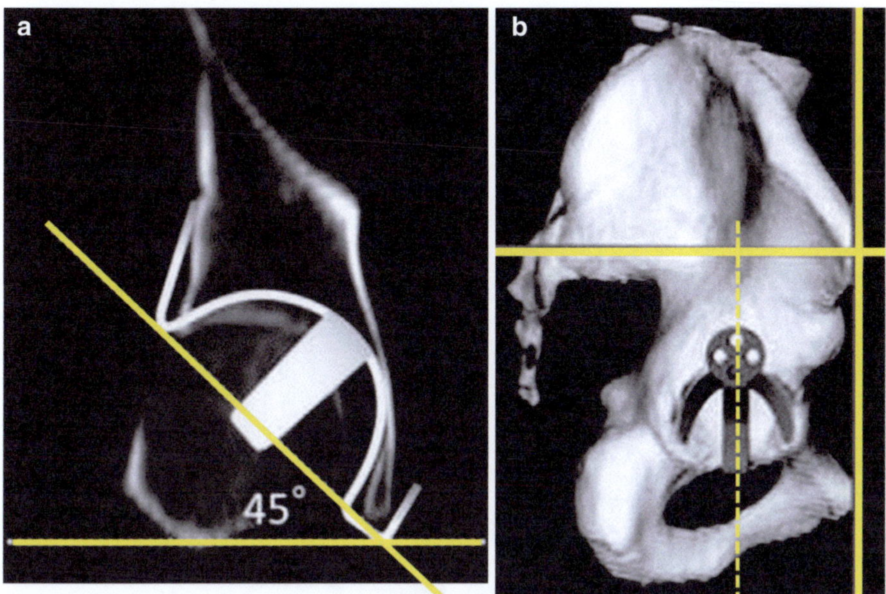


**Fig. 10.4** Sizing of the Kerboull Cross (KC) according to the diameter of the acetabulum. (**a**) The KC is correctly positioned and the size is appropriate. (**b**) The vertical axis must be parallel to the anterior plan of the pelvis

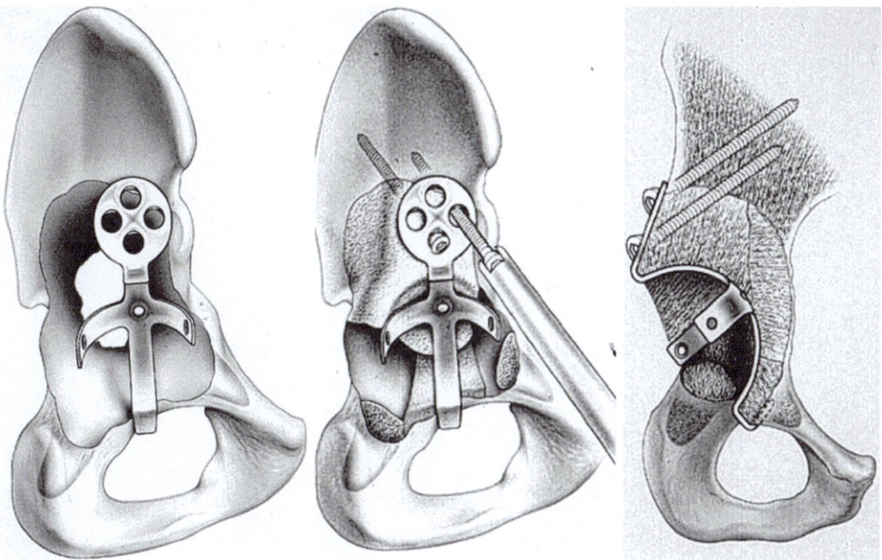

**Fig. 10.5** Positioning of the Kerboull plate and reconstruction of the acetabulum using structural allograft. The inferior hook must be positioned under the inferior margin of the obturator hole and the superior plate must be fixed on the ilium, at 45°of inclination. (From Kerboull et al. [17])

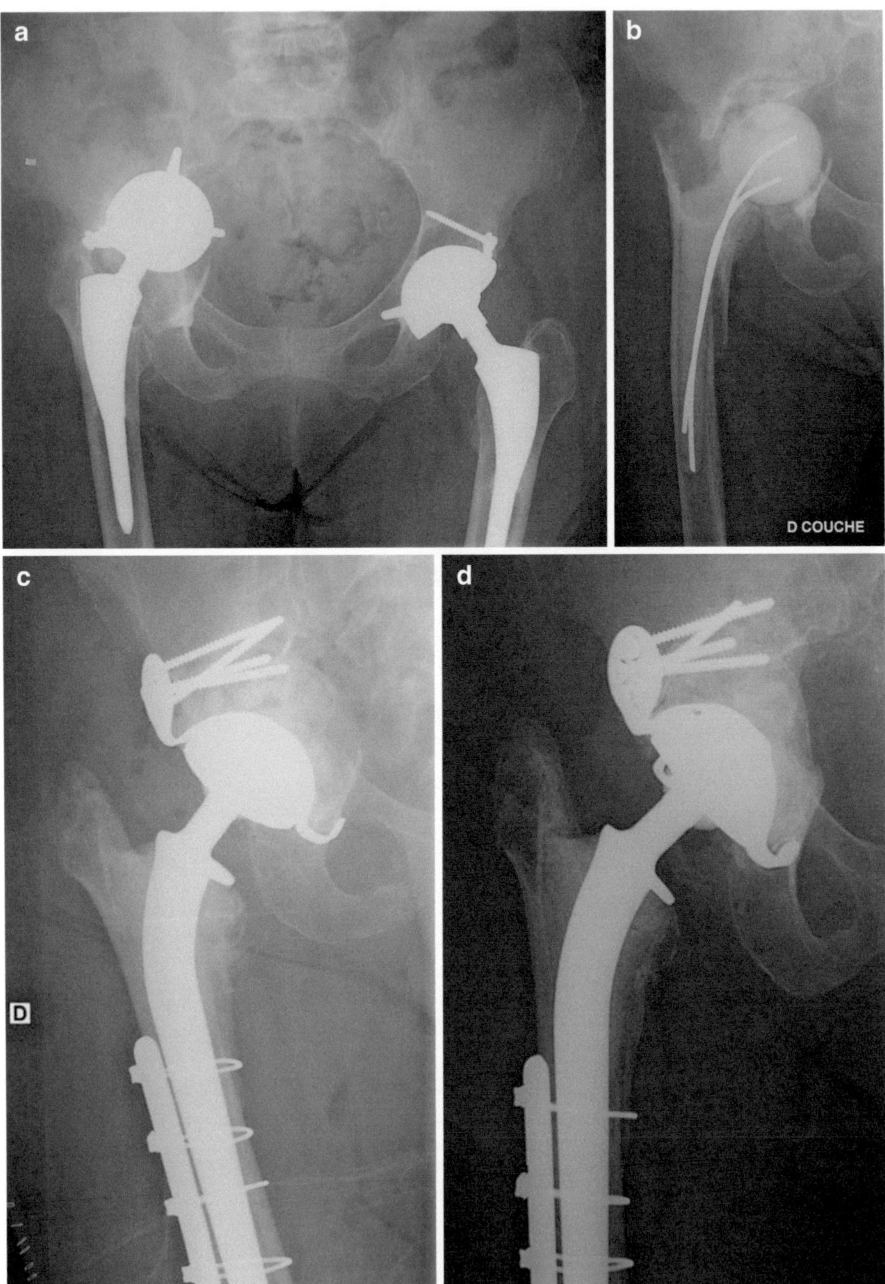


**Fig. 10.6** Women, 86 years old, with Parkinson disease and bilateral uncemented THA. (**a**) Deep infection on the left side with socket pelvic migration. (**b**) Two-stage THA revision. Acrylic spacer. (**c**) THA revision using DM cup cemented into a KC after acetabular reconstruction. (**d**) Excellent result at 1.5 years postoperative

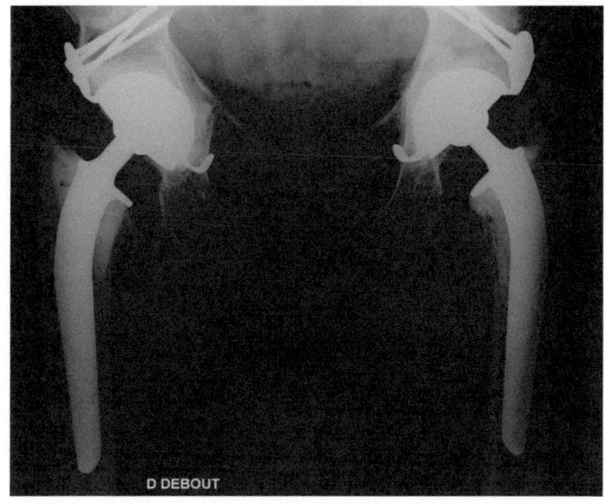


**Fig. 10.7** Bilateral THA bipolar revision in a 75 years old man, using DM cup cemented into a Kerboull plate and a cemented stem. Excellent results on both side at 2-years postoperative

osteolysis (30 hips), infection (2d stage) (4 hips), persistent pain (2 hips), recurrent dislocation (2 hips), and peri-prosthetic fracture (2 hips). All the patients had combined acetabular deficiencies (type III or IV according to the AAOS and Paprosky classifications). There were 6 unipolar and 34 bipolar revisions using 22 cemented and 12 uncemented stems (Fig. 10.7). The acetabular reconstruction has been made with structural femoral head allografts (32 hips) or cement (8 hips). The mean diameter of the DM cup was 49 mm (range 45–55). There were 32 heads of 28 mm (25 metallic, 7 ceramic) and 8 metallic head of 22.2 mm diameter.

Two patients were lost to follow up and one patient deceased from unrelated cause. All the surviving patients were reviewed with clinical and radiological exams. Two patients had a postoperative partial neurological palsy and one patient had a recurrence of deep infection with cup loosening. One patient had a stem exchange to a cemented stem at 1 year, and one patient had an acetabular revision at 5 months for migration of the KC due to an initial malposition. The average follow-up was 36 months. The mean Merle d'Aubigné hip score was 16.6 ± 1.1 at the last follow up. There was one cup migration. No patient had postoperative hip instability.

Our conclusion was that acetabular reconstruction using a DM cup cemented into a KC gave satisfactory results in terms of fixation and joint stability at short term. It becomes, therefore, an interesting option in THA revisions with acetabular reconstruction, especially in patients at risk for instability. However, results need to be confirmed at longer term.

DM cups cemented in a metal reinforcement have been reported in several series (Table 10.1) [6, 21, 22, 28, 30, 34, 36]. The series were very heterogeneous, in terms of patient characteristics, implants designs and surgical technique. They included 37–104 patients, at a mean follow-up ranging from 1.3 to 6.4 years, resulting in a total of 354 patients at a mean of 3.5 years follow-up. The rate of dislocation ranged from 0 to 10.4%, the rate of aseptic loosening from 0 to 6.4%, and the 5–7-year survival was close to 95%. Our series showed comparable, and even better, results

**Table 10.1** Series of dual mobility cups cemented in a metallic reinforcement

| | Hips (n) | Follow up (years) | Dislocation (%) | Aseptic loosening (%) | Aseptic revision (%) | Survival rate (%) |
|---|---|---|---|---|---|---|
| Langlais et al. [21] | 82 | 3 | 1.1 | 2.2 | 8 | 94.6% at 5 years |
| Schneider et al. [34] | 96 | 3.4 | 10.4 | 1 | 4.2 | 95.6% at 8 years |
| Philippot et al. [30] | 104 | 5 | 3.6 | 1.2 | 6.7 | 96.1% at 7 years |
| Civinini et al. [6] | 33 | 2 | 0 | 0 | 0 | 97% at 5 years |
| Pattyn et Audenaert [28] | 37 | 1.3 | 5.4 | 0 | 0 | – |
| Lebeau et al. [22] | 62 | 6.4 | 1.6 | 6.4 | 8.1 | 91.9% at 8 years |
| Wegrzyn et al. [36] | 61 | 7.5 | 0 | 0 | 0 | – |
| Present series | 40 | 3 | 0 | 2 | 2 | – |

in terms of functional scores, postoperative stability and rate of re-revision. Despite different designs of cemented DM cups and metal reinforcements (guided by the surgeon habitus and the severity of the acetabular lesions), a significant reduction of the risk of postoperative dislocation was reported in all series (except in the series of Schneider et al. [34], confirming the advantage of DM cups (cemented or not) as a way to limit, without eliminating, the risk of postoperative dislocation in THA revision [7, 12, 20, 24, 26, 30].

However, the use of DM cup cemented directly into the bone without a reinforcement device has encountered controversies. Although Haen et al. [13] have recently reported a rate of loosening of only 1.5% and a 5-year survival rate of 98%, most of the series have reported a high rate of loosening, ranging from 20% to 40%, and concluded that in case of severe acetabular bone loss, bone graft and reinforcement are recommended [5, 29]. Rates for aseptic loosening of DM cups cemented in a reinforcement have been reported between 0 and 2.2% within 3 years postoperatively [6, 21, 22, 28, 30, 34, 36]. However, Lebeau et al. [22] reported a rate of loosening as high as 6.4% at longer follow-up, considering cementing quality to be a determining factor of assembly stability. In vitro, Wegrzyn et al. [37] reported a good mechanical resistance of DM cups cemented in a reinforcement, greater than in vivo stress levels, and Ebramzadeh et al. [9] found that cement thickness of 2 mm or less between reinforcement and cup incurred greater risk of loosening than thicknesses of 4 mm or more. This may explain the differences reported in the literature in terms of loosening in series of cemented DM cups, illustrating the need for appropriate sizes and designs of cemented cup (transverse and longitudinal grooves on the metal-back, increments of 2 mm) to improve sealing, and a minimum of 2 mm thickness cement to improve the quality of fixation (Figs. 10.2 and 10.3).

## Conclusion

Dual-mobility cup cemented in a Kerboull Cross fulfills the charge-book of revision THA, in terms of reduced instability and bone fixation, at least at midterm. The procedure is indicated in case of poor bone quality and/or insufficient bone stock, in patients at risk for instability (repeat revisions, advanced age, poor medical status, weakness of abductors). The technique offers several potential advantages, by using an unconstrained device which preserves the range of motion of the hip and increases the jump distance while maintaining PE thickness, by automatically restoring the anatomical hip center and allowing bone stock restoration while protecting the graft from overstresses. An appropriate technique is essential, notably as regard the cross positioning (hook) and the cup cementing (with a minimum cement mantel thickness). The results are encouraging at midterm follow up, in terms of bone fixation and stability, but questions remain about long term fixation.

## References


1. Berry DJ. Unstable total hip arthroplasty: detailed overview. Instr Course Lect. 2001;50:265–74.
2. Bonnomet F, Clavert P, Gicquel P, Lefebre Y, Kempf JF. Reconstruction by graft and reinforcement device in severe aseptic acetabular loosening: 10 years survivorship analysis. Rev Chir Orthop. 2001;87(2):135–46.
3. Boyer B, Neri T, Geringer J, Di Iorio A, Philippot R, Farizon F. Long term wear of dual mobility total hip replacement cups: explant study. Int Orthop. 2018;42(1):41–7.
4. Bozic KJ, Kamath AF, Ong K, Lau E, Kurtz S, Chan V, Vail TP, Rubash H, Berry DJ. Comparative epidemiology of revision arthroplasty: failed THA poses greater clinical and economic burdens Than failed TKA. Clin Orthop Relat Res. 2015;473(6):2131.
5. Chen FS, Di Cesare PE, Kale AA, Lee JF, Frnakel VH, Stuchin SA, et al. Results of cemented metal-backed acetabular components. A 10-year-average follow-up study. J Arthroplast. 1998;13:867–73.
6. Civinini R, Carulli C, Matassi F, Nistri L, Innocenti M. A dual-mobility cup reduces risk of dislocation in isolated acetabular revisions. Clin Orthop Relat Res. 2012;470:3542–8.
7. Darrith B, Courtney PM, Della Valle CJ. Outcomes of dual mobility components in total hip arthroplasty: a systematic review of the literature. Bone Joint J. 2018 Jan;100-B(1):11–9.
8. De Martino I, D'Apolito R, Soranoglou VG, Poultsides LA, Sculco PK, Sculco TP. Dislocation following total hip arthroplasty using dual mobility acetabular components: a systematic review. Bone Joint J. 2017 Jan;99-B(ASuppl1):18–24.
9. Ebramzadeh E, Beaulé PE, Culwell JL, Amstutz HC. Fixation strength of an all-metal acetabular component cemented into an acetabular shell: a biomechanical analysis. J Arthroplast. 2004;19:45–9.
10. Fraser GA, Wroblewski BM. Revision of the Charnley low-friction arthroplasty for recurrent or irreducible dislocation. J Bone Joint Surg (Br). 1981;63B:552–5.
11. Gaudin G, Ferreira A, Gaillard R, Prudhon JL, Caton JH, Lustig S. Equivalent wear performance of dual mobility bearing compared with standard bearing in total hip arthroplasty: in vitro study. Int Orthop. 2017;41(3):521–7.
12. Guyen O, Pibarot V, Vaz G, Chevillotte C, Béjui-Hugues J. Use of a dual-mobility socket to manage total hip arthroplasty instability. Clin Orthop Relat Res. 2009;467:465–72.

13. Haen TX, Lonjon G, Vandenbussche E. Can cemented dual mobility cup be used without a reinforcement device in cases of mild acetabular bone stock alteration in total hip arthroplasty? Orthop Traumatol Surg Res. 2015;101:923–7.
14. Hailer NP, Weiss RJ, Stark A, Kärrholm J. Dual-mobility cups for revision due to instability are associated with a low rate of re-revisions due to dislocation: 228 patients from the Swedish hip arthroplasty register. Acta Orthop. 2012 Dec;83(6):566–71.
15. Hamadouche M, Biau DJ, Huten D, Musset T, Gaucher F. The use of a cemented dual-mobility socket to treat recurrent dislocation. Clin Orthop Rel Res. 2010;468:3248–54.
16. Jo S, Jimenez Almonte JH, Sierra RJ. The Cumulative Risk of Re-dislocation After Revision THA Performed for Instability Increases Close to 35% at 15 years. J Arthroplast. 2015 Jul;30(7):1177–82.
17. Kerboull M, Hamadouche M, Kerboull L. The Kerboull acetabular reinforcement device in major acetabular reconstructions. Clin Orthop Rel Res. 2000;378:155–68.
18. Kurtz S, Ong K, Lau E, Mowat F, Halpern M. Projections of primary and revision hip and knee arthroplasty in the United states from 2005 to 2030. J Bone Joint Surg Am. 2007;89(4):780–5.
19. Kurtz S, Ong KL, Lau E, Bozic KJ. Impact of the economic downturn on total joint replacement demand in the United States: updated projections to 2021. J Bone Joint Surg Am. 2014;96(8):624–30.
20. Lange JK, Spiro SK, Westrich GH. Utilizing dual mobility components for first-time revision total hip arthroplasty for instability. J Arthroplast. 2018 Feb;33(2):505–9.
21. Langlais F, Ropars M, Gaucher F, Musset T, Chaix O. Dual-mobility cemented cups have low dislocation rates in THA revisions. Clin Orthop Relat Res. 2008;466:389–95.
22. Lebeau N, Bayle M, Belhaouane R, Chelli M, Havet E, Brunschweiler B, Mertl P. Total hip arthroplasty revision by dual-mobility acetabular cup cemented in a metal reinforcement: A 62 case series at a minimum 5 years follow-up. Orthop Traumatol Surg Res. 2017;103(5):679–84.
23. Lecuire F, Benareau I, Rubini J, Basso M. Intra-prosthetic dislocation of the Bousquet dual-mobility socket. Orthop Traumatol Surg Res. 2004;90:249–55.
24. Leiber-Wackenheim F, Brunschweiler B, Ehlinger M, Gabrion M, Mertl P. Treatment of recurrent THR dislocation using of a cementless dual-mobility cup: a 59 cases series with a mean 8 years' follow-up. Orthop Traumatol Surg Res. 2011;97:8–13.
25. Lübbeke RC, Barea C, Köhnlein W, Hoffmeyer P. Revision total hip arthroplasty in patients 80 years or older. J Arthroplast. 2012;27:1041–6.
26. Massin P, Besnier L. Acetabular revision using a press-fit dual-mobility cup. Orthop Traumatol Surg Res. 2010;96:9–13.
27. Patel PD, Potts A, Froimson MI. The dislocating hip arthroplasty: prevention and treatment. J Arthroplast. 2007;22(suppl 1):86–90.
28. Pattyn C, Audenaert E. Early complications after revision total hip arthroplasty with cemented dual-mobility socket and reinforcement ring. Acta Orthop Belg. 2012;78:357–61.
29. Peraldi P, Vandenbussche E, Augereau B. Bad clinical results of cemented cups with metal-backed acetabular components. 124 cases with 21 months follow-up. Rev Chir Orthop. 1997;83:561–5.
30. Philippot R, Adam P, Reckhaus M, Delangle F, Verdot FX, Curvale G, et al. Post-prosthetic dislocation prevention in total hip revision surgery using a dual-mobility design. Orthop Traumatol Surg Res. 2009;95:505–11.
31. Prudhon JL, Desmarchelier R, Hamadouche M, Delaunay C, Verdier R. SoFCOT: Causes for revision of dual-mobility and standard primary total hip arthroplasty: matched case-control study based on a prospective multicenter study of two thousand and forty-four implants. Int Orthop. 2017;41(3):455–9.
32. Ravi B, Croxford R, Reichmann WM, Losina E, Katz JN, Hawker GA. The changing demographics of total joint arthroplasty recipients in the United States and Ontario from 2001 to 2007. Best Pract Res Clin Rheumatol. 2012;26(5):637–47.

33. Regis SA, Bonetti I, Bortolami O, Bartolozzi P. A minimum of 10-year follow-up of the Burch-Schneider cage and bulk allografts for the revision of pelvic discontinuity. J Arthroplast. 2012;27:1057–63.
34. Schneider L, Philippot R, Boyer B, Farizon F. Revision total hip arthroplasty using a reconstruction cage device and a cemented dual-mobility. Orthop Traumatol Surg Res. 2011;97:807–13.
35. Wachtl SW, Jung M, Jakob RP, Gautier E. The Burch-Schneider antiprotrusion cage in acetabular revision surgery: a mean follow-up of 12 years. J Arthroplast. 2000;15:959–63.
36. Wegrzyn J, Pibarot V, Jacquel A, Carret JP, Béjui-Hugues J, Guyen O. Acetabular reconstruction using a Kerboull cross-plate, structural allograft and cemented dual-mobility cup in revision THA at a minimum 5-year follow-up. J Arthroplast. 2014;29:432–7.
37. Wegrzyn J, Thoreson AR, Guyen O, Lewallen DG, An KN. Cementation of a dual-mobility acetabular component into a well-fixed metal shell during revision total hip arthroplasty. J Orthop Res. 2013;31(6):991–7.

# Chapter 11
# Trabecular Metal in Acetabular Revision Surgery for Severe Bone Defects and Pelvic Discontinuity

**José Sueiro-Fernandez**

## Introduction

Acetabular revision surgery in large bone defects is one of the greatest challenges for the orthopaedic surgeon. It is accepted by all that one of the most important factors affecting the final result of achieving a stable acetabular revision component is the existing bone defect [1]. As a first step in reconstruction, we must identify and classify the bone defect presented to us, even knowing that during the surgical act this will be greater than that initially foreseen. There are multiple classifications that help us identify bone loss at both the acetabular and femoral levels. No one classification can be said to be considered "ideal" and all are subject to controversies either because of incompleteness or because of differences between observers. A large part of the classifications described in the orthopaedic literature have been the result of surgical observations by surgeons who are experts in the subject. In this case, we must exclude the classification called D'Antonio, which emerged as a consensus effort of the American Academy of Orthopaedic Surgeons. Many of these proposed classifications have often not been scrutinised for reliability or validity, and this may be one reason why they have not obtained the support of a large number of surgeons performing these arthroplasty revisions. In the 1990s, when part of these classifications was established, no test of reliability and reproducibility was established either because of imaging test development or surgeon inertia. As Gozard et al. [2] says, Saleh's ranking was the first, and until a few years ago, the only one which was rigorously tested by his own authors, and the only which has demonstrated high inter-observer reliability (Kappa index above 0.8). The first validity and reliability study of the Paprosky classification was published in 2013 [3], obtaining a kappa

J. Sueiro-Fernandez
Orthopaedics Department, Medical School, Cadiz University, Cadiz, Spain

Orthopaedic Surgery Department, Hospital Puerto Real, Cadiz, Spain
e-mail: jose.sueiro@uca.es



E. García-Rey, E. García-Cimbrelo (eds.), *Acetabular Revision Surgery in Major Bone Defects*, https://doi.org/10.1007/978-3-319-98596-1_11

**Table 11.1** Equivalence of acetabular defects according to different classifications taken from Johanson et al. [4] box in red, the defects considered major

MAJOR ACETABULAR DEFECTS

| | | | | | | | | |
|---|---|---|---|---|---|---|---|---|
| Saleh | I | | II | | III | IV | V | |
| Paprosky | 1 | 2a | 2b | 2c | 3a | 3b | | |
| D'Antonio | | | II | | ? ⋮ III | | IV | V |
| Gross | | | Protrussio | | Shelf | Acetabular | | |
| Engh | Mild | | Moderate | | | Severe | | |
| Gustilo | I | | II | | III | IV | | |

index of 0.79 after three learning sessions with it. It also seems interesting that these classifications have scoring guides for the assessment of radiographic characteristics. However, and despite this, as high-degree defects are the least frequent ones, we still need a higher "n" to be able to standardise these classifications.

It is not time in this chapter to list the most used classifications or to make a critique of their weaknesses or recount their strengths. But we need to properly define what we consider a major acetabular bone defect. In this regard, we should highlight the efforts of Johanson et al. [4] in the search for a universal and valid system of classification of acetabular defects. On this basis, we will consider for this chapter major or high-grade defects as follows (Table 11.1 – Red Box):

1. Type III defects of the Paprosky Classification:

   *Superior migration >2 cm and severe medial and ischial osteolysis*
   *IIIA. Köhler's line intact, 30–60% of the component in contact with graft (rim defect: 10–2 o'clock position).*
   *IIIB. Köhler's line is not intact, more than 60% of the component in contact with graft (rim defect – 9–5 o'clock position).*
   Both can be associated to pelvic discontinuity, with more frequent presentation (2/3 of cases) in Type IIIB

2. Type III (Combined) and Type IV (Pelvic Discontinuity) defects of the D'Antonio (AAOS) Classification
3. Type III, IV and V defects of the Saleh Classification:

   - *Type III: Uncontained loss of bone material where there is a less than 50% segmental loss of the acetabulum involving the anterior or posterior column*
   - *Type IV: Uncontained loss of bone material where there is a greater than 50% segmental loss greater of the acetabulum affecting both anterior and posterior columns.*
   - *Type V: Acetabular defect with uncontained bone loss in association with pelvic discontinuity*

4. Acetabular defect of the Gross Classification:

Acetabular defect of one or both columns with a loss of more than 50% of acetabulum

5. Severe defect of the Engh Classification:

The acetabular cavity shows very significant, sclerotic, perforated, and non-hemispheric damage. The edge of the ring is weakened or broken.

6. Gustilo Type III and IV Defect:

*Type III: Local wall defect*

(a) *Anterior*
(b) *Posterior*
(c) *Superior*
(d) *Central*

*Type IV: Collapse or massive global defect affecting one or both columns.*

## Technical Possibilities

When confronted with hip arthroplasty revision on the acetabular side, the orthopaedic surgeon has a wide variety of techniques and implants that should make it easier to restore anatomy and recover hip function. When the acetabular defect is severe, the treatment options are reduced to the use of cups of special designs such as oblong, bilobed, or custom-made triflange cups, reinforcement cages, or the use of trabecular metal augments. Although the use of jumbo-type components for large defects has been proposed, we will not take this into consideration, it is a technical option essentially for moderate defects. Very complete and updated systematic review made by Volpin et al. [5] A total of 50 studies of level IV scientific evidence were included. No randomised controlled trials (RCTs) were available, which was expected given the nature of the study. This pooled analysis suggests that oblong cup components had a lower failure rate compared with other different materials considered in this review. Custom-made triflange cups had one of highest failure rates. However, this may reflect the complexity of revisions and severity of bone loss in the different groups.

In all these high-grade defects, the use of bone graft will always be necessary as a common denominator, preferably an allograft, either structural or fragmented. We will thus first describe the role played by these grafts in acetabular reconstruction with large defects.

Short- and medium-term studies of **structural allograft** have demonstrated "certain success", reporting an overall percentage of good results of 67.1–76% at 5 years [6, 7] and until a few years ago it was the standard [8]. Nevertheless, follow-up from 5 years onwards was affected by complications such as graft resorption, and above all the loss of fixation, leading to great discouragement with its use, while very good short-term results were published with the use of flying buttresses and trabecular metal augments [9]. However, with the improvement in the technique and the indication of its use in revisions of young patients using this structural allograft, a number of benefits have been added which are worth taking into account, and are now achieving full recognition [10].

In order to make their integration as favourable as possible, when using these structured allografts, a stable fixation must be made and a minimum percentage of contact with the host bone, which has been accepted by the majority to be about 50% [11]. However, it is true that other circumstances also need to be considered such as the type of implant metal and the quality of the receiver bone and graft [12, 13].

Regis et al. presented their study of a total of 71 hip arthroplasty revisions, of which 56 were assessed [14]. They had Paprosky IIIA defects in 32% of cases and IIIB in 68%. Large allografts and anti-protrusion cages were used. The reported mean follow-up was 11.7 years, with a total survival of 87.5%. With this percentage, the technique is more favourable compared to others in long-term reconstruction for the treatment of extensive losses of the acetabular bone reserve.

It could be thought that these massive grafts would not be appropriate for revision treatment of infected arthroplasties. Lee et al. [15] conducted a retrospective study of 27 patients reviewed at two times after hip infection. In five patients, moderate or severe acetabular defect was detected. In the overall series, 10-year survival was 93%. Based on this data, they argue that the use of structural allografts is a reasonable option to treat massive bone loss in infected hip arthroplasties in selected patients.

Finally, we should mention the good results reported by Brown et al. with the use of structural distal femoral allograft for the treatment of Paprosky Type IIIA defects [16]. They retrospectively reviewed 31 hips with a mean age of 61 years and a follow-up of 21 years. The acetabular implant was a porous-coated hemispheric dome inserted and secured with screws. They achieved a survival rate of 72%, which means that these massive grafts must continue to be considered in the orthopaedic arsenal for younger patients with type IIIA defects, achieving great improvement in the restoration of the rotation centre and especially of the bone stock with a view to possible future interventions. All this will be clarified after the analysis of trabecular metal that will done further on.

It seems reasonable to use biological techniques, as the **impaction bone grafting (IBG)**, to help restore bone reserve to rebuild acetabular defects in revision surgery. Although there is a history of using bone grafts in arthritic acetabular protrusions, it was not until 1984 that Slooff et al. modified their technique for use in revisions [17]. Since then, the Nimegen' school has shown good clinical outcomes in the medium to long term. In 2001 they published their results with this technique over 20 years of experience [18]. Specifically, they reported 60 hip revisions using their technique, 37 of them with cavitary defects and 23 with combined defects. The reported survival rate for aseptic loosening was 94% at 12 years. They later notified the results between 20 and 25 years, with a favourable survival rate, although it is difficult here to identify the percentage of cases with severe defects, the subject by this chapter, which were registered among those who remained unrevised [19].

Regardless of the more limited diffusion this technique had among American surgeons for minor or medium-sized defects, its efficacy for large defects is doubted. Thus, Van Haaren et al. [20] analysed 71 revisions with an average follow-up of 7.2 years. Forty-one type III and IV cases according to the AAOS classification were identified. Almost all of those in group IV failed (except one case), and a third of all type III cases. This is why they claimed that this high proportion of failures suggests that the IBG technique offers poor results in extensive acetabular defects. These poor results are evident in the study of Gilbody et al. [21], where in a minimum follow-up of 10 years they analysed 304 revisions for aseptic loosening. They reported an overall survival of 85.9% at 13.5 years on average. Significantly, almost half of their failures with this technique occurred in Paprosky type 3A and 3B defects.

Analysing the corresponding data from the previous studies reveals a different behaviour of this technique related to the location of the extensive acetabular defect. This was confirmed by García-Rey et al. who proposed in their study to compare survival between Paprosky type 3A and 3B (large posterolateral versus medial defect) [22]. In their series of 100 hips with type 3A and 104 with type 3B defects, and an average follow-up of 10 years, they observed a significant and favourable survival for medial defects, so they recommend to use an optional aid to rebuild lateral defects. Recently, good results of the IBG technique have been reported in Paprosky type 3B defects, but it should be noted that the average follow-up of 47 months was relatively short, and the authors themselves recommend a longer follow-up so that the potential deterioration of the acetabular fixation can actually be observed [23].

From all the above we can say that the IBG technique is the first choice technique for young patients, as it allows us to recover the bone reserve and the rotation centre, but requires a thorough knowledge of its technical details. It is the first choice in these cases, but not a universal solution, as we must bear in mind that for large acetabular defects affecting the posterolateral zone such as a Paprosky type 3A defect, its survival is limited to the medium and long term, and therefore will require, according to schools, a structural allograft protected by cages, trabecular metal augments or custom-made triflange cup.

Due to this recognised weakness, some better alternative to the IBG technique were proposed, such as inside mesh usage [24]. In the 14 case series, all Paprosky type 3B, no re-revision was recorded. It is an interesting option with still short follow-up (maximum 36 months). Hernigou et al. propose to use irradiated sterilized allograft and over-fed with mesenchymal stem cells is also attractive [25]. They compared two groups of 30 hips each (all, Paprosky type 3A or 3B) with and without mesenchymal cell overload, finding a lower proportion of failures in revitalized grafts. To strengthen assembly in large defects requiring a large containment mesh, a "hybrid" technique has been proposed using trabecular metal augments. This method was first reported in 2012 by the Newcastle Group in Northeast England [26] and also referred to by the Exeter Group in 2013 and in Germany by the

EndoKlinic in 2014. The result in terms of the re-revision rate in these studies was about 4% in the average follow-up of below 5 years [27]. The main virtue of this hybrid technique is that it simplifies surgical technical gestures and adds greater strength to the assembly, being particularly useful for type IIIA defects.

Several acetabular revisions have been reported using uncemented cups after IBG [28, 29], but we will not consider it as it is not considering to be a first line option for severe Paprosky type III defects or AAOS type III and IV defects. The same series reveal that the number of cases with high defects are the fewest.

## Reconstruction Cages

Reconstruction cages combined with structural or fragmented allografts have shown good results, especially in the medium-term follow-up. The literature contains a wealth of work on this technical option, including those related to the **Burch-Schneider cage (BSC)**. The most numerous of these are the many reports in the literature on the use of BSC and their advantages in the treatment of serious acetabular defects, as detailed below [30–32].

BSC was based on the premise of creating a bridge that would at the same time have a protective effect on allograft that helps improve bone reserve. Robert Schneider adopted this concept a year later and among other changes oriented the upper flange towards the sacroiliac joint [33]. The original BSC was made of polished steel, and later in 1986, the developments in titanium began that culminated in rough-blasted titanium in 1999. It was originally intended to screw the bottom flange in the ischium, so it had screw holes. In 2004 a modification of the BSC was introduced, with more anatomical features, a change in the position of the screws, and an unperforated lower flange so that it could be embedded in the ischium [34]. Most authors agree that the most reliable indications for these reinforcement cages would be for larger, usually segmental, acetabular defects that compromise both columns, such as Paprosky types 3A and 3B defects, as well as pelvic discontinuity [34].

Long-term results on the effectiveness of this cage were published as early as 2009. Symeonides et al. conducted a follow-up of 57BSC implants between 5 and 21 years [35]. They reported that there were five Type III cases and 43 Type IV cases according to the AAOS classification. They found only 10.5% of failures between aseptic loosening and mechanical failures. They concluded that the BSC is a durable solution for major acetabular defects.

In this same line is the study of Coscujuela et al. on 96 acetabular revisions treated with BSC, with an average follow-up between 5 and 13 years [31]. These include 25 Type 3A and 11 Type 3B cases according to the Paprosky classification, where the rotational centre is effectively lowered. They confirmed their objective that the BSC has a favourable survival (92.4%) compared to other devices. Combination with structural and/or impaction allograft, the BSC has been a gold standard in acetabular revision of major defects until the arrival of the Trabecular Metal implant.

Another type of reinforcement ring, that we have used has been the ***Graft Augmentation Prosthesis (GAP).*** This type of cage was used in the late nineties and early years of the new millennium. The device launched in its early design was made of sand blasted titanium alloy with a hydroxyapatite coating. Various holes only in the upper pole for the dome and two iliac plates with a single row of three to four holes for the corresponding screws. These highly moldable prolongations can be cut or adapted to the ilium.

There is much less information in the literature about GAP device results compared to the BSC. Duffy et al. studied 17 consecutive cases, of which 11 had a type III acetabular defect according to the AAOS classification, with an average follow-up of 6.5 years [36]. They reported a high percentage of mechanical failure for the GAP-1, so they prefer to use more rigid devices. This GAP-1 was also studied by Hernandez-Vaquero et al. with a slightly shorter follow-up (37 months on average) [37]. Among their cases, seven patients were type 3 and 4 according to the Gross classification. None required revision, and they defend this construct because it allows lowering the rotation centre and recovery of the bone structure reserve early without major complications.

This cage was later modified with multiple holes through the dome for an optional placement of screws, a posterosuperior rim and flanges with five screw holes, this device being known as the GAP II Cage. We collected our experience with this device in 22 cases with an average follow-up of 42 months. Defects were type IIC in 27% of cases and type III in 18%, we experienced three complications with the need for new surgery in two cases, and the other case due to mechanical failure with no clinical significance (Fig. 11.1) [38].

Years later, a high percentage of mechanical failures in severe defects were reported in 2012. Buttaro et al. [39] reviewed 24 patients, 10 Type III patients and 14 Type IV patients according to the AAOS classification, with an average follow-up of 34 months, and observed a 37% rate of catastrophic failures in reconstruction with the GAP II, and particularly in Type IV patients, so they abandoned its use for these advanced defects. More recently, medium-term results with this cage were reported in 2018. Twenty-six cases with an average follow-up of 49 months, of which 12 were type IIIA and 8 were type IIIB, showed a 100% survival rate, although three of them had radiographic failure of the implant without clinical consequences [40]. The mechanical failures related to this type of device have been attributed to its greater malleability, but it can be observed in other series with more rigid implants that the same fatigue was also reported [41].

In summary, in this section we can say that the GAP-type reinforcement cage has been less studied than the BSC, but they meet their objectives of reorienting the rotation centre and restoring bone reserve. Its medium and long-term failures are significant due to the lack of graft integration and osteointegration of the implant, and it is of vital importance for us to explain this, the lack of ischial anchorage, particularly in severe defects such as Paprosky type III.

The ring, plate or cross de **Kerboull (KT)** was designed in 1974 to contain bone allografts placed behind it. This is an implant made of steel, with a lower hook applied to the tear-drop acetabular image and an upper plate fixed to the iliac by four

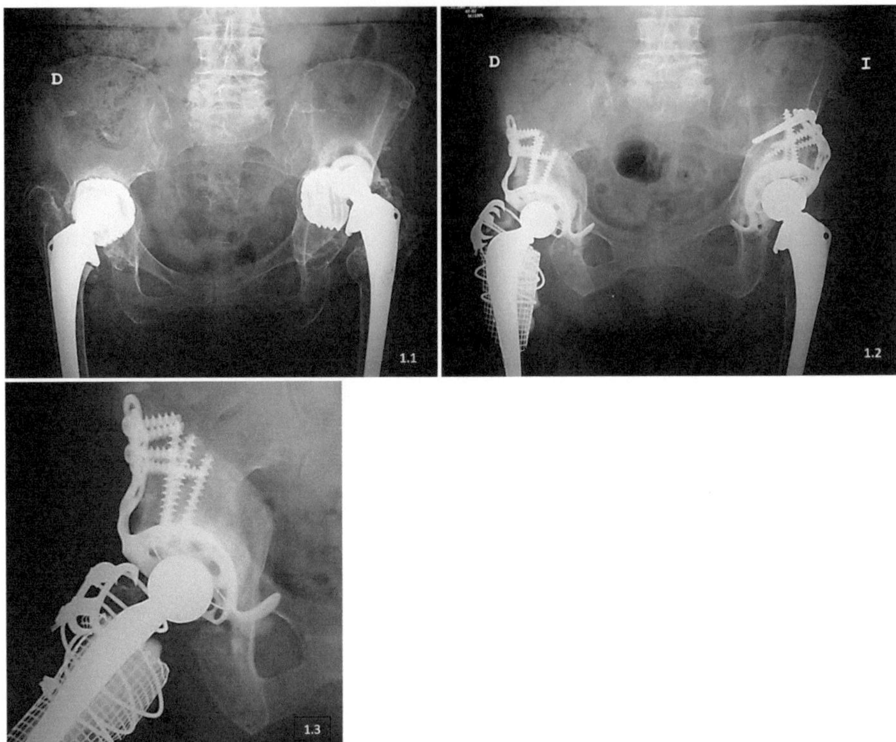


**Fig. 11.1** 1.1: Bilateral acetabular defects. Paprosky type IIC in right side and type IIIB in left. 1.2: Reconstruction with structural and fragmented allograft bone, cage reinforcement GAP II. 1.3: Right hip detail associated to femoral impaction bone grafting

or six screws. It allows large cavities to be filled with allografts and a conventional cup to be cemented, with direct load transmitted to the grafts, as the ring is flexible. The Kerboull plate, KT plate and KT plate for hip replacement are currently distinguished. Its use for acetabular reconstruction has been proposed even in large defects, but failures for severe defects were already reported in 2008. Of 35 cases (34 AAOS Type III and 1 Type IV), 11 failures were found, although three of these did not have clinically significance [42]. Baba and Shitoto reported a survival of 87.5% with a 5-year follow-up in the KT plate group, but only recorded 11 type III and 1 type IV cases according to the AAOS classification [43]. Technical details are emphasised in their application and it is recommended to use a structural graft if the impacted graft layer is greater than 20 mm [44], according to a study of 29 type III defects with a median follow-up of 6.3 years [45], where use of the structural femoral head graft in reconstruction with this device was of great value [46]. A recent series supported by the Kerboull Institute itself performed very well in type 3A and 3B defects, showing a survival of 85.1% at 15.2 years [47]. Other authors has confirmed good results for moderate defects and, conversely, the high rate of revision failures using the Kerboull acetabular reinforcement device with a large skeletal defect of the acetabulum, especially in the cross-plate junction, and its risk factors have been analysed [48].

Sembrano and Cheng performed an analysis of the risk factors related to their failure, using various types of devices [49]. They included in their series 51 Paprosky type III cases, finding an overall survival of 81.3% without any reoperation. Abolghasemian et al. analyse various rings and reinforcement cages for re-revisions with a survival of 75% at 5 years and 56% at 10 years [10]. The use of these structural bone graft reinforcement rings has a very beneficial impact on major defects and discontinuities as preparation for a new revision that is more likely in younger people.

## Special Design Cups

We will not consider jumbo, oblong, bilobed, or asymmetrical cups because, in our opinion, for severe defects with or without pelvic discontinuity, they have their limitations. It is true that the series on these designs also contain a limited number for severe defects [50–53]. Perhaps the greatest success of this type of cups compared to others such as custom-made cups may be due to the fact that their most frequent use is not for such highly severe defects.

Special attention should be given to **Custom-made triflange (CMT)** acetabular components. Already in 2001 a series was presented with these special cups with a follow-up of between 2 and 9 years, which acknowledged 39 pelvic discontinuities and reported a 7.8% rate of dislocation requiring reoperation [54]. DeBoer et al. report that skeletal cement bridges were found in 18 out of 20 hips studied [55] and in the other two implant migration and screw breakage were not observed, but in 5 patients there was one or more postoperative dislocations. Taunton et al. published a large series on pelvic discontinuity with 57 cases which, after a 2-year follow-up, found stability of the component and cure of the discontinuity in 81% [56]. The cost of these implants came to be equivalent to the construct with metal trabecular cup cage, i.e. between 11,000 and 12,000 US dollars. Berasi et al. asked whether these reconstructions were effective, and in their series of 28 hips, all with a 3B defects and an average follow-up of 57 months, they required four subsequent reoperations, and therefore responded that custom triflange components represent a reliable tool in the arsenal of the reconstructive surgeon [57]. There are variations in the strategy of shaping and manufacture, and the preoperative study and preoperative templating are essential with novel three-dimensional reconstructions [58–61].

The CMT tends to lateralize the hip center by approximately 1 cm, and there is a trend toward nearly 2 cm of lateralization in failed construct [62]. In the last year, good results have been reported at 5 and 10 years [63]. Moore et al. reviewed the results of 37 patients undergoing custom triflange revision surgery. Two patients were lost to follow-up, leaving 35 patients with minimum 10-year clinical and radiographic follow-up. Thirty-two (91%) of 35 components were unrevised and functioning well at minimum 10-year follow-up [64].

Although there are few studies describing clinical outcomes (most common complications include dislocation and infection), the rates of revision of the implants for other reasons are low [65]. Clinical results are promising given the challenging problem. We think these devices can be helpful in catastrophic bone loss situations such as type IIIB defects and chronic pelvic discontinuities with the disadvantage that their preparation and manufacture may take a few months [56]. Ries report that CMT would be indicated for massive bone loss with or without discontinuity and when other reconstructive options are not feasible [66]. We believe that in the coming years this technique will become more readily available for more widespread use by the reconstructive surgeon.

## Trabecular Metal (TM)

The first studies with hopeful results in acetabular revision surgery by combining tantalum cups with the first "augments" and "restrictors" for moderate and severe defects were published in 2005 [67, 68]. Compared with other commonly used materials, tantalum has been shown to have a substantially higher friction coefficient on cancellous bone and higher bone interface shear strength compared to other fixation surfaces. This metal, due to its reduced stiffness, may also provide a more favourable environment for the remodelling of morsellised or structural bone graft in comparison with other material [69].

We published our experience with trabecular metal augments and cup-cage constructs [70]. Of 35 patients undergoing acetabular reconstruction with a TM acetabular revision system, 19 acetabular revisions associated with major bone loss in which we reconstructed the acetabulum with buttress tantalum augments or cup-cage construct combined with a TM shell, were available for evaluation. Mean follow-up was 26 months (range 18–43 months). Mean patient age was 63 years, and 12 patients were women. All defects were classified according to Paprosky and Saleh classifications; there were 13 type IIIA and 6 type IIIB acetabular defects. Five chronic pelvic discontinuities were preoperatively or intraoperatively assessed (Saleh type 5) and a cup-cage construction was employed. The centre of the femoral head was relocated from a mean of 1.4 cm (range, −3–2.6 cm) lateral from the vertical at the teardrop to 3 cm (range 0.2–4 cm). No mechanical failure has occurred in any hip, and all patients have radiographically stable cups (Figs. 11.2 and 11.3).

Different studies in the early years of this decade defended the use of TM. When the reconstruction ring fails, it performs better and delivers better TM and cup-cage results compared to treatment with a second reinforcement ring [71]. Operative reports, radiographs, and clinical data were evaluated. Minimum follow-up was 24 months (average 57 months; range 24–209 months). They get as a result that 33 failed first reinforcement rings were converted to one of three types of acetabular reconstruction, TM cup in 14, cup-cage in seven and a second reinforcement rings in 12. The TM cup group (TM cup and cup-cage) had a significantly longer survival than the second reinforcement rings group.

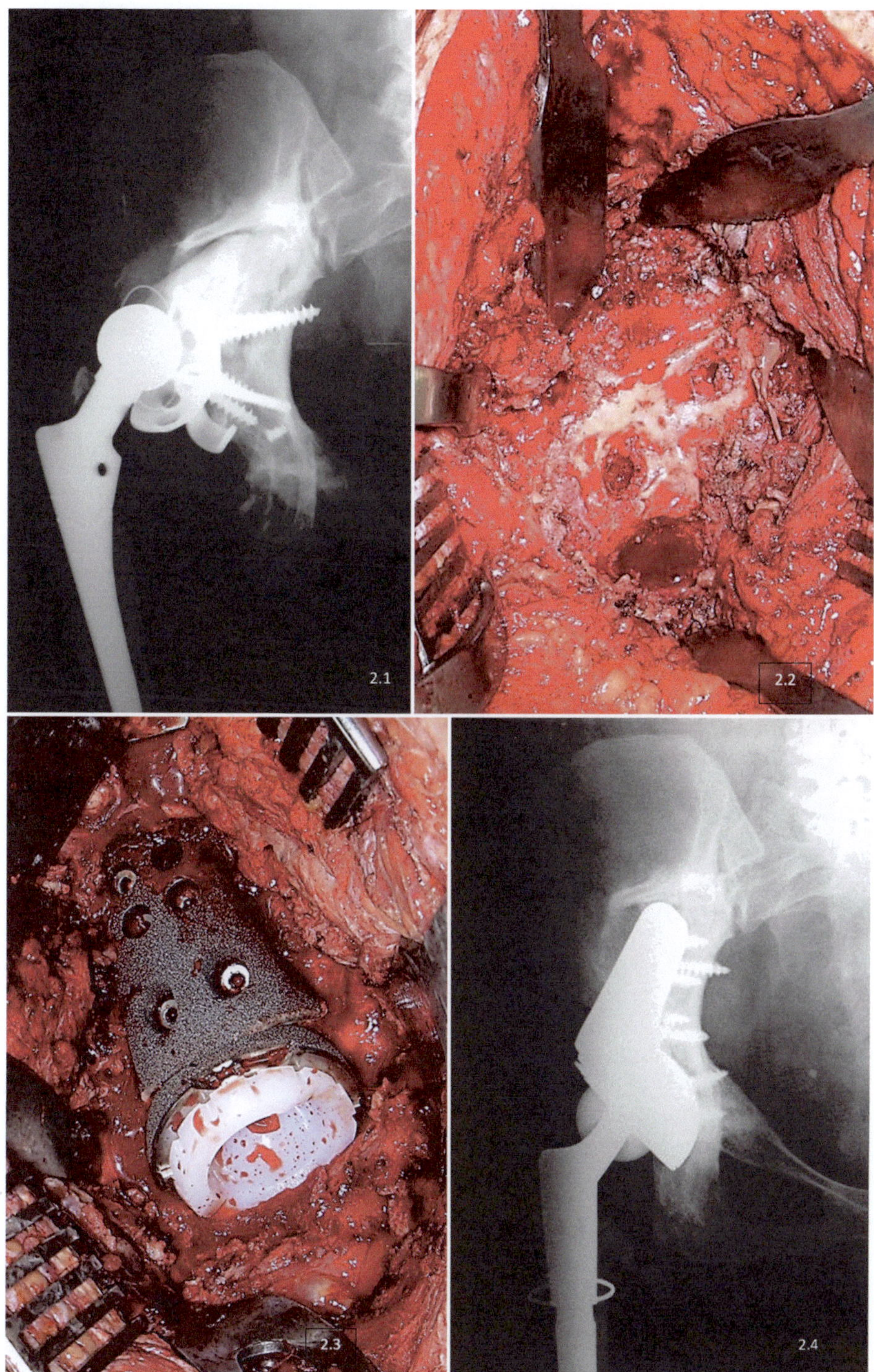


**Fig. 11.2** 2.1: Acetabular defects Paprosky type IIIA. 2.2: Intraoperative view. 2.3: Iliac butress. 2.4: Postoperative radiograph at 7 years

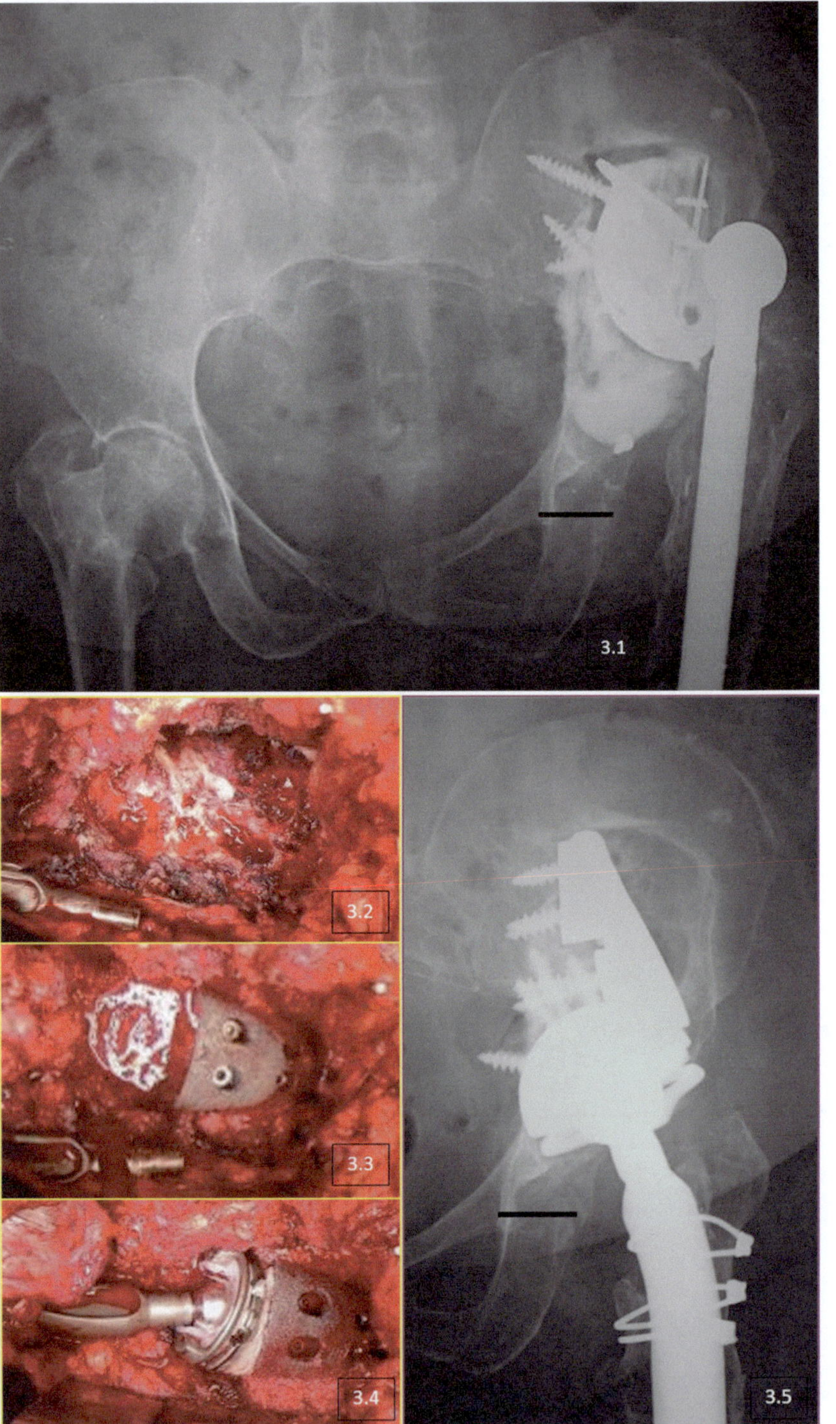


**Fig. 11.3** 3.1: Acetabular defects Paprosky type IIIA without pelvic discontinuity. 3.2–3.4: Intraoperative views. 3.5: Postoperative radiograph reconstruction: trabecular metal and iliacs augments with supplements blocks

Banerjee et al. did a systematic review of 25 studies of four electronic databases [72]. There was lack of high quality evidence (level I and level II studies) and only two studies with level III evidence, while the remainder were all level IV studies. In addition, a majority of the studies had small sample sizes and had short to mid-term follow-up. The mean age of the patients was 65 years (range, 58–72 years) and the mean follow-up was 3.6 years (range, two to six years). They allowed him to conclude that the short-term clinical and radiographic results of highly-porous metals in revision hip arthroplasty are excellent with a low rate of loosening in the presence of both major and minor bone loss. Jain et al. focuses their attention on the group of patients with severe acetabular losses [73]. A literature search of multiple databases applying specific criteria revealed a total of 50 articles of level IV scientific evidence comprising 2415 patients (2480 hips) managed with reinforcement devices, custom-made triflanged acetabular components, jumbo cups and tantalum metal (TM) systems. Overall, patients had improved postoperative hip scores for each technique. The use of reinforcement devices resulted in a mean revision rate of 8.2% and a mean complication rate of 29.21%. Custom-made were associated with a revision rate of 15.9% and had a complication rate of 24.5%. Jumbo cups were revised in 8.8% of patients and had a complication rate of 18.4%. TM systems had an overall revision rate of 8.5% with complications seen in 18.5% of patients. Custome made had considerably higher revision rates compared to the other techniques.

Similarly, Beckman et al. in another study based on a systematic literature review compared treatment for acetabular revision with trabecular metal and reinforcement rings with an average follow-up between 3 and 5 years [74]. They review the literature on the treatment of revision acetabular arthroplasty using revision rings (1541 cases) and TM, implants (1959 cases) to determine if a difference with regard to revision failure could be determined. In the study, TM shows statistically significant decreased loosening rates relative to revision rings for all grades including severe acetabular defects and pelvic discontinuity. The severe defects appear to benefit the most from TM.

The clinical and radiological results at 5 years of follow-up were better than those offered by reinforcement rings. All this is confirmed with the recent work de López-Torres et al. [75]. They compare in 94 hips the clinical and radiological outcomes, complications, and survival of two systems commonly used in complex acetabular revisions (AAOS types II, III, and IV), (TM) and BSC. The mean follow-up was 4.77 years, and TM implants afforded better clinical outcomes and greater patient satisfaction than antiprotrusion cages in the treatment of severe acetabular defects. Numerous articles have been communicated in recent years highlighting the good results of the use of trabecular metal with a 5–7 year follow-up for severe defects. The percentage of survival reflected is very high in relation to the severity of the defect (between 91.2% and 94.7%) [76–79].

In 2017 the Mayo Clinic Department reported on its series of 58 hips with a minimum follow-up of 5 years [80]. The defects studied were Paprosky type IIIA in 48% and type IIIB in 38%, including 11 cases of discontinuity. The mean preoperative Mayo hip score was 35.7, which improved to 61.9 at 3 months and was 61.7 at the minimum 5-year follow-up. They demonstrated a 97% survival rate and satisfactory function maintenance, but six failures of 11 discontinuities make it advisable to reinforce its fixation or use alternative techniques.

One of the main weaknesses offered by the MT system and its augments is that they do not improve the bone stock. Interesting proposal that makes Prieto et al. of the same previous Orthopedic Department to make compatible MT and structural allograft [81]. They identify 58 hips where a trabecular metal revision cup was supported by structural allograft. Mean follow-up was 5.4 years. Preoperatively acetabular bone defects were classified as Paprosky 3A in 11 hips (19%), and 3B in 17 hips (29%). All hips showed evidence of union between the allograft and host bone at latest follow-up, 14 hips had partial resorption of the allograft that did not affect cup stability. Three acetabular components demonstrated failure of ingrowth. Survivorship-free from radiographic acetabular loosening as end point was 94% at 5 years. The 5-year survivorship with revision for any reason as end point was 90%. Therefore, another positive aspect of trabecular metal is that these acetabular components combined with structural bone allograft show excellent survival (94%) over the medium term (5 years). Allograft restored bone reserve with minimal resorption and when it occurred, it did not alter the survival of the acetabular component.

## Pelvic Discontinuity

Pelvic discontinuity (PD) is a loss of integrity or continuity between the inferior pelvis and the superior pelvis considering the acetabulum the centre thereof. PD is a complex problem in orthopaedic surgery and can be defined as a complication of hip arthroplasty in which there is a massive loss of structural bone through the anterior and posterior columns of the acetabulum [82]. This discontinuity that separates the ilium from the ischium results in internal rotation of the lower segment and external rotation of the upper segment.

This situation can be reached as a result of a progressive resorption of the bone secondary to periprosthetic osteolysis that results in a combined segmental and cavity bone defect. However, discontinuity may also appear acutely due to trauma, infection, fracture during the excessive impactation of a primary or revision cup or over reaming of the acetabulum [83, 84]. This differentiation is important as the treatment strategy will be very different.

The estimated incidence in hip revision calculated according to different publications is between 1% and 8% of all acetabular revisions preformed [85], although it should be agreed that this figure could be higher if they did not go undetected in certain cases. Risk factors for PD include female sex, rheumatoid arthritis, prior pelvic radiation, and a massive loss of bone that predisposes it [86].

Pelvic discontinuities were not initially taken into account in the different classifications. It was Berry et al. who extended the AAOS type IV classification for PD according to the associated type of bone defect and the ability to repair the remaining bone after acetabular preparation in the surgical intervention [82]. Type IVa includes pelvic discontinuity with cavitary or moderate segmental bone defect; in type IVb, pelvic discontinuity is associated with severe segmental loss or combined segmental and massive cavitary bone defect; type IVc refers to pelvic discontinuity in a pelvis previously subjected to radiation. Similarly, pelvic discontinuity was not an independent group in the Paprosky classification. The author currently (pending publication) creates a separate group with PD, which in turn subdivides it into four subgroups according to their treatment option.

In order to try to reduce to the least the number of discontinuities that go undetected in the preoperative study, we must perform a careful quality radiographic study including AP, lateral, and oblique views [87]; paying special attention to some in the false profile view for their detection [88]. Preoperative evaluation with a combination of AP pelvic X-ray, plus true lateral hip X-ray, plus oblique Judet view, allowed Martin et al. to identify PD in all patients [89]. Once diagnosed, 3D printer usage is increasingly permeable to further understand anatomical alteration and to more accurately establish possible solutions [90–92].

Regarding the treatment strategy, it will be necessary to distinguish between acute and chronic (3 months). They have different biology, different biomechanical concept and different healing potential. The technique that best exploits the biological potential for bone repair will be to insert a compression, one or two pelvic reconstruction plates on the posterior column [93]. Success of this technique depends on both adequate bone stock and a favorable biologic environment necessary for primary bone healing, although there are authors who biomechanically recommend bicolumnar osteosynthesis [94, 95]. These injuries were usually treated years ago with reconstruction rings plus structural and/or fragmented allograft as mentioned above and with ht. usual problems and complications [96]. Kosahsvili et al. reported the relatively novel treatment of 26 PDs with trabecular metal cups, allograft, and an anti-protrusion ilio-ischial cage called **Cup-Cage (CC)**, for severe acetabular bone loss associated with pelvis discontinuity [97]. Later, with an average follow-up of 44.6 months, 88.55% of implant stability was found, so this technique is reliable for the treatment of PD in the medium term [98]. However, it may be inappropriate for use in patients who have previously undergone irradiation or a tumor resection involving the acetabulum. It will be recommended to build a more rigid construction, while at the same time acting as a bridge between the ilium and ischium in the most effective way [99]. There are even authors who ensure a better biomechanical response of the anterior plate than the posterior [100].

We published our unit's experience with eleven reconstructed pelvic discontinuities using the trabecular metal revision system. The mean follow-up was 30 months. The mean age was 69, and 8 patients were women. In ten hips (91%), there was no radiological evidence of loosening at the end of the follow-up, with discontinuity cure according to Berry criteria. The Harris scale improved from an average of 39.8–75.6 points. The modified Merle d'Aubigné-Postel scale improved from 4.3 to 8.6 points. Complications included acute infection and paralysis of the external popliteal sciatic nerve. We had no dislocations. For us the early results indicate that Trabecular Metal revision cup-cage construct may be a reliable alternative for the pelvic discontinuity treatment [101] (Figs. 11.4, 11.5, and 11.6).

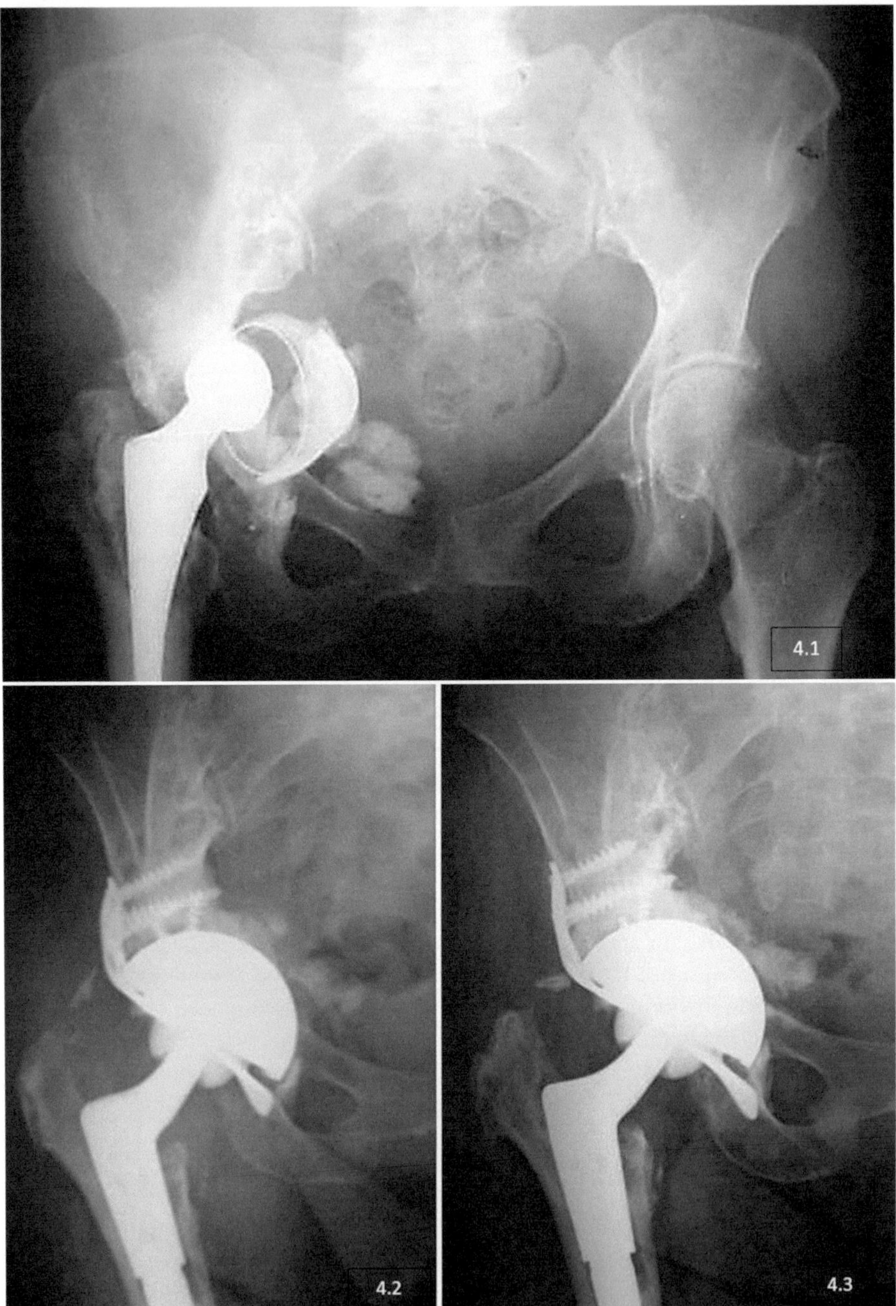


**Fig. 11.4** 4.1: Pelvic discontinuity post-mieloma 4.2: Postoperative radiograph one year after. 4.3: Postoperative radiograph three year after

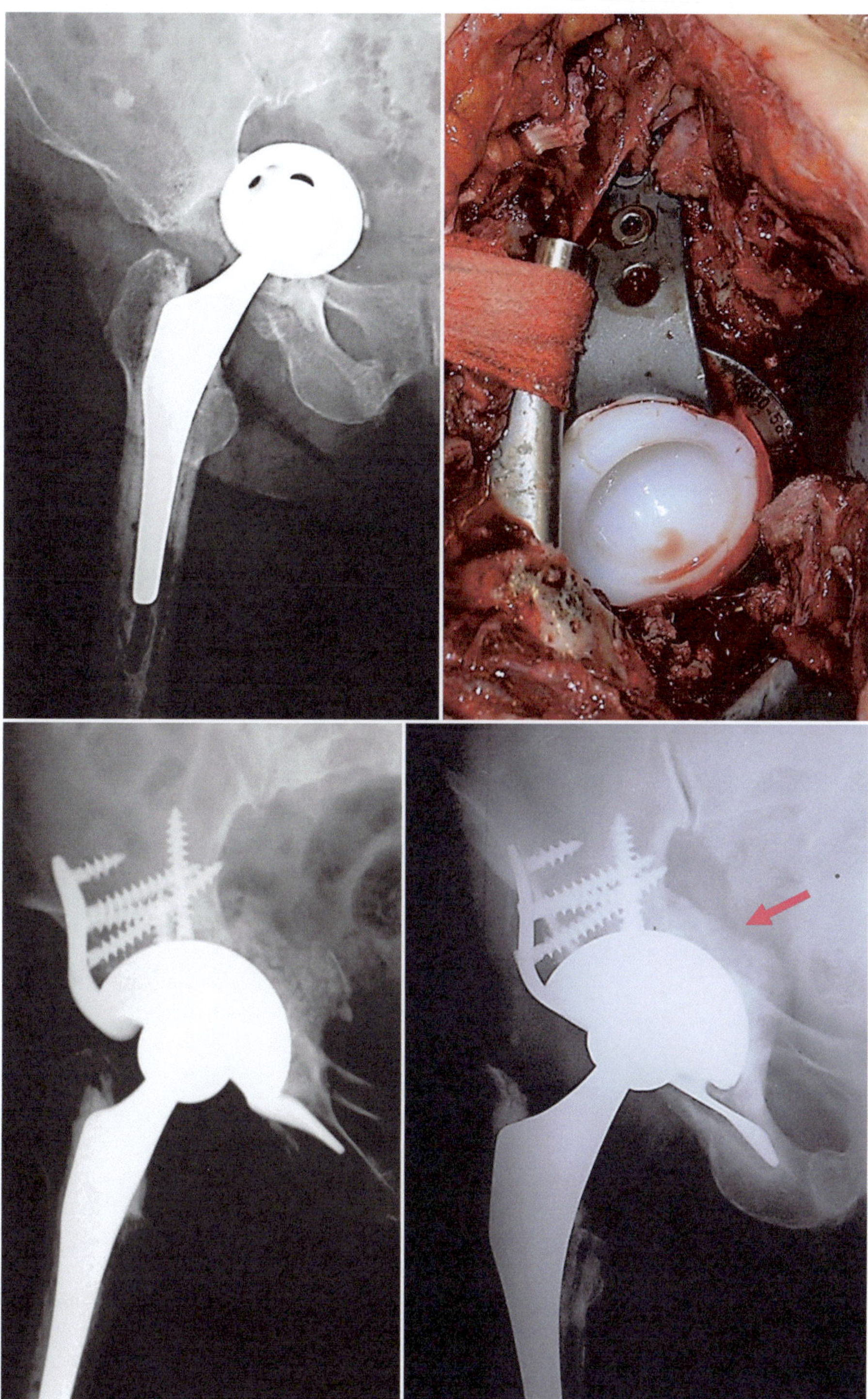

**Fig. 11.5** Acetabular defects Paprosky type IIIB with pelvic discontinuity. Trabecular metal with cup-cage. Remodeling and incorporation of the bone graft at 5 years

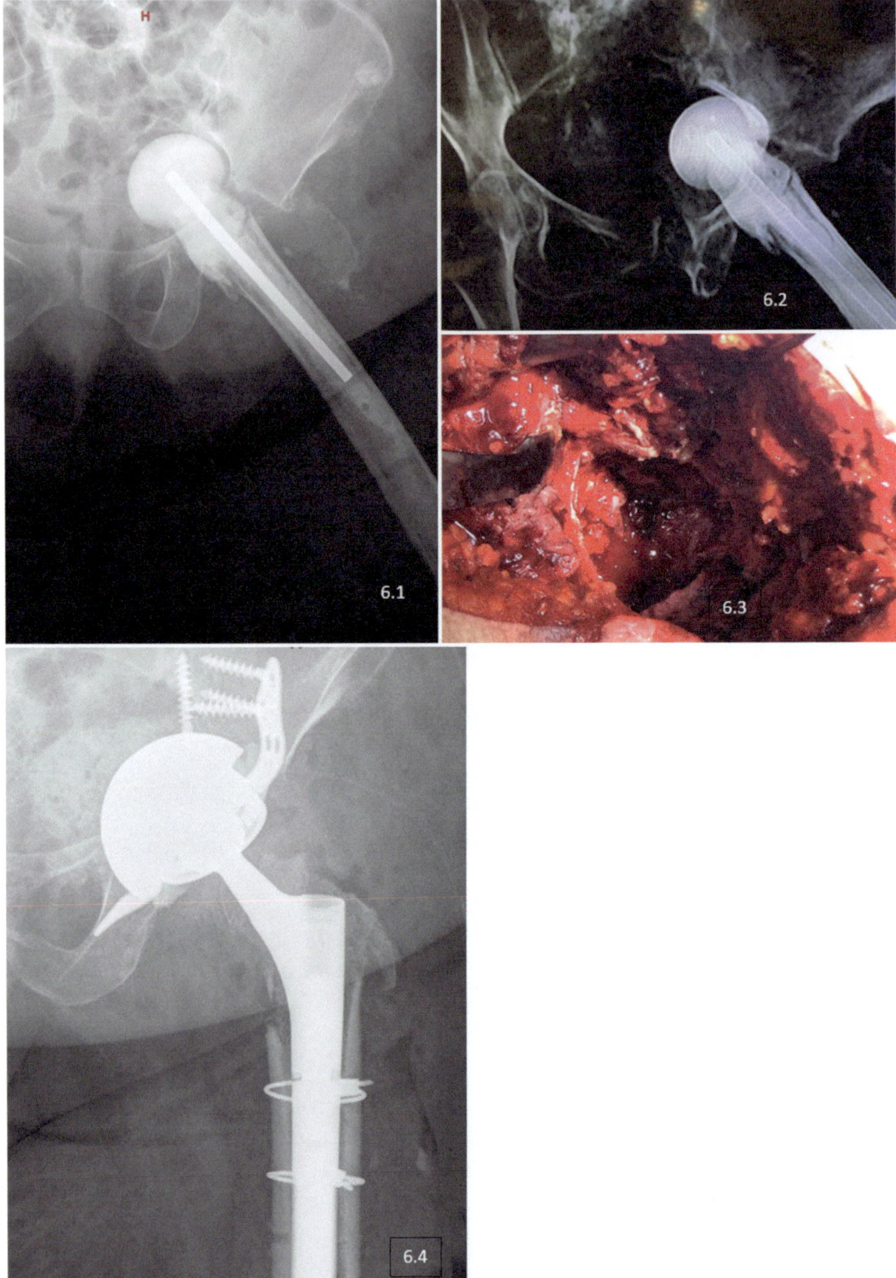


**Fig. 11.6** 6.1 and 6.2: Intrapelvic spacer. Acetabular defects Paprosky type IIIB with pelvic discontinuity. 6.3: Intraoperative view 6.4: Postoeprative radiograph reconstruction with trabecular metal and cup-cage

Sporer et al. asked whether pelvic distraction could be an alternative for these PDs [102]. They presented a series of 20 cases with an average follow-up of 4.7 years with a single infection failure. They claimed that acetabular distraction with porous tantalum components provides predictable pain relief and durability of two to seven years of follow-up when severe defects with associated PD are reconstructed. These authors presumed this method would provide adequate initial mechanical stability for bone ingrowth to occur into the prosthesis both superiorly and inferiorly to bridge the discontinuity in a biologic fashion. Thus, they anticipate a decreased incidence of mechanical failure with our method of acetabular distraction. This would also be confirmed later in various articles where the technical details of acetabular distraction are explained as an alternative reliable to pelvic discontinuity in failed total hip replacement [103–107].

The CC technique provides very promising results, protecting the titanium cage that acts as a bridge for graft incorporation and integration of the revision tantalum cup, delimiting the indications, surgical techniques and outcomes of various methods which use acetabular reconstruction cages for revision total hip arthroplasty [108]. Amenabar et al. analyze sixty-seven CC procedures with an average follow up of 74 months [109]. Acetabular bone loss and presence of pelvic discontinuity were assessed according to the Gross classification, 39% type IV and 61% type V (Pelvic discontinuity). The 5-year Kaplan-Meier survival rate of revision for any cause was 93%. They believe that the CC construct is a suitable choice to treat chronic pelvic discontinuity; it also remains a reliable option for the treatment of severe acetabular bone defects if stable fixation cannot be obtained through the use of a trabecular metal cup with or without augments.

Other possibilities have evolved for the treatment of the most difficult defects in recent years, but longer-term follow-up will be required to determine the durability of these atypical variants. It has been proposed to associate a reconstruction cage and porous metal augment. The augments were used in place of structural allografts. In this series all patients had segmental defects involving more than 50% of the acetabulum and seven hips had an associated pelvic discontinuity Acceptable early survivorship can be achieved using this novel technique, but it may be unsuitable for use in patients who have previously undergone the resection of a tumour involving the acetabulum [110].

Also, it has been proposed to implant the cage as such or to create a half cup-cage (a metal-cutting carbide-tipped burr is used to remove the inferior portion of the cage through the central hemispherical section). The half cup-cage technique avoids wider exposure and may result in a lower risk of soft-tissue damage including sciatic nerve palsy or the creation of an iatrogenic dissociation from cage impaction when the acetabulum is deficient but still intact [111]. Both techniques were used in a series of 57 cases with major acetabular defects graded as Paprosky Type 2B through 3B, with 34 (60%) having an associated pelvic discontinuity. Short-term survivorship free from re-revision for any cause or reoperation was 89%. Both full and half cup-cage constructs demonstrated successful clinical outcomes and survivorship in the treatment of major acetabular defects and pelvic discontinuity. Each method is utilized on the basis of individual intraoperative findings, including the extent and pattern of bone loss, the quality and location of host bone remaining after preparation, and the presence of pelvic discontinuity. Longer-term follow-up is required to understand the durability of these constructs in treating major acetabular defects and pelvic discontinuity [111]. The comparative study about DP of the mentioned Toronto group is very interesting. Patients treated with CC (mean follow-up of 88 months) with other cases treated with conventional rings (mean follow-up of 69 months), where it is claimed that CC reconstruction performs better in the medium term than conventional rings in pelvic discontinuities [112].

Based on the above, we can state that trabecular metal marks a new era in the treatment in acetabular revisions, particularly with regard to major defects and discontinuities. This is supported by the good published results and systematic reviews of the aforementioned literature. But can we say that reinforcement rings have been relegated to history? In this regard, we must answer that we agree with the conclusions of Abolghasemian et al. [10], who claimed that the use of the rings accompanied by structural allograft for the treatment of defects not contained in the acetabular revision surgery helps us restore bone reserve and facilitates subsequent re-revision, which is of particular interest in younger people.

## References


1. García-Cimbrelo E, García-Rey E. Bone defect determines acetabular revision surgery. Hip Int. 2014;24(Suppl 10):s33–6.
2. Gozzard C, Blom A, Taylor A, Smith E, Learmonth I. A comparison of the reliability and validity of bone stock loss classification systems used for revision hip surgery. J Arthroplast. 2003;18(5):638–42.
3. Yu R, Hofstaetter JG, Sullivan T, Costi K, Howie DW, Solomon LB. Validity and reliability of the paprosky acetabular defect classification hip. Clin Orthop Relat Res. 2013;471(7):2259–65.
4. Johanson NA, Driftmier KR, Cerynik DL, Stehman CC. Grading acetabular defects. The need for a universal and valid system. J Arthroplast. 2010;25(3):425–31.
5. Volpin A, Konan S, Biz C, Tansey RJ, Haddad FS. Reconstruction of failed acetabular component in the presence of severe acetabular bone loss : a systematic review. Musculoskelet Surg. 2018; https://doi.org/10.1007/s12306-018-0539-7. Abr 13
6. Schelfaut S, Cool S, Mulier M. The use of structural periacetabular allografts in acetabular revision surgery: 2.5–5 years follow-up. Arch Orthop Trauma Surg. 2009;129(4):455–61.
7. Garbuz D, Morsi E, Gross AE. Revision of the acetabular component of a total hip arthroplasty with a massive structural allograft. J Bone Joint Surg Am. 1996;78–A(5):693–7.
8. O'Rourke MR, Paprosky WG, Rosenberg AG. Use of structural allografts in acetabular revision surgery. Clin Orthop. 2004;420:113–21.
9. Flecher X, Sporer SM, Paprosky WG. Management of severe bone loss in acetabular revision using a trabecular metal shell. J Arthroplast. 2008;23(7):949–55.
10. Abolghasemian M, Sadeghi Naini M, Tangsataporn S, Lee P, Backstein DJ, Safir O, et al. Reconstruction of massive uncontained acetabular defects using allograft with cage or ring reinforcement: an assessment of the graft's ability to restore bone stock and its impact on the outcome of re-revision. Bone Joint J. 2014;96–B(3):319–24.
11. Gross AE, Wong P, Saleh KJ. Don't throw away the ring: indications and use. J Arthroplast. 2002;17(4):162–6.

12. García-Anaya LE, Negrete-Corona J, Jiménez-Aquino J. Utilidad del aloinjerto óseo estructurado para defectos acetabulares en prótesis de revisión. Acta Ortopédica Mex. 2014;28(4):212–7.
13. Gross AE, Goodman S. Importancia actual de los injertos estructurales y las cajas en la artroplastia de revisión de la cadera. Clin Orthop Relat Res. 2004;429:193–200.
14. Regis D, Magnan B, Sandri A, Bartolozzi P. Long-term results of anti-protrusio cage and massive allografts for the management of periprosthetic acetabular bone loss. J Arthroplast. 2008;23(6):826–32.
15. Lee PTH, Clayton RA, Safir OA, Backstein DJ, Gross AE. Structural allograft as an option for treating infected hip arthroplasty with massive bone loss. Clin Orthop Relat Res. 2011;469:1016–23.
16. Brown NM, Morrison J, Sporer SM, Paprosky WG. The use of structural distal femoral allograft for acetabular reconstruction of paprosky type IIIA defects at a mean 21 years of follow-up. J Arthroplast. 2016;31(3):680–3.
17. Slooff TJJH, Huiskes R, van Horn J, Lemmens AJ. Bone grafting in total hip replacement for acetabular protrusion. Acta Orthop Scand. 1984;55(6):593–6.
18. Schreurs BW, Slooff TJJH, Gardeniers JWM, Buma P. Acetabular reconstruction with bone impaction grafting and a cemented cup. Clin Orthop Relat Res. 2001;393:202–15.
19. Schreurs BW, Keurentjes JC, Gardeniers JWM, Verdonschot N, Slooff TJJH, Veth RPH. Acetabular revision with impacted morsellised cancellous bone grafting and a cemented acetabular component: a 20- to 25-year follow-up. J Bone Joint Surg Br. 2009;91–B:1148–53.
20. van Haaren EH, Heyligers IC, Alexander FGM, Wuisman PIJM. High rate of failure of impaction grafting in large acetabular defects. J Bone Jt Surg Br. 2007;89–B(3):296–300.
21. Gilbody J, Taylor C, Bartlett GE, Whitehouse SL, Wilson, Hubble MJ, Timperley AJ, et al. Clinical and radiographic outcomes of acetabular impaction grafting without cage reinforcement for revision hip replacement: a minimum ten-year follow-up study. Bone Joint J. 2014;96–B(2):188–94.
22. García-Rey E, Madero R, García-Cimbrelo E. THA revisions using impaction allografting with mesh is durable for medial but not lateral acetabular defects. Clin Orthop Relat Res. 2015;473(12):3882–91.
23. Waddell BS, Boettner F, Gonzalez Della Valle A. Favorable early results of impaction bone grafting with reinforcement mesh for the treatment of paprosky 3B acetabular defects. J Arthroplast. 2017;32(3):919–23.
24. Buckup J, Alvarez Salinas E, Gonzalez Della Valle A, Boettner F. Treatment of large acetabular defects: a surgical technique utilizing impaction grafting into a metallic mesh. HSS J. 2013;9(3):242–6.
25. Hernigou P, Pariat J, Queinnec S, Homma Y, Flouzat Lachaniette CH, Chevallier N, et al. Supercharging irradiated allografts with mesenchymal stem cells improves acetabular bone grafting in revision arthroplasty. Int Orthop. 2014;38:1913–21.
26. Borland WS, Bhattacharya R, Holland JP, Brewster NT. Use of porous trabecular metal augments with impaction bone grafting in management of acetabular bone loss. Acta Orthop. 2012;83(4):347–52.
27. Jones SA. Impaction grafting made easy. J Arthroplast. 2017;32(9):S54–8.
28. Della Valle CJ, Berger RA, Rosenberg AG, Galante JO. Cementless acetabular reconstruction in revision total hip arthroplasty. Clin Orthop. 2004;420:96–100.
29. Lee JM, Nam HT. Acetabular revision total hip arthroplasty using an impacted morselized allograftand a cementless cup. Minimum 10-year follow-up. J Arthroplast. 2011;26(7):1057–60.
30. Winter E, Piert M, Volkmann R, Maurer F, Eingartner C, Weise K, et al. Allogeneic cancellous bone graft and a burch-schneider ring for acetabular reconstruction in revision hip arthroplasty. J Bone Joint Surg Am. 2001;83–A(6):862–7.
31. Coscujuela-Mañá A, Angles F, Tramunt C, Casanova X. Burch-Schneider antiprotrusio cage for acetabular revision: a 5- to 13-year follow-up study. Hip Int. 2010;14(20 Suppl 7):112–8.

32. Jones L, Grammatopoulos G, Singer G. The Burch-Schneider cage: 9-year survival in paprosky type 3 acetabular defects. Clinical and radiological follow-up. Hip Int. 2012;22(1):28–34.
33. Lamo-Espinosa J, Duart Clemente J, Díaz-Rada P, Pons-Villanueva J, Valentí-Nín JR. The Burch-Schneider antiprotrusio cage: medium follow-up results. Musculoskelet Surg. 2013;97(1):31–7.
34. Fink B, Grossmann A. Recambio acetabular con anillos antiprotrusión en defectos de mayor tamaño. Tec Quirúrgicas en Ortop y Traumatol. 2011;20(4):216–27.
35. Symeonides PP, Petsatodes GE, Pournaras JD, Kapetanos GA, Christodoulou AG, Marougiannis DJ. The effectiveness of the Burch-Schneider antiprotrusio cage for acetabular bone deficiency. Five to twenty-one years' follow-up. J Arthroplast. 2009;24(2):168–74.
36. Duffy GP, O'Connor MI, Brodersen MP. Fatigue failure of the GAP ring. J Arthroplast. 2007;22(5):711–4.
37. Hernández-Vaquero D, Gava R, Suárez-Vázquez A, Pérez-Hernández D, Fernández-Lombardía J. Anillos de reconstrucción en la cirugía de revisión de las artroplastias de cadera. Rev Ortop y Traumatol. 2006;50:93–9.
38. Ballester Alfaro J, Sueiro-Fernández J. Reconstrucción acetabular con sistema GAP II. En: SATO, editor. Alteraciones acetabulares displásicas, postraumáticas y postprotésicas. Sevilla; 2008. p. 119–34.
39. Buttaro MA, Muñoz de Rosa D, Comba F, Piccaluga F. High failure rate with the GAP II ring and impacted allograft bone in severe acetabular defects. Clin Orthop Relat Res. 2012;470:3148–55.
40. Hosny HAH, El-Bakoury A, Fekry H, Keenan J. Mid-term results of graft augmentation prosthesis II cage and impacted allograft bone in revision hip arthroplasty. J Arthroplast. 2018;33(5):1487–93.
41. Pieringer H, Auersperg V, Böhler N. Reconstruction of severe acetabular bone-deficiency. The Burch-Schneider antiprotrusio cage in primary and revision total hip arthroplasty. J Arthroplast. 2006;21(4):489–96.
42. Buttaro M, Nuñez L, Lopez Ovenza J, Comba F, Piccaluga F. Falla mecánica precoz de un anillo de reconstrucción acetabular tipo Kerboull. Rev Asoc Argent Ortop Traumatol. 2008;73(3):285–9.
43. Baba T, Shitoto K. Revision of total hip arthroplasty using the Kerboull and KT plates. Int Orthop. 2010;34:341–7.
44. Matsumoto M, Baba T, Ochi H, Ozaki Y, Watari T, Homma Y, et al. Kerboull-type plate in a direct anterior approach for severe bone defects at primary total hip arthroplasty: technical note. Sicot-J. 2017;3:21.
45. Okano K, Miyata N, Enomoto H, Osaki M, Shindo H. Revision with impacted bone allografts and the kerboull cross plate for massive bone defect of the acetabulum. J Arthroplast. 2010;25(0):594–9.
46. Inoue D, Kabata T, Maeda T, Kajino Y, Yamamoto T, Takagi T, et al. The value of bulk femoral head allograft in acetabular reconstruction using Kerboull-type plate. Int Orthop. 2015;39(9):1839–44.
47. Makita H, Kerboull M, Inaba Y, Tezuka T, Saito T, Kerboull L. Revision total hip arthroplasty using the kerboull acetabular reinforcement device and structural allograft for severe defects of the acetabulum. J Arthroplast. 2017;32(11):3502–9.
48. Hayashi S, Nishiyama T, Hashimoto S, Matsumoto T, Takayama K, Ishida K, et al. Risk factors for failure of revision total hip arthroplasty using a Kerboull-type acetabular reinforcement device. BMC Musculoskelet Disord. 2017;18(1):4–9.
49. Sembrano JN, Cheng EY. Acetabular cage survival and analysis of factors related to failure. Clin Orthop Relat Res. 2008;466:1657–65.
50. Moskal JT, Higgins ME, Shen J. Type III acetabular defect revision with bilobed components: five-year results. Clin Orthop Relat Res. 2008;466:691–5.
51. Desai AS, Dramis A, Board TN, Hekal W, Farhan MJ. Acetabular revision surgery with the uncemented oblong BOFOR cup – early to midterm results. Hip Int. 2012;22(3):280–5.

52. Lachiewicz PF, Watters TS. The jumbo acetabular component for acetabular revision: curtain calls and caveats. Bone Joint J. 2016;98–B(1 Supple A):64–7.
53. McLaughlin JR, Lee KR. Acetabular revision arthroplasty using an uncemented deep profile jumbo component: a ten to sixteen year follow-up study. J Arthroplast. 2018;33(2):496–9.
54. Christie MJ, Barrington SA, Brinson MF, Ruhling ME, DeBoer DK. Bridging massive acetabular defects with the triflange cup. Clin Orthop Relat Res. 2001;393:216–27.
55. DeBoer DK, Christie MJ, Brinson MF, Morrison JC. Revision total hip arthroplasty for pelvic discontinuity. J Bone Joint Surg Am. 2007;89–A:835–40.
56. Taunton MJ, Fehring TK, Edwards P, Bernasek T, Holt GE, Christie MJ. Pelvic discontinuity treated with custom triflange component: a reliable option. Clin Orthop Relat Res. 2012;470:428–34.
57. Berasi CC, Berend KR, Adams JB, Ruh EL, Lombardi AV. Are custom triflange acetabular components effective for reconstruction of catastrophic bone loss? Clin Orthop Relat Res. 2015;473(2):528–35.
58. Colen S, Harake R, De Haan J, Mulier M. A modified custom-made triflanged acetabular reconstruction ring (MCTARR) for revision hip arthroplasty with severe acetabular defects. Acta Orthop Belg. 2013;79(1):71–5.
59. Hogan C, Ries M. Treatment of massive acetabular bone loss and pelvic discontinuity with a custom triflange component and ilio-sacral fixation based on preoperative CT templating. A report of 2 cases. Hip Int. 2015;25(6):585–8.
60. Schwarzkopf R, Ihn HE, Ries MD. Pelvic discontinuity: modern techniques and outcomes for treating pelvic disassociation. Hip Int. 2015;25(4):368–74.
61. Berend ME, Berend KR, Lombardi AV, Cates H, Faris P. The patient-specific Triflange acetabular implant for revision total hip arthroplasty in patients with severe acetabular defects: planning, implantation, and results. Bone Joint J. 2018;100–B(1 Supple A):50–4.
62. Barlow BT, Oi KK, Yu LY, Carli AV, Choi DS, Bostrom MP. Outcomes of custom flange acetabular components in revision total hip arthroplasty and predictors of failure. J Arthroplast. 2016;31(5):1057–64.
63. Gladnick BP, Fehring KA, Odum SM, Christie MJ, DeBoer DK, Fehring TK. Midterm survivorship after revision total hip arthroplasty with a custom triflange acetabular component. J Arthroplast. 2017;33(2):500–4.
64. Moore KD, McClenny MD, Willis B. Custom triflange acetabular components for large acetabular defects: minimum 10-year follow-up. Orthopedics. 2018;16:1–5.
65. Goodman GP, Engh CA. The custom triflange cup. Build it and they will come. Bone Joint J. 2016;98–B(1 Supple A):68–72.
66. Ries MD. The triflange cup: build it and they will wait. Semin Arthroplast. 2017;28:264–6.
67. Paprosky WG, O'Rourke MR, Sporer SM. The treatment of acetabular bone defects with an associated pelvic discontinuity. Clin Orthop Relat Res. 2005;441:216–20.
68. Gross AE, Goodman SB. Rebuilding the skeleton: the intraoperative use of trabecular metal in revision total hip arthroplasty. J Arthroplast. 2005;20(4):91–3.
69. Burns AWR, McCalden RW. (ii) Current techniques and new developments in acetabular revision surgery. Curr Orthop. 2006;20(3):162–70.
70. Ballester Alfaro JJ, Sueiro-Fernández J. Trabecular metal buttress augment and the trabecular metal cup-cage construct in revision hip arthroplasty for severe acetabular bone loss and pelvic discontinuity. Hip Int. 2010;20(Suppl 7):S119–27.
71. Tangsataporn S, Abolghasemian M, Kuzyk PR, Backstein DJ, Safir OA, Gross AE. Salvaged failed roof rings and antiprotrusion cages: surgical options and implant survival. Hip Int. 2013;23:166–72.
72. Banerjee S, Issa K, Kapadia BH, Pivec R, Khanuja HS, Mont MA. Systematic review on outcomes of acetabular revisions with highly-porous metals. Int Orthop. 2014;38:689–702.
73. Jain S, Grogan RJ, Giannoudis PV. Options for managing severe acetabular bone loss in revision hip arthroplasty. A systematic review. Hip Int. 2014;24(2):109–22.

74. Beckmann NA, Weiss S, Klotz MCMM, Gondan M, Jaeger S, Bitsch RG. Loosening after acetabular revision: comparison of trabecular metal and reinforcement rings. A systematic review. J Arthroplast. 2014;29(1):229–35.
75. López-Torres II, Sanz-Ruíz P, Sánchez-Pérez C, Andrade-Albarracín R, Vaquero J. Clinical and radiological outcomes of trabecular metal systems and antiprotrusion cages in acetabular revision surgery with severe defects: a comparative study. Int Orthop. 2018;42(8):1811–8.
76. Clement RGE, Ray AG, MacDonald DJ, Wade FA, Burnett R, Moran M. Trabecular metal use in paprosky type 2 and 3 acetabular defects: 5-year follow-up. J Arthroplast. 2016;31(4):863–7.
77. Grappiolo G, Loppini M, Longo UG, Traverso F, Mazziotta G, Denaro V. Trabecular metal augments for the management of paprosky type III defects without pelvic discontinuity. J Arthroplast. 2015;30(6):1024–9.
78. Lopez-Torres II, Sanz-Ruiz P, Sánchez-Pérez C, Andrade-Albarracín RL, León-Román VE, Vaquero-Martín J. Resultados clínicos y funcionales de los sistemas de metal trabecular en la cirugía de revisión acetabular con defectos severos. Resultados a 5 años. Rev Latinoam Cir Ortop. 2016;1(3):77–82.
79. O'Neill CJ, Creedon SB, Brennan SA, O'Mahony FJ, Lynham RS, Guerin S, et al. Acetabular revision using trabecular metal augments for paprosky type 3 defects. J Arthroplast. 2018;33(3):823–8.
80. Jenkins DR, Odland AN, Sierra RJ, Hanssen AD, Lewallen DG. Minimum five-year outcomes with porous tantalum acetabular cup and augment construct in complex revision total hip arthroplasty. J Bone Joint Surg Am. 2017;99–A(10):e49. 1-7
81. Prieto HA, Kralovec ME, Berry DJ, Trousdale RT, Sierra RJ, Cabanela ME. Structural allograft supporting a trabecular metal cup provides durable results in complex revision arthroplasty. J Arthroplast. 2017;32(11):3488–94.
82. Berry DJ, Lewallen DG, Hanssen AD, Cabanela ME. Pelvic discontinuity in revision total hip arthroplasty. J Bone Joint Surg Am. 1999;81–A(12):1692–702.
83. Springer BD, Berry DJ, Cabanela ME, Hanssen AD, Lewallen DG. Early postoperative transverse pelvic fracture: a new complication related to revision arthroplasty with an uncemented cup. J Bone Joint Surg Am. 2005;87–A(12):2626–31.
84. Takigami I, Ito Y, Mizoguchi T, Shimizu K. Pelvic discontinuity caused by acetabular overreaming during primary total hip arthroplasty. Case Rep Orthop. 2011;2011:1–4.
85. Abdelnasser MK, Klenke FM, Whitlock P, Khalil AM, Khalifa YE, Ali HM, et al. Management of pelvic discontinuity in revision total hip arthroplasty: a review of the literature. Hip Int. 2015;25(2):120–6.
86. Abdel MP, Trousdale RT, Berry DJ. Pelvic discontinuity associated with total hip arthroplasty: evaluation and management. J Am Acad Orthop Surg. 2017;25(5):330–8.
87. Giori NJ, Sidky AO. Lateral and high-angle oblique radiographs of the pelvis aid in diagnosing pelvic discontinuity after total hip arthroplasty. J Arthroplast. 2011;26(1):110–2.
88. Wendt MC, Adler MA, Trousdale RT, Mabry TM, Cabanela ME. Effectiveness of false profile radiographs in detection of pelvic discontinuity. J Arthroplast. 2012;27(7):1408–12.
89. Martin JR, Barrett IJ, Sierra RJ, Lewallen DG, Berry DJ. Preoperative radiographic evaluation of patients with pelvic discontinuity. J Arthroplast. 2016;31(5):1053–6.
90. Hughes AJ, Debuitleir C, Soden P, O'Donnchadha B, Tansey A, Abdulkarim A, et al. 3D printing aids acetabular reconstruction in complex revision hip arthroplasty. Adv Orthop. 2017;2017:1–7.
91. Wyatt MC. Custom 3D-printed acetabular implants in hip surgery -innovative breakthrough or expensive bespoke upgrade? Hip Int. 2015;25(4):375–9.
92. Citak M, Kochsiek L, Gehrke T, Haasper C, Suero EM, Mau H. Preliminary results of a 3D-printed acetabular component in the management of extensive defects. Hip Int. 2017;00(00):000–0. https://doi.org/10.5301/hipint.5000561.
93. Rogers BA, Whittingham-Jones PM, Mitchell PA, Safir OA, Bircher MD, Gross AE. The reconstruction of periprosthetic pelvic discontinuity. J Arthroplast. 2012;27(8):1499–506.

94. Stiehl JB, Saluja R, Diener T. Reconstruction of major column defects and pelvic discontinuity in revision total hip arthroplasty. J Arthroplast. 2000;15(7):849–57.
95. Gililland JM, Anderson LA, Henninger HB, Kubiak EN, Peters CL. Biomechanical analysis of acetabular revision constructs: is pelvic discontinuity best treated with bicolumnar or traditional unicolumnar fixation? J Arthroplast. 2013;28(1):178–86.
96. Regis D, Sandri A, Bonetti I, Bortolami O, Bartolozzi P. A minimum of 10-year follow-up of the burch-schneider cage and bulk allografts for the revision of pelvic discontinuity. J Arthroplast. 2012;27(6):1057–63.
97. Kosashvili Y, Backstein DJ, Safir O, Lakstein D, Gross AE. Acetabular revision using an anti-protrusion (ilio-ischial) cage and trabecular metal acetabular component for severe acetabular bone loss associated with pelvic discontinuity. J Bone Joint Surg Br. 2009;91–B:870–6.
98. Abolghasemian M, Tangsataporn S, Kuzyk PRT, Safir OA, Backstein DJ, Gross AE. Cup-cage solution for pelvic discontinuity. Semin Arthroplast. 2012;23(3):171–5.
99. Martin JR, Barrett I, Sierra RJ, Lewallen DG, Berry DJ. Construct rigidity: keystone for treating pelvic discontinuity. J Bone Joint Surg Am. 2017;99(9):e43. 1-6
100. Ribes-Iborra J, Atienza C, Sevil-De la Torre J, Gómez Pérez A. Biomechanical study of pelvic discontinuity in failed total hip arthroplasty. Lessons learnt from the treatment of pelvic fractures. Injury. 2017;48(Suppl 6):S34–9.
101. Ballester Alfaro JJ, Sueiro-Fernández J, Domínguez F, Valero J, Ayerbe P. Tratamiento de la discontinuidad pélvica periprotésica. Rev S And Traum y Ort. 2012;29(1/2):73–88.
102. Sporer SM, Bottros JJ, Hulst JB, Kancherla VK, Moric M, Paprosky WG. Acetabular distraccion. An alternative for severe defects with chronic pelvic discontinuity? Clin Orthop Relat Res. 2012;470(11):3156–63.
103. Brown NM, Hellman M, Haughom BH, Shah RP, Sporer SM, Paprosky WG. Acetabular distraction: an alternative approach to pelvic discontinuity in failed total hip replacement. Bone Joint J. 2014;96–B(11 Suppl A):73–7.
104. Sheth NP, Melnic CM, Paprosky WG. Acetabular distraction: an alternative for severe acetabular bone loss and chronic pelvic discontinuity. Bone Joint J. 2014;96–B(11 Suppl A):36–42.
105. Melnic CM, Sheth NP. Operative technique: acetabular distraction for severe acetabular bone loss with associated chronic pelvic discontinuity. UPOJ. 2015;25(6):68–70.
106. Sheth NP, Paprosky WG. Acetabular distraction technique—an alternative for the treatment of chronic pelvic discontinuity. Semin Arthroplast. 2015;26(3):190–4.
107. Hasenauer MD, Paprosky WG, Sheth NP. Treatment options for chronic pelvic discontinuity. J Clin Orthop Trauma. 2017;9(1):58–62.
108. Mäkinen TJ, Fichman SG, Watts E, Kuzyk PRT, Safir OA, Gross AE, et al. The role of cages in the management of severe acetabular bone defects at revision arthroplasty. Bone Joint J. 2016;98–B(1 Suppl A):73–7.
109. Amenabar T, Rahman WA, Hetaimish BM, Kuzyk PR, Safir OA, Gross AE. Promising mid-term results with a cup-cage construct for large acetabular defects and pelvic discontinuity. Clin Orthop Relat Res. 2016;474(2):408–14.
110. Mäkinen TJ, Abolghasemian M, Watts E, Fichman SG, Kuzyk P, Safir OA, et al. Management of massive acetabular bone defects in revision arthroplasty of the hip using a reconstruction cage and porous metal augment. Bone Joint J. 2017;99–B(5):607–13.
111. Sculco PK, Ledford CK, Hanssen AD, Abdel MP, Lewallen DG. The evolution of the cup-cage technique for major acetabular defects full and half cup-cage reconstruction. J Bone Joint Surg Am. 2017;99–A(13):1104–10.
112. Abolghasemian M, Tangsataporn S, Drexler M, Barbuto R, Backstein DJ, Safir O, et al. The challenge of pelvic discontinuity: cup-cage reconstruction does better than conventional cages in mid-term. Bone Joint J. 2014;96–B(2):195–200.

# Chapter 12
# Acetabular Bone Defect in Infected Total Hip Arthroplasty

**Jose Cordero-Ampuero and Eduardo García-Rey**

## Introduction

Periprosthetic joint infection (PJI) is the most severe complication in terms of mortality, morbidity and functional disability. The cost of a septic revision surgery is 3–4 times greater than primary total hip arthroplasty, and double that of an aseptic revision surgery [1, 2]. Frequency varies depending on different etiopathogenic factors such as local contamination, hematogenous contamination and well as patient-associated factors. Local contamination is related with the type of surgical theater (laminar air flow and space suits, less than 1%), the existance of previous surgery [3], dislocations, surgical wound secretion [4], skin coverage defect [5], and antibiotic prophylactic non-use that can multiply the infection risk by seven [6]. Hematogenous contamination is related with the existance of distant septic foci (urinary, dental), and multiplies the risk of infection by three [6]. In regard to patient-associated risk factors, the existance of associated diseases, such as diabetes, rheumatoid arthritis, tuberculosis etc.; the abuse of some drugs and toxic-substances, such as corticotherapy, alcoholism, or drug addiction can also increase the risk of infection [7]. Older ages can also produce immunodepresion associated to progressive thymus gland atrophy (the site of T cell maduration), delayed hypersensibility and weaker lymphocyte response [8]. Nutritional alterations including obesity or deficiencies are also related with higher infection rates.

Diagnosis is challenging and it is a frequent cause of repeated surgeries that affect not only soft-tissues around a joint but also bone. Prosthetic joint infection is less frequent in the hip than in the knee, management is significantly different. Systemic antibiotic therapy after positive intraoperative cultures subsequent to a

J. Cordero-Ampuero (✉)
Orthopaedic Surgery Department, Hospital Universitario La Princesa, Madrid, Spain

E. García-Rey
Orthopaedic Surgery Department, Hospital Universitario La Paz-IdiPaz, Madrid, Spain



E. García-Rey, E. García-Cimbrelo (eds.), *Acetabular Revision Surgery in Major Bone Defects*, https://doi.org/10.1007/978-3-319-98596-1_12

revision procedure, single- or two-stage procedures depending on the general status of the patient, the bone status (stock) receiving the new implant, and the microbiology analysis, all affect outcome. Controversial issues like temporary spacer use, have been reported. The low number of cases and the differences in patient's characteristics make the analysis of clinical studies the surgeon's decision very difficult.

## Diagnosis of Infection

### *Risk Factors and Clinical Suspicion*

During the last decades, many studies have reported some clinical and laboratory issues to help to identify risk factors in individual patients and enable post-operative evaluation of failed arthroplasty, determining the probability of infection in high versus low risk patients or situations; this information should help the surgeon decide on a more or less aggressive response to of possible infection [9].

### *Symptoms: Pain*

When the surgeon evaluates a patient with a painful hip arthroplasty all important questions should be replanted including whether the pain had presented recently arises, if it is different than before surgery, or whether it could be related to other sites of infection. Pain in infection is not always "inflammatory", many times "mechanical" pain occurs, when walking and standing, particularly if there is loosening, or a continuous pain that is not alleviated by rest. At this point, it is important to identify "over-demanding" patients (those expecting complete absence of pain and unlimited walking/activity) through the quantity and quality of analgesics, life style, their actual functional limitations, by the use of internationally-accepted patient reported outcomes.

### *Signs*

During physical examination most International Scientific Societies and Consensus Systems include some signs as major criteria of infection like persistent drainage and a chronics in us with or without the abscence of associated issues such as edge necrosis or wound dehiscence [10, 11]. Most authors agree that these signs are critical even a case shows a negative culture. To date, some controversial studies have reported that simply culturing fistula samples is inadequate while others supports the 80% agreement between cultures of fistula and deep tissue infection [12]. Other inflammatory changes (redness, swelling, and/or increase of local temperature) are less specific and require confirmation. When inflammatory changes appear the clinician will have doubts; these signs need confirmation further study.

## *Blood Analysis*

The most commonly-used laboratory markers are increases in of white cells blood counts, erithrocyte sedimentation rate (ESR) and C-reactive protein (CRP). Erithrocyte sedimentation rate is usually higher than 30 in theses patients, but ESR sensitivity is between 66% and 82%, and the specificity between 85% and 90%. A CRP above one has with a sensitivity between 77% and 96%, and specificity between 84% and 92% for infection. However, sensitivity and specificity increase when are combined showing a high positive (83%) and negative (92–100%) predictive value [13–15].

The normal elevation of CRP usually decreases after three weeks and ESR after 6 or even 12 weeks. Other comorbidity problems like another infection affecting the urinary or teeth or rheumatological conditions may also elevate these parameters, so the clinician needs to be aware. Other serum markers like procalcitonin or IL-6 have been investigated but further evidence and cost-efectiveness studies are recommended to confirm their usefulnes. Bottner et al. report a not high sensitivity for these markers: 87% for IL6, 33% for Procalcitonin, and 43% for TNF [16]. Recently, D-dimer seems to be another promising and easy to evaluate marker when compared to combined ESR and PCR values [17].

## *Imaging assessment*

Imaging assessment is also controversial, since simple radiographs can show signs of prosthetic radiographic loosening, such as migration of the components, subsidence of the stem, radiolucent lines wider 2 mm around all the contour of the socket and the stem. Suspicion of infection arises when these signs appear early, present a fast progression, and/or there is an absence of mechanical explanation. The appearance of bone cysts and osteolysis unrelated to radiographic polyethylene wear strongely suggest infection when they are focal, rapidly progressive and massive. Early periosteal reaction (periostitis) is also frequent in these patients [18, 19] (Fig. 12.1).

The use of Computed tomography(CT) associated with radiographs can be useful in helping to confirm acetabular and femoral bone loss particularly when combined with other signs like secuestrum and cortical defects. Periprosthetic fluid collections can also be diagnosed using ultrasound, CT, or MRI [10, 19].

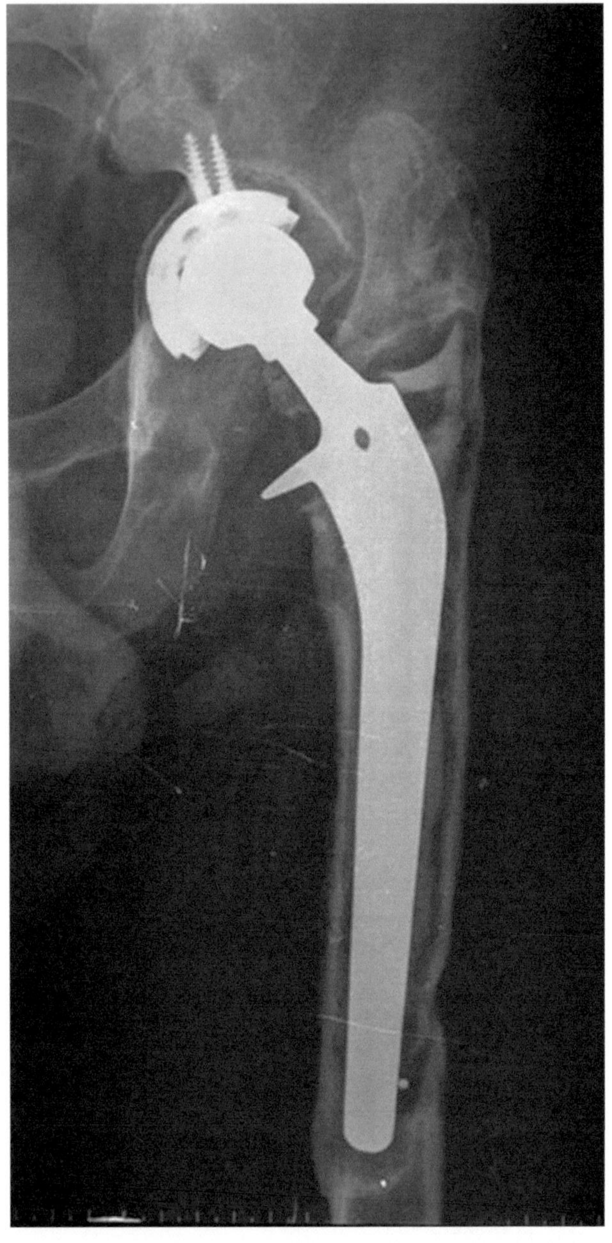

**Fig. 12.1** Anteroposterior radiographs of hip. Early signs of prosthetic radiographic loosening, such as component migration, stem subsidence, radiolucent lines wider than 2 mm all around the contour of the socket and the stem strongly suggest infection. Bone cysts and osteolysis are unrelated to significant radiographic polyethylene wear

An even more controversial topic is the use of conventional scintigraphy [20, 21]. Tecnecium and Galium scintigraphy become positive when bone turnover is increased and remain high during first year after any arthroplasty due to secondary implant fixation. Labeled leukocytes [21, 22] have shown high specificity but low sensitivity. Galium scintigraphy is positive when inflammation is present, so it is always positive during secondary fixation of THA. It has high sensitivity (95%) but very poor specificity (20%). This makes it useful for negative diagnosis (to confirm no infection is present). CT images of bone marrow with labeled leukocytes shows increased in sensitivity and specificity (accuracy: 89–98%).

The accuracy of fluorodeoxyglucose positron emission tomography (PET) in detecting differences between aseptic and septic failure has lead to an increased use of this technique, although it is still difficult to access and expensive [10, 23]. There also are doubts about its accuracy, which may be less than that of CT combined with labeled leukocytes.

## *Articular aspiration*

A preoperative analysis of articular liquid has been also recommended. Some technical issues make this management somewhat difficult, requiring an aseptic preparation (operation room), and these are some imaging techniques like radiographs, ultrasonography or CT that can help determine the best sample [14]. A liquid sample in a blood-culture bottle is much better than a swab [24]. Another controversial issue with articular aspiration is that a needle can only obtain planctonical bacteria, and the biofilm is not analyzed.

The leukocyte level diagnostic ranges are quite controversial and many authors have proposed very different thresholds: >1800 [10, 11], >2700, >3000 in chronic cases [25], or >4350. The sensitivity of this parameter is 90% (>1800) and the specificity: 99% (>1800). The proportion of polymorphonuclear(PMN) cells is also very controversial because many authors again have proposed quite different thresholds: >73% [10, 11], >77%, >80%in chronic cases [25], and >85%. PMN level sensitivity is 83% (>73%), and its specificity 93% (>73%). The use of leukocyte esterase reagent strips, offers a good sensitivity (93%) with low specificity (77%), but 33% of the samples are unuseful because of blood or debris [26]. Alpha-defensin determination has a sensitivity of 97–100% and specificity of 95–97% [27, 28]. These new markers are not significantly better than the more traditional ESR, CRP, leukocyte count and/or PMN [27].

Gram staining has a very low sensitivity (50–75%). Aspirate cultures only show a sensitivity of 56–92%. The specificity is 95%, but very low with skin contaminants (*S epidermidis, Propionibacterium sp*) [14, 29–34].

## *Biopsy. Culture and Diagnosis of Infection*

So, biopsy appears to be a better option than aspiration, offering a sensitivity and specificity ranging between 82% and 98% [35], which increases with the use of arthroscopic basketsup to 88–100% [36].

## Intraoperative Diagnosis of Infection

### Macroscopical Observations. Are They Useful?

An intraoperative diagnosis will usually confirm the preoperative diagnoses. Subjective, macroscopic observations based on the surgical teams experience and sensorial perceptions (eyes and noses) are important. Photographs ought to be taken. The Musculoskeletal Infection Diseases Society criteria includes gross purulence, great amount of liquid, necrotic and devitalized tissues or smell characteristics as signs of infection [10, 25]. To date, some types of bacteria can be suspected based on the appearance of the purulence. For example, a creamy, yellowish-white, abundant pus, suggests *S. Aureus; s*carce purulence, dirty interfaces, no smell, and undefinite color suggest *S. Epidermidis; a*bundant exudation and "urine-like" smell suggest *E Coli, Proteus* spp.; a fecal appearance and/or smell suggest *Enterobacter, Enterococcus, Klebsiella* and *Serratia; a*sewer smell, *Pseudomonas* spp.; *and s*trong acid/sour smell: *Streptococcus* spp.

Gram staining has a sensitivity below 17%, so, itis not useful at all [30]. The use of frozen sections can supply the number of PMN cells per high-power microscopic field [37–45]. A figure higher than 10 PMN suggest probable infection (implant extraction). From 5 to less than 10 PMN: possible infection. A figure below than 5 PMN: very low probability of infection. However, Gram staining has very low sensitivity in suspected aseptic loosening (50%) and reimplantation surgery (second stage of two-stage exchange) (29%) [38].

## Postoperative Diagnosis of Infection

### Conventional Cultures

Conventional recommendations for culturing include samples obtained from synovial fluid and tissues (synovial, devitalized soft-tissues, periprosthetic membranes, intramedullary bone content) [31]. Liquids only have planctonic bacteria, while tissuescan provideintracellular as well as sessile (from biofilm) bacteria [46, 47]. At least three periprosthetic tissue specimens, ideally five to six samples must be taken before irrigation is started [11, 14, 30, 31, 48].

### Sonication of Retired Implants

Sonication of retired implants has been reported to be of great value due to its sensitivity, specificity and ability to supply material for quantitative cultures and culture-media for slow-growing microorganisms. It is always recommended and the resulting cultures show a sensitivity of 78%, and specificity of 99% [15]. Associated with quantitative cultures and culture-media for slow-growing microorganisms, sensitivity improves but specificity is worse [47]. There is no consensus if as yet on usually-non-pathogenic bacteria obtained by sonication are actually responsible for clinical syndromes? [49, 50].

### Pathology of Intraoperative Samples

Pathologists can be very helpful since frozen sections are still probably the most accurate intraoperative test giving the number of PMN cells per high-power microscopic field [51]. Also quantification of sinovial CRP hace been reported to be evaluable as study of frozen sections [52].There are some doubts as to when the neutrophils are the immune response against plantonic bacteria, and macrophages are the immune response against biofilm. But, how do we differentiate between macrophages against wear particles and those against biofilm?. The pathological report on intraoperative samples is affected by the macrophage response to wear particles and biofilm.

### Infection Criteria

Different infection criteria have been postulated based on an International Consensus in order to clearly define this complication [25]. Any of the following will indicate a deep infection: (1) There is a sinus tract communicating with the prosthesis; (2) A pathogen is isolated by culture from at least two separate tissue or fluid samples obtained from the affected prosthetic joint; or (3) Four of the following six criteria exist:

1. Elevated serum erythrocyte sedimentation rate (ESR) and serum C-reactive protein (CRP) concentration,
2. Elevated sinovial leukocyte count,
3. Elevated sinovial neutrophil percentage (PMN%),
4. Presence of purulence in the affected joint,
5. Isolation of a microorganism in one culture of periprosthetic tissue or fluid, or
6. More than five neutrophils per high-power field in five high-powe fields observed from histologic analysis of periprosthetic tissue at ×400 magnification.

The presence of a sinus tract, visible pus surrounding the joint without other explanation (e.g. no crystals), acute inflammation on histopathological examination (>5 neutrophils/high-powerfield), >4200 leukocyte per μl and/or >80% polymorphonuclear leukocytes in synovial fluid, growth of the same microorganism in at least two cultures of synovial fluid, peri-prosthetic issue and/or sonication fluid. Patients were classified into acute postoperative (≤1 month after implantation), acute hematogenous (≤3 weeks of infectious symptoms), and chronic PJI (all other situations).

Major criteria are two positive periprosthetic cultures with identical microroganisms, and sinus tract communication with the joint. Minor criteria are: elevated serum ESR and CRP, elevated synovial fluid white blood cell count or leucocyte esterase test strip, elevated PMN synovial fluid, positive histological analysis, a single positive culture.

This complex problem is critically important to making the right decision regarding management.

## Treatment of the Infected Total Hip Arthroplasty

Once the infection is diagnosed, the surgeon must keep several considerations in mind. Particularly is important the time element (early or late), the severity of the infection according to the microbiological analysis and the comorbidity and medical situation of the patient. Once surgery is decided, the question of a single- or two-stage procedure, the local status of soft tissues, surgical and hospital environment must be taken into account in order to manage the most important aspect in hip revision reconstruction: bone loss.

A multidisciplinary approach with the Microbiology and Infectious Disease Department is recommended to properly manage the antibiotherapy. In a few cases a suppressive therapy (unexpected intraoperative cultures in an aseptic revision procedure or very fragile patients with previous repeated surgeries) may be indicated, but, in most cases surgery should be done.

According to the origin of infection and biofilm formation, the implant must be removed whenever possible. A single surgical debridement is often considered controversial due to its inefficacy because bacteria create biofilm in less than 24 h, and thus a single- or two-stage procedure may be indicated. Even more controversial, the surgeon must decide which components should be changed: First it was the polyethylene, then the femoral head, more recently all the uncemented and loose components (it is supposed that in the first 2–4 weeks they are not biologically fixed, but this may be not true with hydroxyapatite-coated pieces). The question arises immediately from a formal point of view: Is it a debridement, or is its a "one-stage" exchange?

Despite deciding on whether to do a single- or a two-stage procedure the management of bone loss is critical for the success of the problem. The surgeon must be aware that a bone defect is created after the implant's removal so while preoperative planning may be helpful it is not definitive. Currently, aggressive debridement is recommended to remove all membranes from the bone as well as all necrotic and devitalized tissue so the infection can be healed before re-implanting the new prosthesis.

### *Acetabular Bone Defect in an Infected Total Hip Arthroplasty*

As previously mentioned, it is critical to remove all necrotic soft-tissue and membranes. The bone defect will be determined after explanting the acetabular and femoral components, a point that will determine the re-implantation stage [53]. Another issue, when a two-stage procedure is performed is the use of spacer.

Although widely used for their theoretical advantages in terms of soft tissue management and infection control [54–60], the high number of intrinsic complications can make considering the good results of not using attractive. The possibility of acetabular erosion when the spacer is left over long times is also a matter for concern [61, 62].

Girdlestone resection-arthoplasty (RA) can be a useful procedure to solve difficult cases such as severe infections with very severe bone defects, however, numerous studies have reported some unsatisfactory outcomes, including painful hips, the necessity of crutch use, severe limps, hip instability, leg length discrepancy (LLD) and increased oxygen consumption.

Considering the published results, the indications for RA of the hip must be strictly limited to non-ambulatory patients, intravenous drug abuse and impossible reimplantation because of new medical comorbidities or technical difficulties in medically compromised patients. Given these difficulties, some patients do not accept their condition as definitive and request conversion of their RA to a THA, hoping to alleviate symptoms and enhance their quality of life. The clinical outcome after conversion to a THA is unpredictable, so patients must be well informed regarding the expected results of this kind of complex procedure. It is uncommon, technically demanding and frequently associated with difficulties that can lead to complications resulting from some preoperative conditions like severe bone defects, osteoporotic bone, or LLD, which may make a shortening femoral osteotomy necessary, and abductor weakness.

Although the surgery may be technically demanding and the number of complications is not low, the clinical outcome for conversion from RA to THR is comparable to conventional revision surgery. Since the surgery is adapted to the bone defect in both groups, the defect may influence outcome more than the conversion procedure itself.

In fact, conversion of an RA, even after several years, can be done with an acceptable rate of complications (Fig. 12.2). Although dislocation is one of the concerns [63], this complication may be the result of inadequate cup positioning or soft tissue tension or both; at conversion, the soft tissues have invariably tightened, making proper testing of hip instability difficult and thus reconstruction of the hip rotation centre and proper management of the bone defect are more determinant of outcome rather than the use of constraint or dual mobility cups [64]. The number of periprosthetic fractures is usually low, and limited to intraoperative proximal cracks, which can be solved during the surgery. The circumstance that there is no need to remove a previous implant in an RA conversion may be one of the explanations for the relatively low number of complications, particularly for intraoperative fractures.

Functional outcome is commonly affected in many patients. Limp is frequent due to destruction of the soft tissue and poor active joint movement that may result in only fair improvement after re-implantation. When compared by bone defect and age the clinical outcome can be similar to that of an aseptic revision surgery, but nevertheless, pain, function, and motion are improved after conversion in most series [63, 65].

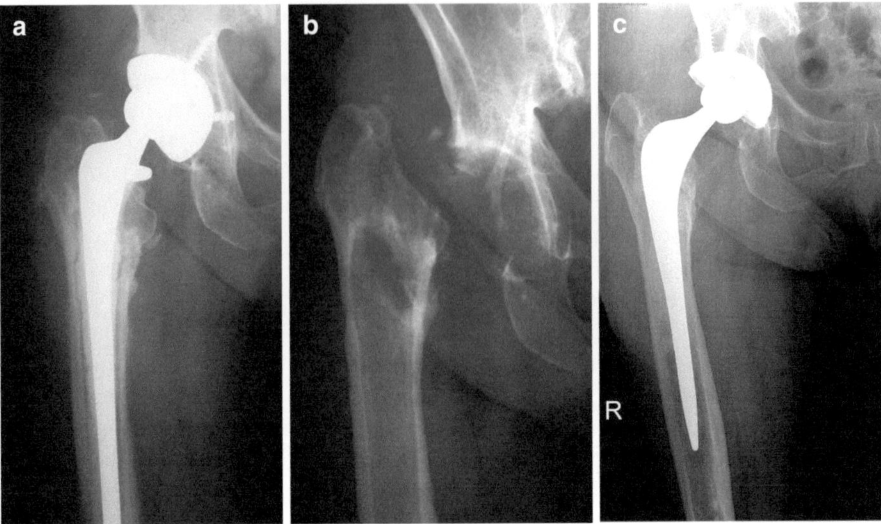


**Fig. 12.2** (**a**) Anteroposterior radiograph of a hip in a 72 year-old woman shows an infected cementless hip prosthesis. (**b**) Resection-arthroplasty. (**c**) Three months later, the hip was reconstructed using a cementless cup and impacting bone grafting with a cemented femoral long-stem showing a good outcome at 10 years

Age and bone defect, and/or physical status determine acetabular and femoral reconstruction [53, 66, 67]. RA in older low-demand patients may be adequate for some years, but muscular weakness and excessive oxygen consumption can be very disabling in this population [63]. Acetabular bone defect is the most important factor to affect postoperative clinical outcome, function, range of mobility and LLD so adequate reconstruction is critical to improve results in this complex situation. The low number of cases in most series makes it difficult to recommend the optimal interval between RA and conversion [68–72].

Despite THA after RA showing a clinical outcome and radiographic results similar to those obtained in aseptic revision surgery when the hips have similar bone defects, preoperative counseling must stress the influence of the intraoperative bone defect that will determine the surgical procedure and the risk of complications. Nevertheless, the fact that the functional level will be related to any resulting limp and LLD, mean a patients' high expectations of improved hip function should be tempered to a realistic level.

## *Reconstruction of the Acetabular Bone Defect in the Infected Hip*

Although an infected THA has been considered as a contraindication for bone graft due to the possibility of a potential sequestrum [73], many series have reported

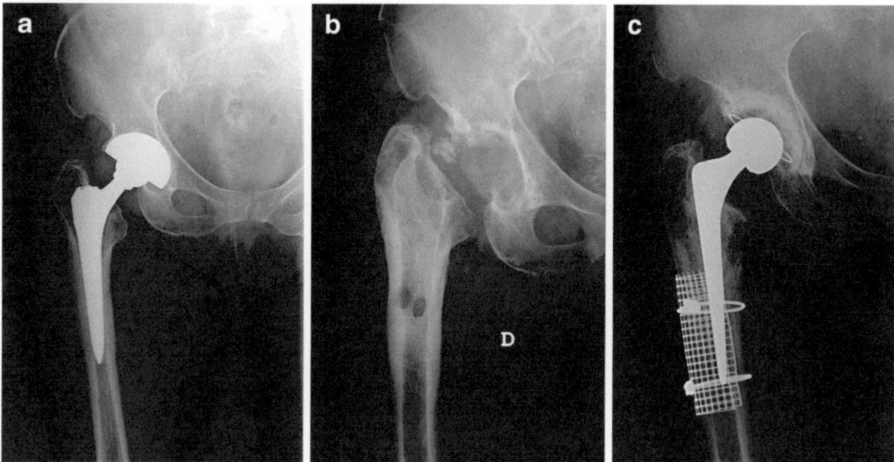


**Fig. 12.3** (**a**) Anteroposterior radiograph of the hip of a 70-year-old woman shows an infected cementless total hip arthroplasty. (**b**) Resection arthroplasty. (c). The hip was reconstructed using impacting bone grafting with cemented components., with a good clinical outcome at 5 years

acceptable results and contributed to this option now being considered in some cases.

Filling with antibiotic-loaded cement should be recommended only for small cavitary defects and low-demand patients. Despite its efficacy in controlling infection, mechanically done filling can be less safe in a more active population.

Cementless implants are more widely used for small or moderate acetabular bone defects of less than 30% [67] since they provide better mechanical fixation in most cases. Infection healing has been reported to be similar to cemented fixation with contemporary cups, including "Jumbo" cups, and hemispherical tantalum cups (Fig. 12.3); tantalum supplements [19, 74–78]; and antiprotrusio cage plus tantalum augments [79]. Currently, It is not yet established how much healthy bone is necessary for integration using tantalum prosthesis [80].

The most serious cases with large bone acetabular defects will be managed with similar techniques in infected cases and aseptic cases (Fig. 12.4). Reconstruction of large bone defects with impacting bone grafting technique associated with a cemented cup has obtained very good results and low recurrence figures (from 0% to 8%) (Fig. 12.5) [47, 75, 81]. Antibiotic-loaded cements and vancomycin-loaded graft chips are recommended by the original and other centres [82, 83]. As in aseptic cases, the biological restoration of bone stock makes this technique very attractive, particularly in the most active and young patients. Other options like the use of reinforcement rings, trabecular metal augments or custom-made implants along with the allograft have also provided acceptable early results in patients with infection [84].

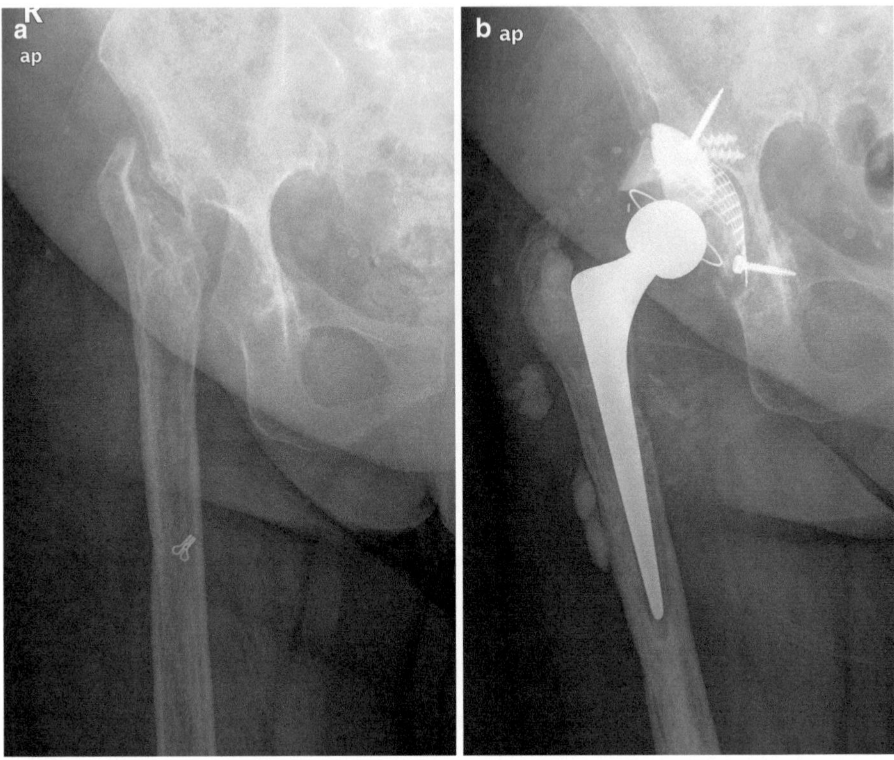


**Fig. 12.4** (**a**) Anteroposterior radiograph of the pelvis of a 83 year-old woman shows a resection-arthroplasty done 28 years earlier due to infection of a total hip arthroplasty. (**b**) The hip was reconstructed using a tantalum augment associated to bone impacting grafting technique with a cemented cup and bone impacting technique in the femur

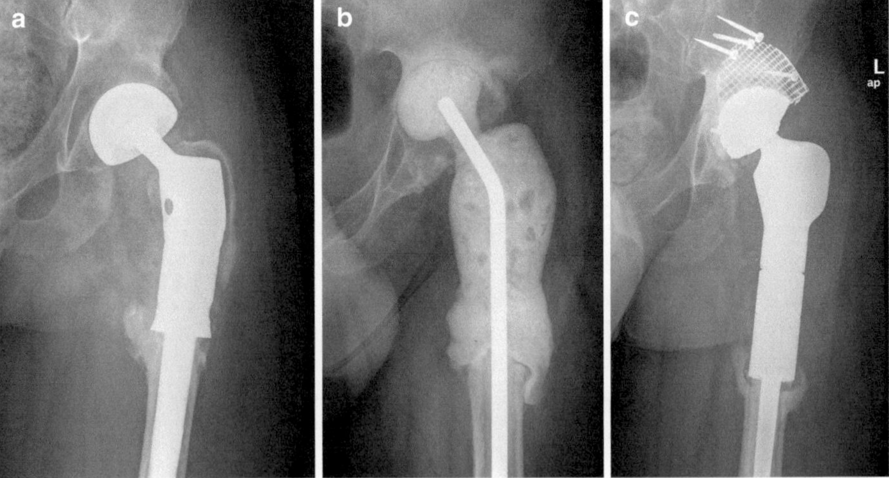


**Fig. 12.5** (**a**) Radiograph shows an infected bipolar tumoral femoral stem. (**b**) The prosthesis was removed and a spacer implanted. (**c**) A new femoral stem was implanted associated with a cup using impacting bone grafting technique

## References


1. Herbert CK, Williams RE, Levy RS, Barrack RL. Cost of treating of a total knee replacement. Clin Orthop Relat Res. 1996;331:140–5.
2. Bozic KJ, Ries MD. The impact of infection after total hip arthroplasty on hospital and surgeon resource utilization. J Bone Joint Surg Am. 2005;87:1746–51.
3. Tsukayama DT, Estrada R, Gustilo RB. Infection after total hip arthroplasty. A study of the treatment of one hundred and six infections. J Bone Joint Surg Am. 1996;78-A:512–23.
4. Ure KJ, Amstutz HC, Nasser S, Schmalzried TP. Direct exchange arthroplasty for the treatment of of infection after total hip replacement. An average tenýear follow-up. J Bone Joint Surg Am. 1998;80:961–8.
5. Lieberman JR, Callaway GH, Salvati EA, Pellicci PM, Brause BDI. Treatment of the infected total hip arthroplasty with a two-stage reimplantation protocol. Clin Orthop Relat Res. 1994;301:205–12.
6. Surin VV, Sundholm K, Bäckman L. Infection after total hip replacement. With special reference to a discharge from the wound. J Bone Joint Surg (Br). 1983 Aug;65(4):412–8.
7. Canner GC, Stenberg ME, Heppenstall RB, Balderstorn R. The infection hip after total hip arthroplasty. J Bone Joint Surg Am. 1984;66:1393–9.
8. Garvin KL, Evans BG, Salvati EA, Brause BD. Palacos gentamicin for the treatment of deep periprosthetic hip infections. Clin Orthop Relat Res. 1994;298:97–105.
9. Cordero-Ampuero J, de Dios M. What are the risk factors for infection in hemiarthroplasties and total hip arthroplasties? Clin Orthop. 2010;468:3268–77.
10. Parvizi J, Zmistowski B, Berbari EF, Bauer TW, Springer BD, Della Valle CJ, Garvin KL, Mont MA, Wongworawat MD, Zalavras CG. New definition for periprosthetic joint infection: from the workgroup of the musculoskeletal infection society. Clin Orthop Relat Res. 2011;469:2992–4. https://doi.org/10.1007/s11999-011-2102-9.
11. Zimmerli W, Trampuz A, Ochsner PE. Prosthetic-joint infections. N Engl J Med. 2004;351:1645–54.
12. Cuñé J, Soriano A, Martínez JC, García S, Mensa J. A superficial swab culture is useful for microbiologic diagnosis in acute prosthetic joint infections. Clin Orthop Relat Res. 2009;467(2):531–5.
13. Sanzén L, Carlsson AS, Josefsson G, Lindberg LT. Revision operations on infected total hip arthroplasties. Clin Orthop Relat Res. 1988;229:165–72.
14. Spangehl J, Masri BA, O'Connell JX, Duncan CP. Prospective analysis of preoperative and intraoperative investigations for the diagnosis of infection of the sites of two hindred and teo revision total hip arthroplasties. J Bone Joint Surg Am. 1999;81:672–83.
15. Trampuz A, Hanssen AD, Osmon DR, Mandrekar JR, Steckelberg JM, Patel R. Synovial fluid leukocyte count and differential for the diagnosis of prosthetic knee infection. Am J Med. 2004;117:556–62.
16. Bottner E, Wegner A, Winkelmann W, Becker K, Erren M, Götze C. Interleukin-6, procalcitonin and TNF-alpha. Markers of peri-prosthetic infection following total hip replacement. J Bone Joint Surg (Br). 2007;89:94–9.
17. Shahi A, Kheir MM, Tarabichi M, Hosseinzadeh HRS, Tan TL, Parvizi J. Serum D-Dimer test is promising for the diagnosis of periprosthetic joint Infection and timing of reimplantation. J Bone Joint Surg Am. 2017;99(17):1419–27.
18. Della Valle C, Zuckerman JD, Di Cesare PE. Periprosthetic sepsis. Clin Orthop Relat Res. 2004;420:26–31.
19. Toms AD, Davidson D, Masri BA, Duncan CP. The management of peri-prosthetic infection in total joint arthroplasty. JBJS-Br. 2006;88-B:149–55.
20. Levitsky KA, Hozack WJ, Balderston RA, Rothman RH, Gluckman SJ, Maslack MM, Booth RE Jr. Evaluation of the painful prosthetic joint. Relation value of bone scan, sedimentation rate, and joint aspiration. J Arthroplast. 1991;6:237–44.

21. Stumpe KD, Nötzli HP, Zanetti M, Kamel EM, Hany TF, Görres GW, von Schulthess GK, Hodler J. FDG PET for differentiation of infection and aseptic loosening in total hip replacements: comparison with conventional radiography and three-phase bone scintigraphy. Radiology. 2004;231(2):333–41.
22. Fuster D, Duch J, Soriano A, García S, Setoain X, Bori G, Rubí S, Rodríguez D, Doménech B, Piera C, Mensa J, Pons F. Potential use of bone marrow scintigraphy in suspected prosthetic hip infection evaluated with 99mTc-HMPAO-leukocytes. Rev Esp Med Nucl. 2008;27(6):430–5.
23. Chryssikos T, Parvizi J, Ghanem E, Newberg A, Zhuang H, Alavi A. FDG-PET imaging can diagnose periprosthetic infection of the hip. Clin Orthop Relat Res. 2008;466(6):1338–42.
24. Geller JA, MacCallum KP, Murtaugh TS, Patrick DA Jr, Liabaud B, Jonna VK. Prospective comparison of blood culture bottles and conventional swabs for microbial identification of suspected periprosthetic joint infection. J Arthroplast. 2016;31(8):1779–83.
25. Parvizi J, Gehrke T, Chen AF. Proceedings of the international consensus on periprosthetic joint infection. Bone Joint J. 2013;95-B(11):1450–2.
26. Wetters NG, Berend KR, Lombardi AV, Morris MJ, Tucker TL, Della Valle CJ. Leukocyte esterase reagent strips for the rapid diagnosis of periprosthetic joint infection. J Arthroplast. 2012;27(Suppl 1):8–11.
27. Bingham J, Clarke H, Spangehl M, Schwartz A, Beauchamp C, Goldberg B. The alpha defensin-1 biomarker assay can be used to evaluate the potentially infected total joint arthroplasty. Clin Orthop Relat Res. 2014;472(12):4006–9.
28. Bonanzinga T, Zahar A, Dütsch M, Lausmann C, Kendoff D, Gehrke T. How reliable is the alpha-defensin immunoassay test for diagnosing periprosthetic joint infection? A prospective study. Clin Orthop Relat Res. 2017;475(2):408–15.
29. Lachiewicz PF, Rogers GD, Thomason HC. Aspiration of the hip joint before revision total hip arthroplasty. Clinical and laboratory factors influencing attainment of a positive culture. J Bone Joint Surg Am. 1996;78(5):749–54.
30. Atkins BL, Athanasou N, Deeks JJ, Crook DW, Simpson H, Peto TE, McLardy-Smith P, Berend AR. Prospective evaluation of criteria for microbiological diagnosis of prosthetic joint infection at revision arthroplasty. The OSIRIS collaborative study group. J Clin Microbiol. 1998;36:2932–9.
31. Patel R. Biofilms and antimicrobial resistance. Clin Orthop Relat Res. 2005;437:41–7.
32. Deirmengian C, Hallab N, Tarabishy A, Della Valle C, Jacobs JJ, Lonner J, Booth RE Jr. Synovial fluid biomarkers for periprosthetic infection. Clin Orthop Relat Res. 2010;468:2017–23.
33. McArthur BA, Abdel MP, Taunton MJ, Osmon DR, Hanssen AD. Seronegative infections in hip and knee arthroplasty: periprosthetic infections with normal erythrocyte sedimentation rate and C-reactive protein level. Bone Joint J. 2015;97-B(7):939–44.
34. ShanmugasundaramS RBF, Briggs TW, Sussmann PS, Bostrom MP. Evaluation and management of periprosthetic joint infection-an international, multicenter study. HSS J. 2014;10(1):36–44.
35. Fink B, GrossmanA FM, Schäfer P, Frommelt L. Two-stage cementless revision of infected hip endoprostheses. Clin Orthop. 2009;467:1848–58.
36. Corona P, Gil E, Guerra E, Soldado F, Amat C, Flores X, Pigrau C. Percutaneous interface biopsy in dry-aspiration cases of chronic periprosthetic joint infections: a technique for preoperative isolation of the infecting organism. Int Orthop. 2012;36(6):1281–6.
37. Bori G, Soriano A, Garcia S, Gallart X, Casanova L, Mallofre C, Almela M, Martinez JA, Riba J, Mensa J. Low sensitivity of histology to predict the presence of microorganisms in suspected aseptic loosening of a joint prosthesis. Mod Pathol. 2006;19:874–7.
38. Bori G, Soriano A, Garcia S, Mallofré C, Riba J, Mensa J. Usefulness of histological analysis for predicting the presence of microorganisms at the time of reimplantation after hip resection arthroplasty for the treatment of infection. J Bone Joint Surg Am. 2007;89:1232–7.
39. Mirra JR, Amstutz HC, Matos M, Gold R. The pathology of the joint tissues and its clinical relevance in prostheses failure. Clin Orthop Relat Res. 1976;117:221–40.

40. Fehring TK, McAlister JRJA. Frozen histologic section as a guide to sepsis in revision joint arthroplasty. Clin Orthop Relat Res. 1994;304:229–37.
41. Feldman DS, Lonner JH, Desai P, Zuckerman JD. The role of intraoperative frozen section in revision total hip arthroplasty. J Bone Joint Surg Am. 1995;77:1807–13.
42. Athanasou NA, Pandey R, de Steiger R, Crook D, Smith PM. Diagnosis of infection by frozen section during revision arthroplasty. J Bone Joint Surg Br. 1995;77:28–33.
43. Lonner JH, Desai P, Di Cesare PE, Steiner G, Zuckerman JD. The reliability of analysis of intraoperative frozensections for identifiying active infection during revision hip or knee arthroplasty. J Bone Joint Surg Am. 1996;78:1553–8.
44. Della Valle CJ, Bogner E, Desai P, Lonner JH, Adler E, Zuckerman JD, Di Cesare PE. Analysisof frozen sections of intraoperative specimens obtained at the time of reoperation after hip or knee resection arthroplasty for the treatment of infection. J Bone Joint Surg Am. 1999;81:684–9.
45. Pandey R, Drakoulakis E, Athanasou NA. An assessment of the histological criteria used to diagnose infection in hip revision arthroplasty tissues. J Clin Pathol. 1999;52:118–23.
46. Costerton JW. Biofilm theory can guide the treatment of device-related orthopaedic infections. Clin Orthop Relat Res. 2005;437:7–11.
47. Esteban J, Molina-Manso D, Spiliopoulou I, Cordero-Ampuero J, Fernández-Roblas R, Foka A, Gómez-Barrena E. Biofilm development by clinical isolates of Staphylococcus spp. from retrieved orthopaedic prosthesis. Acta Orthop. 2010;81:674–9.
48. Kamme C, Lindberg L. Aerobic and anaerobic bacteria in deep infections after total hip arthroplasty: differential diagnosis between infectious and non-infectious loosening. Clin Orthop Relat Res. 1981;154:201–7.
49. Nelson CL, McLarec AC, McLaren SG, Johnson JW, Smeltzer MS. Is aseptic loosening truly aseptic. Cllin Orthop Rel Res. 2005;437:25–30.
50. Esteban J, Gómez-Barrena E, Cordero J, Zamora N, Kinnari TJ, Fernández-Roblas R. Evaluation of quantitative analysis of cultures from sonicated retrieved orthopaedic implants in diagnosis of orthopaedic infection. J Clin Microbiol. 2008;46:488–92.
51. Kwiecien G, George J, Klika AK, Zhang Y, Bauer TW, Rueda CA. Intraoperative frozen section histology: matched for musculo skeletal infection society criteria. J Arthroplast. 2017;32(1):223–7.
52. Buttaro MA, Martorell G, Quinteros M, Comba F, Zanotti G, Piccaluga F. Intraoperative synovial C-reactive protein is as useful as frozen section to detect periprosthetic hip infection. Clin Orthop Relat Res. 2015;473(12):3876–81.
53. García-Cimbrelo E, García-Rey E. Bone defect determines acetabular revision surgery. Hip Int. 2014;24(Suppl 10):S33–6. https://doi.org/10.5301/hipint.5000162.
54. Gustilo RB, Tsukayama D. Treatment of infected cemented total hip arthroplasty with tobramycin beads and delayed revision with a cementless prosthesis and bone grafting. Orthop Trans. 1988;12:739.
55. Duncan CP, Beauchamp C. A temporary antibiotic-loaded joint replacement system for management for complex infection involving the hip. Orthop Clin North Am. 1993;24:751–9.
56. Masri BA, Duncan CP, Beauchamp CP. Long-term elution of antibiotics from bone cement an in vitro study using the prosthesis of antibiotic-loaded acrylic cement (PROSTALAC) system. J Arthroplast. 1998;13:331–8.
57. Hsieh PH, Shih CH, Chang YH, Lee MS, Yang WE, Shih HN. Treatment of deep infection of the hip associated with massive bone loss: two-stage revision with an antibiotic-loaded interim cement prosthesis followed by reconstruction with allograft. J Bone Joint Surg (Br). 2005;87B:770–5.
58. Degen RM, Davey JR, Davey JR, Howard JL, McCalden RW, Naudie DD. Does a prefabricated gentamicin-impregnated, load-bearing spacer control periprosthetic hip infection? Clin Orthop Relat Res. 2012 Oct;470(10):2724–9.
59. Neumann DR, Hofstaedter T, List C, Dorn U. Two-stage cementless revision of late total hip arthroplasty infection using a premanufactured spacer. J Arthroplast. 2012;27(7):1397–401.

60. Romanò CL, Romanò D, Albisetti A, Meani E. Preformed antibiotic-loaded cement spacers for two-stage revision of infected total hip arthroplasty. Long-term results Hip Int. 2012;22(S8):46–53. https://doi.org/10.5301/HIP.2012.9566.
61. Macheras GA, Koutsostathis S, Kateros K, Papadakis S, Anastasopoulos P. A two stage reimplantation protocol for the treatment of deep periprosthetic hip infection. Mid to long-term results. Hip Int. 2012;22(S8):54–61. https://doi.org/10.5301/HIP.2012.9571.
62. Cordero-Ampuero J, Esteban J, García-Cimbrelo E. Oral antibiotics are effective for highly resistant hip arthroplasty infections. Clin Orthop. 2009;467:2335–42.
63. Charlton WPH, Hozack WJ, Teloken MA, Rao R, Bissett GA. Complications associated with reimplantation after Girdlestone arthroplasty. Clin Orthop Relat Res. 2003;407:119–26.
64. Garcia-Rey E, Cruz-Pardos A, Madero R. Clinical outcome following conversion of Girdlestone's resection arthroplasty to total hip replacement: a retrospective matched case-control study. Bone Joint J. 2014;96-B(11):1478–84. https://doi.org/10.1302/0301-620X.96B11.33889.
65. Dallari D, Fini M, Carubbi C, Giavaresi G, Rani N, Del Piccolo N, Sartori M, Masso A. Total hip arthroplasty after excision arthroplasty: indications and limits. Hip Int. 2011;21: 436–40.
66. García-Cimbrelo E, García-Rey E, Cruz-Pardos A. The extent of the bone defect affects the outcome of femoral reconstruction in revision surgery. J Bone Joint Surg (Br). 2011;93-B:1457–64. 24
67. Garcia-Cimbrelo E. Porous-coated cementless acetabular cups in revision surgery: a 6- to 11-year follow-up study. J Arthroplast. 1999;14:397–406.
68. Castellanos J, Flores X, Llusà M, Chiriboga C, Navarro A. The Girdlestone pseudoartrosis in the treatment of infected hip replacements. Int Orthop. 1998;22:178–81.
69. Grauer JD, Amstutz HC, O'Carroll PF, Doray FG. Resection arthroplasty of the hip. J Bone Joint Surg Am. 1989;71-A:669–78.
70. McElwaine JP, Colville J. Excision arthroplasty or infected total hip replacement. J Bone Joint Surg (Br). 1984;66-B:168–71.
71. Schröder J, Saris D, Besselaar PP, Marti RK. Comparison of the results of the Girdlestone pseudoartrosis with reimplantation of a total hip replacement. Int Orthop. 1998;22:215–8.
72. Rittmeister ME, Manthei L, Hailer NP. Prosthetic replacement in secondary Girdlestone artthroplasty has an unpredictible outcome. Int Orthop. 2005;29:145–8.
73. Salvati EA, Chekofski KM, Brause BD, Wilson PD. Reimplantation in infection. A 12-year experience. Clin Orthop Relat Res. 1982;170:62–75.
74. Jeong M, Kim HJ, Lim SJ, Moon YW, Park YS. Revision total hip arthroplasty using tantalum augment in patients with Paprosky III or IV acetabular bone defect: a minimum 2-year follow-up study. Hip Pelvis. 2016;28:98–103.
75. Rowan FE, Gorenchtein M, Aslam S, Condon F, Masterson EL. A comparison of acetabular impaction grafting and trabecular metal for revision arthroplasty. Hip Int. 2016;26:350–4.
76. Kraay MJ, Goldberg VM, Fitzgerald SJ, Salata MJ. Cementless two-staged total hip arthroplasty for deep periprosthetic infection. Clin Orthop Relat Res. 2005;441:243–9.
77. Haddad FS, Muirhea-Allwood SK, Manktelow ARJ, Bacarese-Hamilton I. Two-stage uncemented revision hip arthroplasty for infection. J Bone Joint Surg (Br). 2000;82:689–94.
78. Fehring TK, Calton TF, Griffin WL. Cementless fixation in 2-stage reimplantation for periprosthetic sepsis. J Arthroplast. 1999;14(2):175–81.
79. Gunther KP, Wegner T, Kirschner S, Hartmann A. Modular reconstruction in acetabular revision with antiprotrusio cages and metal augments: the cage-and-augment system. Oper Orthop Traumatol. 2014;26:141–55.
80. Kim WY, Greidanus NV, Duncan CP, Masri BA, Garbuz DS. Porous tantalumuncemented acetabular shells in revision total hip replacement: two to four year clinical and radiographic results. Hip Int. 2008;18:17–22.
81. Petheram TG, Howell JR. The Exeter method-acetabular impaction grafting with cemented reimplantation. Oper Orthop Traumatol. 2014;26:114–25.

82. Witso E, Persen L, Loseth K, Bergh K. Cancellous bone as an antibiotic carrier. Acta Orthop Scand. 2000;71:80–4.
83. Buttaro MA, Pusso R, Piccaluga F. Vancomycin-supplemented impacted bone allografts in infected hip arthroplasty. Two-stage revision results. J Bone Joint Surg (Br). 2005;87-B: 314–9.
84. Abolghasemian M, Tangsataporn S, Sternheim A, Backstein D, Safir O, Gross AE. Combined trabecular metal acetabular shell and augment for acetabular revision with substantial bone loss: a mid-term review. Bone Joint J. 2013;95:166–72.

# Index





E. García-Rey, E. García Cimbrelo (eds.), *Acetabular Revision Surgery in Major Bone Defects*, https://doi.org/10.1007/978-3-319-98596-1